Handbook on
Neonatal ICU

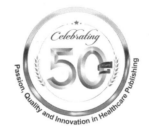

Celebrating 50

Passion, Quality and Innovation in Healthcare Publishing

Handbook on
Neonatal ICU

Editors

Neelam Kler
MBBS MD (Ped)
Chairperson
Department of Neonatology
Institute of Child Health
Sir Ganga Ram Hospital
New Delhi, India
Padma Bhushan 2014

Pankaj Garg
MBBS MD (Ped) DNB (Ped)
Senior Consultant
Department of Neonatology
Institute of Child Health
Sir Ganga Ram Hospital
New Delhi, India

Anup Thakur
MBBS MD (Ped) DNB (Neonatology)
Consultant
Department of Neonatology
Institute of Child Health
Sir Ganga Ram Hospital
New Delhi, India

Forewords

Ann R Stark
DeWayne M Pursley
Ashok Deorari
VK Bhutani
ON Bhakoo

JAYPEE BROTHERS MEDICAL PUBLISHERS
The Health Sciences Publisher
New Delhi | London

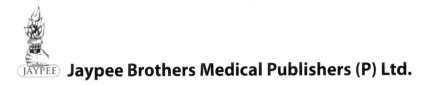

Jaypee Brothers Medical Publishers (P) Ltd.

Headquarters
Jaypee Brothers Medical Publishers (P) Ltd.
4838/24, Ansari Road, Daryaganj
New Delhi 110 002, India
Phone: +91-11-43574357
Fax: +91-11-43574314
Email: jaypee@jaypeebrothers.com

Overseas Office
JP Medical Ltd.
83, Victoria Street, London
SW1H 0HW (UK)
Phone: +44 20 3170 8910
Fax: +44 (0)20 3008 6180
E-mail: info@jpmedpub.com

Website: www.jaypeebrothers.com
Website: www.jaypeedigital.com

Inquiries for bulk sales may be solicited at: jaypee@jaypeebrothers.com

Handbook on Neonatal ICU

First Edition: **2020**

ISBN: 978-93-89587-23-4

Printed at: Sterling Graphics Pvt. Ltd. India.

Dedicated to

*Sidharth Kler, Aditya Kler, Tanmay Garg, Paavni,
Atharv Sachdeva Thakur, Anika Sachdeva Thakur*

CONTRIBUTORS

Aakriti Soni MBBS
Intern
Sir Ganga Ram Hospital
New Delhi, India

Abdul Razak MD
Associate Professor
Department of Pediatrics
Division of Neonatology
McMaster University
Hamilton, ON, Canada

Amrit Jeevan
DCH MD (Ped) MRCPCH (UK) DNB (Neonatology)
Consultant
Department of Neonatology
Surya Mother and Child Superspecialty Hospital
Mumbai, Maharashtra, India

Anita Singh MD (Ped) DNB (Neonatology)
Associate Professor
Department of Neonatology
Sanjay Gandhi Postgraduate Institute
of Medical Sciences
Lucknow, Uttar Pradesh, India

Anumodan Gupta MD (Ped) DNB (Neonatology)
Consultant Pediatrics
Department of Pediatrics
Government Medical College
Kathua, Jammu, India

Anup Thakur MD (Ped) DNB (Neonatology)
Consultant
Department of Neonatology
Sir Ganga Ram Hospital
New Delhi, India

Anurag Fursule DNB (Ped) DNB (Neonatology)
Fellow
Department of Neonatology
Sir Ganga Ram Hospital
New Delhi, India

Arpita Gupta
Assistant Professor
Developmental and Behavioral Pediatrics
Department of Pediatrics
Maulana Azad Medical College
New Delhi, India

Arti Maria MD DM (Neonatology)
Consultant and Head
Department of Neonatology
Dr Ram Manohar Lohia Hospital
New Delhi, India

Arun Soni DNB (Ped)
Senior Consultant
Department of Neonatology
Sir Ganga Ram Hospital
New Delhi, India

Arvind Shenoi MD DM (Neonatology)
Chief Neonatologist and Medical Director
Department of Neonatology
CloudNine Hospital, Bengaluru, Karnataka, India

Ashish Jain MD DM
Associate Professor
Department of Neonatology
Maulana Azad Medical College
New Delhi, India

Ashish Mehta MD
Director and Consultant
Department of Neonatology
Fellow in Neonatal
Medicine College of Pediatrics, Australia
ARPAN Newborn Care Centre Pvt Ltd
Ahmedabad, Gujarat, India

B Adhisivam DCH DNB PhD
Additional Professor and HOD
Department of Neonatology
Jawaharlal Institute of Postgraduate Medical
Education and Research (JIPMER)
Puducherry, India

B Vishnu Bhat MD
Director-Medical Research
Professor of Pediatrics and Neonatology
Aarupadai Veedu Medical College (AVMC)
Puducherry, India
Former Director
Senior Professor and Head
Department of Neonatology
Jawaharlal Institute of Postgraduate Medical
Education and Research (JIPMER)
Puducherry, India

Brajesh Jha MD
Senior Resident (DM Neonatology)
Department of Neonatology
Maulana Azad Medical College
New Delhi, India

Deblina Dasgupta MD (Ped) FNB Pediatric Nephrology
Fellow
Division of Pediatric Nephrology and
Renal Transplantation
Institute of Child Health
Sir Ganga Ram Hospital
New Delhi, India

Geeta Gathwala DCH MD (Ped) DM (Neonatology)
Senior Professor and Head
Department of Pediatrics and Neonatology
Pandit Bhagwat Dayal Sharma Postgraduate
Institute of Medical Sciences
Rohtak, Haryana, India

Harish Chellani MD DCH
Additional DGHS and Professor
Department of Pediatrics
Vardhman Mahavir Medical College and
Safdarjung Hospital
New Delhi, India

Harish Nayak DOMS MS FRCS FRC (Ophth)
Consultant Pediatric Ophthalmologist
CloudNine Hospital
Bengaluru, Karnataka, India
Alderhey Children's Hospital
Liverpool, UK

Jaswinder Kaur MD (Ped)
Clinical Associate
Division of Pediatric Gastroenterology
Hepatology and Liver Transplantation
Institute of Child Health
Sir Ganga Ram Hospital
New Delhi, India

Jogender Kumar DM (Neonatology)
Assistant Professor
Division of Neonatology
Department of Pediatrics
Postgraduate Institute of Medical Education and
Research, Chandigarh, India

Kanav Anand MD (Ped) FPN
Consultant Pediatric Nephrologist
Division of Pediatric Nephrology and
Renal Transplantation
Institute of Child Health
Sir Ganga Ram Hospital
New Delhi, India

Karthik Nagesh N MD FRCPCH (UK) FNNF
Neonatal Intensive Care Fellowship (UK)
Chairman
Neonatology and NICUs
Manipal Group of Hospitals
Head Department of Neonatology
Chairman, Manipal Advanced Children's Center
Manipal Hospitals, Professor of Neonatology and
Pediatrics, Manipal University
Bengaluru, Karnataka, India

Kavitha Rao DNB (Ophth)
Fellowship in VR Surgery
Consultant Vitreo-Retinal Surgeon
Retina Institute of Karnataka
Bengaluru, Karnataka, India

Koshy Marucoickal George MBBS
Neonatologist
Rapides Regional Medical Center
Alexandria, Louisiana, USA

Kumari Gunjan MD (Ped)
DNB Neonatology Fellow
Department of Neonatology
Sir Ganga Ram Hospital
New Delhi, India

M Jeeva Sankar MD DM
Associate Professor
WHO Collaborating Centre for Training and
Research in Newborn Care
Department of Pediatrics
All India Institute of Medical Sciences
New Delhi, India

Maneesha PH DNB
Fellowship in Neonatology
Department of Neonatology
Consultant Neonatologist
People Tree @ Meenakshi Hospitals
Bengaluru, Karnataka, India

Nandkishor S Kabra
DM (Neonatology) MD (Ped) DNB (Ped) MSc (Clinical
Epidemiology)
Director and Head
Department of Neonatology
Surya Children's Medicare Pvt Ltd
Mumbai, Maharashtra, India

Naveen Jain DM (Neonatology)
Head
Department of Neonatology
Kerala Institute of Medical Sciences
Thiruvananthapuram, Kerala, India

Naveen Parkash Gupta MD (Ped) DNB (Neonatology)
Fellowship in Neonatal Perinatal Medicine (Canada)
Senior Consultant
Department of Neonatology
Rainbow Children's Hospital
New Delhi, India

Nirupama Laroia MD (Ped)
Professor
Department of Pediatrics
Division of Neonatology
University of Rochester, NY, USA

Nishad Plakkal MD (Ped)
Fellowship in Neonatal Perinatal Medicine (Canada)
Associate Professor
Department of Neonatology
Jawaharlal Institute of Postgraduate Medical
Education and Research (JIPMER)
Puducherry, India

Nishant Wadhwa MBBS DCH (Ped) DNB
Consultant and Chief
Division of Pediatric Gastroenterology
Hepatology and Liver Transplantation
Institute of Child Health
Sir Ganga Ram Hospital
New Delhi, India

Pankaj Garg DNB MBBS MD
Senior Consultant
Department of Neonatology
Sir Ganga Ram Hospital
New Delhi, India

Pradeep Kumar Sharma MD (Ped) DM (Neonatology)
Senior Consultant Neonatologist
Department of Neonatology
Satguru Partap Singh (SPS) Hospitals
Ludhiana, Punjab, India

Praveen Kumar MD (Ped) DM (Neonatology)
Professor
Department of Pediatrics, Division of Neonatology
Postgraduate Institute of Medical Education and
Research, Chandigarh, India

Raktima Chakrabarti
MD (Ped) Fellowship (Neonatology)
Consultant Pediatrician and Neonatologist
Department of Neonatology
Cloudnine Hospitals
Gurugram, Haryana, India

Ranjan Kumar Pejaver FRCPCH (UK) FRCPI FIAP FNNF
Professor
Department of Pediatrics
Kempegowda Institute of Medical Sciences
Bengaluru, Karnataka, India
Chief Neonatologist
People Tree @ Meenakshi Hospitals
Bengaluru, Karnataka, India

Sachin Kumar Dubey (Maj)
MD (Ped) DNB (Neonatology)
Consultant Neonatology
Department of Pediatrics
Yashoda Superspecialty Hospital
Ghaziabad, Uttar Pradesh, India

Sanjay Wazir DM (Neonatology)
Director
Department of Neonatology and Pediatrics
Cloudnine Hospitals
Gurugram, Haryana, India

Sanjiv B Amin MD MS
Professor
Department of Pediatrics
University of Rochester School of Medicine
Rochester, NY, USA

Shiv Sajan Saini DM (Neonatology)
Assistant Professor
Department of Pediatrics
Division of Neonatology
Postgraduate Institute of Medical Education and
Research (PGIMER), Chandigarh, India

Shridevi S Bisanalli MD DM
Faculty
Department of Neonatology
St John's Medical College
Bengaluru, Karnataka, India

Sindhu Sivanandan MD DM
Assistant Professor
Department of Neonatology
Jawaharlal Institute of Postgraduate Medical
Education and Research (JIPMER)
Puducherry, India

Sonalika Mehta MBBS MD
Consultant Neonatologist
Department of Neonatology
Rainbow Hospitals
New Delhi, India

Suman Rao PN MD (Ped) DM
Professor and Head of Department
Department of Neonatology
St John's Medical College
Bengaluru, Karnataka, India

Supreet Khurana MD (Ped) DM (Neonatology)
Assistant Professor
Department of Neonatology
Government Medical College Hospital
Chandigarh, India

Susanta Kumar Badatya
MD (Ped) DNB (Neonatology)
Consultant Neonatologist
Department of Neonatology
Apollo Cradle
New Delhi, India

Swarna Rekha Bhat MD
Former Professor
Department of Pediatrics
Division of Neonatology
St John's Medical College
Bengaluru, Karnataka, India

Tapas Bandyopadhyay
MD (Ped) DM (Neonatology)
Assistant Professor
Department of Neonatology
Dr Ram Manohar Lohia Hospital
New Delhi, India

Umesh Vaidya MBBS DNB
Consultant and Head
Division of Neonatology
King Edward Memorial (KEM) Hospital
Pune, Maharashtra, India

Venkataseshan Sundaram DM (Neonatology)
Additional Professor
Division of Neonatology
Department of Pediatrics
Postgraduate Institute of Medical Education and
Research, Chandigarh, India

Vivek Choudhury MD (Ped) DNB (Neonatology)
Consultant Neonatologist
Department of Neonatology
Apollo Cradle, New Delhi, India

Wg Cdr (Dr) Ajoy Kumar Garg
MD (Ped) DNB (Neonatology)
Assistant Professor
Department of Pediatrics
Army Hospital Research and Referral (R&R)
New Delhi, India

FOREWORD

We were very pleased to learn that our distinguished colleague Professor Neelam Kler and her associates, Drs Pankaj Garg and Anup Thakur, have collaborated to develop a new and much needed *Handbook on Neonatal ICU*. Drawing on national experts in neonatology and supplemented by their own decades of experience providing neonatal care at the renowned Sir Ganga Ram Hospital in New Delhi, India, the editors have developed an important resource for neonatal care providers in India.

A key characteristic of the handbook is that it is easy-to-use and can be applied directly at the bedside. Thirty-three individual chapters focus on the important issues in providing contemporary neonatal care. Rather than providing a long narrative, each chapter is organized with clear headings that include relevant information noted with bullet points. Ample tables, flowcharts, diagrams, illustrations, and photos provide additional well-organized information and supplement the text. At the end of each chapter, bulleted Key Points emphasize the "take home" messages. The self-assessment questions that follow will be helpful to students at every level, from residents and fellows to practicing neonatologists. Finally, a list of carefully selected articles provides a handy resource for more extensive reading.

The importance of high quality neonatal care cannot be overstated. The newborn period— the first 28 days of life—is the most vulnerable time for a child's survival. In India, deaths during this period represent more than half of the deaths occurring among children under 5 years of age. The interventions that are effective in the care of preterm and medically fragile newborns are unique to that period and require substantial training and mastery. Textbooks such as *Handbook on Neonatal ICU* can be effective tools in improving outcomes for this most vulnerable of populations. Combined with public health measures, improved clinical outcomes facilitated by making current knowledge readily accessible can contribute to improved survival and help minimize sequelae of neonatal illness.

Another potential benefit of this handbook would be that neonatal care is standardized within a facility or perhaps across several in a region, since reducing variation tends to improve clinical outcomes. Standardization also provides a platform for quality improvement, allowing incremental tests of change. Finally, recognizing where evidence is limited may stimulate readers to pursue research and expand our knowledge.

We are confident that the *Handbook on Neonatal ICU* will be increasingly found in NICUs throughout India, contribute to optimizing care of our fragile patients, and provide a study guide to a new generation of learners in our field. We look forward to further editions as knowledge continues to expand.

Ann R Stark MD
DeWayne M Pursley MD MPH
Department of Neonatology
Beth Israel Deaconess Medical Center
Harvard Medical School, USA

FOREWORD

Ensuring healthy survival of all neonates is among the highest priorities of our times. The global community has committed itself to attain an under-five child mortality rate of less than 20 per 1,000 live births in all countries by 2035. This would only be achieved if the neonatal mortality rate declines to less than 10 per 1,000 live births. For India, this would be nearly halving the current neonatal mortality rate of 23 per 1,000 live births.

India's success in reduction of neonatal mortality since the launch of the National Rural Health Mission has been modest. Nonetheless, the country mounted a spectacular effort in establishing newborn care corners and special newborn care units, thus creating an impressive neonatal care infrastructure in the public sector. There has also been a concomitant expansion of neonatal care services in the private sector. This massive expansion of neonatal care services has also brought to the fore an extraordinary need for skilled nurses and doctors. Sir Ganga Ram Hospital, New Delhi, India, which runs one of the best tertiary care, newborn units for more than three decades in the city of Delhi, has been in the forefront of training healthcare providers in neonatal care. The unit has tried to capture the best learnings in neonatology in the current handbook. This compilation is a timely step towards filling the gap for knowledge translation for ensuring quality of care for sick newborns. The handbook has 33 chapters on common issues faced while caring a sick newborn. It provides comprehensive, systematic approach in identification and management of sick neonates. The evidence-based practices are tailored to day-to-day needs of neonatology fellows, resident doctors, and practicing pediatricians. I am confident that the effort of updating chapters of the handbook in the future will continue with the energetic next generation leadership of the unit.

I would like to congratulate the contributors, reviewers, and the editorial team for an outstanding product. The credit goes to a very large team of neonatologists trained in India who have contributed in this endeavor. I am glad to see many young neonatologists, most of whom I know personally, contributing to this book. They are exceptional up-to-date educators with hands-on experience in managing sick neonates. My special congratulations to Dr Neelam Kler for taking, leadership role in this endeavor.

I am sure this handbook will help in providing safe, affordable care with focus on quality in neonatal units in the country and beyond.

Ashok Deorari
MD FAMS FNNF
Professor and Head
Department of Pediatrics
In-charge
WHO Collaborating Center for Education and Research in Newborn Care
Chairman, Skills Center
Lead for QI in SEARO
All India Institute of Medical Sciences
New Delhi, India
President (2020)
National Neonatology Forum (NNF), India

FOREWORD

Padma Bhushan Dr Neelam Kler leads her team Dr Pankaj Garg and Dr Anup Thakur to take the key steps that will help develop a national "standard of care" for neonatal medicine for Indian families. Collaboration with national experts provides a unique insight that bridges the gap between academic knowledge and practical realties that burden practicing front-line clinicians. The algorithms and tables categorizing neonatal conditions should be used as guidelines for judgment-driven disease management.

This handbook deals with the current state of neonatology and provides a comprehensive, systematic approach in the identification and management of sick neonates to make evidence-based decisions in clinical practice for both public and private sectors. Sections on follow-up care deserve special mention. Future publications could include individual attention to antibiotic stewardship, breastfeeding, small-for-dates neonates, phototherapy, hyperammonemia syndromes and NICU-based neurodevelopmental protection and maturation. Other novel areas on the horizon in future editions include prenatal and perinatal cardiac disorders and other fetal disorders that require specific neonatal care.

The handbook is directed for use by the bedside clinician who is still a student of neonatal diagnosis and disorders before the results of laboratory tests are available. It is well structured and easy-to-read. Editors are specifically congratulated for attempting to provide a forum for families who are likely to be readers.

Content in this handbook should be updated periodically (more than annually). Hopefully this will be achieved through a web-based portal for rapid alerts, novel approaches and newer sections. These are exciting prospects and speak to the mission of the handbook as a knowledge resource that governs national intensive neonatal care patterns for safer care of vulnerable infants.

Contributions of Drs Neelam Kler, Pankaj Garg and Anup Thakur are significant and over the years will help clinicians and families to develop sound as well as safe judgment.

Well done and well-read.

VK Bhutani
Professor of Pediatrics (Neonatology)
Lucile Salter Packard Hospital
Standford University, USA

FOREWORD

Neonatal intensive care has become more rewarding because of the improving intact survival rates of high-risk neonates. This has been possible because of better understanding of neonatal physiology, new technology, and improved skills of collating the two.

The current book uses this amalgam to describe the practical approach to evaluation and management of a sick neonate. The text is kept to minimum and there is liberal use of tables and illustrations. Flowcharts and algorithms make the decision making easy.

To keep the book small and easily portable recent literature has been condensed, but provides adequate evidence for appropriate decision making. Additional highlight of this book is that each chapter closes with key points which highlight the take home message. The self-assessment questions following the key points should be helpful to the student for self evaluation. This book can be carried to the bedside in a pocket and should be a boon for the residents, fellows, consultants, and the senior nursing staff involved in neonatal intensive care.

I congratulate Dr Neelam Kler and her editorial staff along with expert contributors to various chapters for bringing out a very useful and timely publication. In fact, going through this book one felt like a student once again.

ON Bhakoo
MD FIAP FAMS FNNF
Former Professor and Head
Department of Pediatrics and Neonatology
Postgraduate Institute of Medical Education and Research
Chandigarh, India

PREFACE

I do not know what I may appear to the world, but to myself I seem to have been only like a boy playing on the seashore, and diverting myself in now and then finding a smoother pebble or a prettier shell than ordinary, whilst the great ocean of truth lay all undiscovered before me.

—**Isaac Newton**

The confines of knowledge are limitless. How much sand can we hold from the vast shores of knowledge? As we begin this *Handbook on Neonatal ICU*, we attempt to unravel the art and science of neonatology in a comprehensive manner, understanding that it is a tall order. Well! It is not just a compendium of 33 chapters covering most practical aspects of neonatal intensive care, but a treasury of recent evidence-based literature accrued and turned into an elixir by a team of experts from India and abroad in an easy-to-read format with ample numbers of figures, tables, and diagrams. The cardinal points at the end of each chapter and self-assessment questions further add up to the potion. The realms of neonatology are vast and the book being limited by its volume does not encompass some of its aspects such as drugs, procedures, quality improvement and perinatal medicine, which we intent to include in the future editions. While the pursuit for excellence may be eluding, we the editors and the authors have put into our hard work with unfeigned passion to make this book a small treatise for medical students, residents, pediatricians, nurses and neonatologists to assist them in management of critical and sick neonates ultimately helping them to save these little angels, who are our *tomorrow*.

Walt Disney aptly said, "There is more treasure in books than in all the pirate's loot on Treasure Island." We hope the readers not only enjoy reading the book but also practice its principles of management in neonatal intensive care.

विद्यां ददाति विनयं विनयाद् याति पात्रताम्।
पात्रत्वात् धनमाप्नोति धनात् धर्मं ततः सुखम्।।

Neelam Kler
Pankaj Garg
Anup Thakur

ACKNOWLEDGMENTS

We are indebted to our teachers for the knowledge and skills imparted to us to take care of sick and vulnerable neonates.

We are extremely thankful to our colleagues Drs Satish Saluja, Arun Soni, Manoj Modi, team of residents and nurses for providing an environment of clinical and academic excellence in the department. We are grateful to our institution Sir Ganga Ram Hospital New Delhi, India for nurturing a culture of humanitarian care and stand by its ethos to provide world class healthcare in a safe, comfortable and caring environment at an affordable cost to all sections of the society.

We are thankful to Dr Naveen Parkash Gupta for reviewing some important sections of the book and providing us with important feedbacks to improve its content and readability. We sincerely acknowledge the secretariat help provided by Ms Renu Bisht. We thank Shri Jitendar P Vij (Group Chairman), Mr Ankit Vij (Managing Director), Ms Chetna Malhotra Vohra (Associate Director–Content Strategy) of M/s Jaypee Brothers Medical Publishers (P) Ltd, New Delhi, India, who invited us to edit the textbook and guided its framework throughout the period of writing.

Our heartfelt gratitude goes to the neonates in the neonatal intensive care unit (NICU) and their families who have always inspired us to practice the art of compassionate neonatal care. Last but not least, we thank our families for bearing with us.

CONTENTS

Chapter 1

Neonatal Resuscitation

Koshy Marucoickal George, Nirupama Laroia

INTRODUCTION

- Of approximately 4 million neonatal deaths globally, 23% are accounted by birth asphyxia.
- The outcome of thousands of newborns born each year can be improved by widespread use of resuscitation taught and practiced appropriately and systematically. Studies show that resuscitation training has significantly reduced neonatal and perinatal mortality and morbidity.
- About 8–10% of the newborns require some assistance at birth and less than 1% need extensive resuscitative measures including chest compressions or emergency medications **(Fig. 1)**.
- It is difficult to predict requirement of assistance at birth; therefore, teams capable of performing neonatal resuscitation should be prepared to act promptly and efficiently in providing lifesaving interventions at every birth.
- At the time of delivery, focus should be on providing interventions such as drying, keeping the baby warm, clearing the airway, stimulation to breathe, and providing positive pressure breaths. These simple interventions can save many babies.

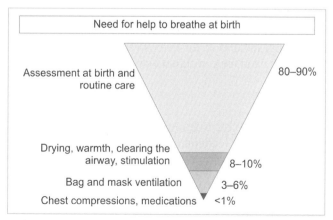

Fig. 1: Requirement of resuscitation.
Source: Adapted from Wall SN, Lee AC, Niermeyer S, et al. Neonatal resuscitation in low-resource settings: what, who, and how to overcome challenges to scale up? Int J Gynaecol Obstet. 2009;107:S47-62, S63-4.

PATHOPHYSIOLOGY

- Ventilation of the baby's lung is the most important and effective step in neonatal resuscitation. The most common cause for need of resuscitation is inability to breathe effectively at birth leading to inadequate gas exchange. This can result in respiratory failure before, during or after birth.
- In utero, respiratory function is performed by the placenta. The placenta functions in transfer of oxygen from the mother to fetus and removal of CO_2. In case placental diffusion fails, there is insufficient transfer of oxygen to fetus causing inability to support normal cellular functions and CO_2 cannot be removed. Fetal monitoring may show a decrease in fetal activity, loss of heart rate (HR) variability, and HR decelerations.
- Before birth only a small quantity of blood flows to the lungs because of the increased resistance to flow [increased pulmonary vascular resistance (PVR)] in the pulmonary vessels. There is no gas exchange in the lung and lung sacs are filled with fluid. Blood returning to the right side of the heart from the umbilical vein has the highest oxygen saturation.
- After birth, baby breathes and the umbilical cord is clamped (loss of the placenta—low resistance circuit), systemic vascular resistance (SVR) increases, fluid in alveoli absorbed and replaced by air, blood vessels in lung relax (decreased PVR) with dramatic increased blood flow and reversal of shunt occurs through ductus arteriosus leading to increased left atrial pressure resulting in functional closure of foramen ovale.
- If this transition does not happen smoothly then infant could present with irregular respiratory effort, tachypnea, respiratory depression with apnea, bradycardia, tachycardia, hypotonia, low oxygen saturation, persistent cyanosis, or hypotension.

PREPARING FOR RESUSCITATION

Resuscitation Team

- Every birth should be attended by at least one individual trained in neonatal resuscitation.
- In case of presence of any of the risk factors **(Table 1)**, minimum two qualified persons should attend the resuscitation.
- The number and qualifications of personnel will increase if higher risk such as an extremely premature birth or high likelihood for extensive resuscitation such as cord prolapse is present. Always identify need for additional help.

Behavioral Skills

Behavioral skills which are key to resuscitation include anticipated preparation, prebriefing, effective communication, assumed leadership role, delegation of roles, proper documentation, and identification of additional help and resources. The role of effective communication is extremely essential.

Four Prebirth Questions

- At every delivery, following four prebirth questions should be asked to the obstetrics care provider:

Table 1: Risk factors that increase the likelihood for need of resuscitation.

Antepartum risk factors

GA <36 0/7 weeks or >41 0/7 weeks	Polyhydramnios, oligohydramnios
Preeclampsia, eclampsia, gestational hypertension	Fetal macrosomia, prior history of shoulder dystocia
Gestational diabetes	Intrauterine growth restriction
Multiple gestation	Fetal malformations or anomalies
Premature rupture of membranes	Inadequate prenatal care
Previous preterm delivery	Maternal infections
Previous neonatal/fetal deaths	Maternal systemic diseases
Bleeding in second or third trimester	Maternal medications
Placental abnormalities	Lack of maternal steroids use for fetal lung maturation
Fetal anemia	Adrenergic agonists
Isoimmunization	Decreased fetal movements
Hydrops	Fetal heart tracing and duration

Intrapartum risk factors

Reason for emergency cesarean delivery	Maternal blood loss
Precipitous delivery	Placental abruption
Prolonged labor	Placenta previa/percreta/accreta
Instrument-assisted delivery	Maternal abdominal trauma
Breech or other abnormal presentations	PROM >18 hrs
Shoulder dystocia	Chorioamnionitis
Category II or III fetal heart rate pattern and duration	Meconium staining of fluid
Maternal general anesthesia	Prolapsed cord
Maternal narcotic administration	Nuchal cord
Maternal magnesium therapy	Cord avulsion

(GA: general anesthesia; PROM: premature rupture of membranes)

1. Expected gestational age
2. Amniotic fluid clear or not
3. Number of babies expected
4. Any other additional risk factors.

- Importance of prenatal counseling in the presence of risk factors is also pertinent for improved resuscitation.

Delayed Cord Clamping

- Current evidence suggests delayed cord clamping (DCC) for at least 30–60 seconds is beneficial for vigorous term and preterm newborns.
- Delayed cord clamping is not performed in cases of maternal hemorrhage, placental abruption, bleeding placenta previa, bleeding vasa previa, uterine rupture, cord avulsion,

severe intrauterine growth restriction (IUGR) with abnormal cord Doppler studies, suspected twin-to-twin transfusion, hydrops, severe chromosomal, or structural anomalies.
- Benefits include improved transitional circulation hemoglobin levels, improved iron stores, decreased need for blood transfusions, lower incidence of necrotizing enterocolitis, intraventricular hemorrhage (IVH), and neurodevelopmental outcome.

INITIAL STEPS OF NEWBORN CARE

Evaluation at Birth (Neonatal Resuscitation Program Algorithm—Flowchart 1)

- All neonates should have a prompt evaluation at birth on three questions to decide if they can stay with their mother for transition or moved under warmer for further assessment and initial steps.
  1. Does the baby appear to be term?
  2. Does the baby have good muscle tone?
  3. Is the baby breathing or crying?
- If answer to all three is yes, then baby can transition to skin-to-skin care with the mother (routine care). If answer to any of the questions is NO, one should move the baby under radiant warmer and perform initial steps of resuscitation.

Initial Steps

- *Providing warmth:* Place the baby under radiant warmer. For preterm infants <32 weeks, additional warming methods like thermal blanket, covering the head with a hat and placing a plastic wrap over the body without drying can be used. Maintaining the temperature between 36.5°C and 37.5°C in the delivery room is associated with better perinatal outcome.
- *Position the head and neck to open the airway:* Slightly extend the head in sniffing position to open the airways and allow unrestricted air entry. One may place a small rolled towel under the baby's shoulder.
- *Clear airway (if necessary):* Clear secretions, if baby is not breathing/gasping/has poor tone/secretions are obstructing the airways or when positive pressure ventilation (PPV) is anticipated. Suction only when visible secretions are present. Suction pressure should not exceed 80–100 mm Hg. Suction mouth before nose (remember M comes before N). Routine tracheal suction is no longer recommended for nonvigorous babies with meconium stained fluid.
- *Dry:* The baby should be thoroughly dried to decrease evaporative heat loss and wet linen should be discarded. Preterm infants <32 weeks should be covered immediately in a polyethylene plastic to decrease heat loss.
- *Stimulate:* The initial steps provided so far will frequently provide enough stimulation for the baby to breathe. If the newborn does not have adequate respiration, providing brief stimulation by gently rubbing of back, trunk or extremities will stimulate breathing. One should begin PPV immediately if the newborn remains apneic despite brief stimulation. Vigorous use of tactile stimulation in a baby, who is not breathing, wastes valuable time.

POSITIVE PRESSURE VENTILATION

The most important effective action in resuscitating a compromised newborn is assisted ventilation.

Flowchart 1: Neonatal Resuscitation Program (NRP) algorithm.

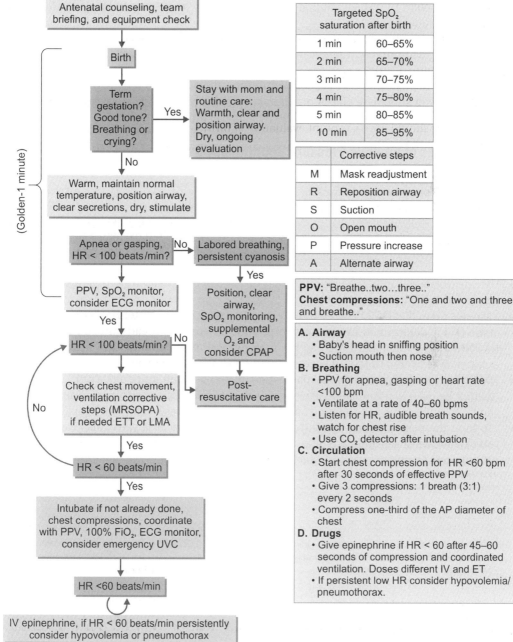

Indication

- After initial steps of resuscitation, if the baby is apneic or gasping or has HR <100 beats/min, PPV should be started.
- Additional indication is if baby is breathing and has HR >100 beats/min but baby is not maintaining saturations in target range despite free flow oxygen or continuous positive airway pressure (CPAP).

Whenever indicated, it should be started within 1 minute of birth called the golden minute.

Pulse oximeter should be placed on right wrist (preductal). Probe is attached first to hand and then cable is attached to monitor for better signal acquisition.

Different Types of Positive Pressure Ventilation Devices (Figs. 2 to 4)

Self-inflating Bag

- Unless squeezed, a self-inflating bag remains in a fully expanded state. It recoils and re-expands drawing fresh air on its release. When the bag is connected to a source of oxygen, it gets filled with the gas that depends on the supplied oxygen concentration. In case an oxygen source is not attached to the bag, it gets refilled by drawing room air (21% oxygen).
- Because of its self-inflating nature, there is no need of compressed gas or a tight seal at the outlet to keep it inflated.
- The rate of ventilation is decided by how frequently you squeeze the bag and the inspiratory time (IT) is determined by the duration of the squeeze. Peak inspiratory pressure (PIP) is controlled by how hard the bag is squeezed. Positive end expiratory pressure (PEEP) cannot be delivered unless an accessory PEEP valve is attached.
- Because gas only flows out of the mask when the bag is being squeezed, a self-inflating bag cannot be used to administer CPAP or free-flow oxygen. It is possible to administer free-flow oxygen in some self-inflating bags through the open reservoir ("tail") on them.
- To limit the peak inflating pressure, there is a pressure-release valve, also called a pop-off valve in most self-inflating bags. The limiting pressure in these valves is usually set at 30–40 cm H_2O pressure beyond which they are released. However, at times, they may not be

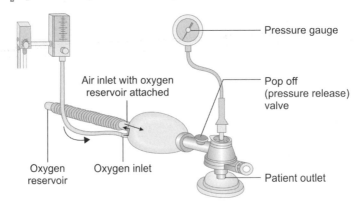

Fig. 2: Parts of self-inflating bag.
Parts: Air inlet and attachment site for oxygen reservoir, oxygen inlet, patient outlet, valve assembly, oxygen reservoir, pressure-release pop-off valve, and pressure gauge.

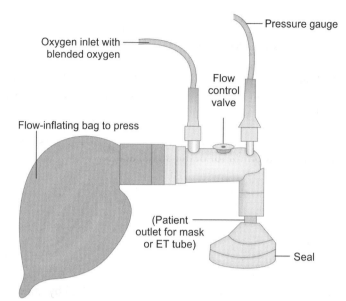

Fig. 3: Parts of flow-inflating bag. (ET: endotracheal tube)
Parts: Oxygen inlet from blender, patient outlet, flow control valve, and pressure gauge.

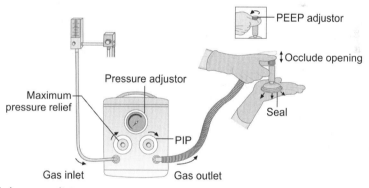

Fig. 4: Parts of T-piece resuscitator.
Parts: Gas inlet, patient outlet PIP (peak inspiratory pressure), control, PEEP (positive end expiratory pressure), cap, circuit pressure gauge reading, and maximum pressure relief.

very reliable and may not release until higher pressures are achieved. In some self-inflating bags, the pressure-release valve can be temporarily occluded, to allow higher pressures to be delivered.

- It can be used even in the absence of compressed air or oxygen source.

Flow-inflating Bag

- It requires source of compressed gas and gets inflated only when the gas is flowing into it and the outlet is sealed, such as when the mask is tightly applied to a baby's face. In the absence of a compressed gas source or improper seal, the bag will collapse and look like a deflated balloon. In case the bag fails to inflate or gets partially inflated, it indicates that the seal is not tight.

- The ventilation rate will depend on how many times one squeezes the bag and how fast is the bag squeezed and released will determine the IT. PIP is controlled by how hard the bag is squeezed to ensure that the appropriate pressure is used. To measure the delivered PIP, one should use a manometer with a self-inflating or a flow-inflating bag.
- Can be used to deliver 100% free-flow oxygen.
- Positive end expiratory pressure is adjusted using a flow control valve adjustment.
- Cannot be used outside the setting of delivery room as it fills only when compressed air flows into it.
- Needs practice and the importance of a good seal is extremely important for use for this device.

T-piece Resuscitator

- It is a mechanical device that uses valves to regulate the compressed gas flowing toward the patient. A compressed gas source is needed for this device.
- A finger is used to alternately occlude and release an opening on the top of the T-piece cap to deliver a breath. On occlusion of the opening, gas flows through the device toward the baby and on releasing the opening, some gas will escape through the cap.
- The ventilation rate will depend on how often the opening on the cap is occluded and how long the cap is occluded will decide the IT.
- Peak inspiratory pressure during each assisted breath is limited by the inspiratory pressure control.
- To prevent inadvertent delivery of PIP beyond predetermined preset value, the device has a maximum pressure relief control.
- Inspiratory and expiratory pressure are measured by a built-in manometer. Hence PEEP and free-flow oxygen can be given and a predetermined consistent PIP can be provided to prevent over inflation.
- Disadvantage of the device is that it cannot be used outside the delivery room setting.

Important Considerations during PPV

- Indicators of successful PPV are rising HR, chest rise, bilateral breath sounds, and improvement in oxygen saturation.
- Effective seal with the mask is one of the key elements missed. Mask should be applied on the face such that the pointed edge is over the nose and mask covers the mouth and nose and the tip of the chin rests within the rim of the mask. The thumb and the index fingers encircle the rim of the mask and the other three fingers are snugly placed under the bony angle of the jaw to gently lift the jaw upward toward the mask. When the correct position of the mask is ensured, one should apply even downward pressure on the rim of the mask to obtain an airtight seal with the head held in sniffing position. In a large baby, it may be difficult to achieve a correct head position and a good seal using one hand. In such a scenario, one can use both hands to hold the mask with the jaw thrust technique by gently lifting the jaw toward the mask.
- *Timing of PPV:* Use the rhythm, "Breathe, two, three... Breathe, two, three.... breathe, two, three." During PPV, 40 to 60 breaths per minute should be delivered. Count out loudly to help maintain the correct rate.

Table 2: Ventilation corrective steps.

	Corrective steps	Actions
M	Mask readjustment	Reapply mask to assure good seal, consider two-hand technique
R	Reposition airway	Head in sniffing position
	Reattempt PPV and reassess chest movements	
S	Suction	Suction mouth then nose, use bulb/suction catheter
O	Open mouth	Open mouth, lift jaw forward
	Reattempt PPV and reassess chest movements	
P	Pressure increase	Increase pressure in slow increments, maximum of 40 for adequate chest movements
	Reattempt PPV and reassess chest movements	
A	Alternate airway	Place an ET/LMA
	Reattempt PPV and reassess chest movements	

(ET: endotracheal tube; LMA: laryngeal mask airway; PPV: positive pressure ventilation)

- Initial PIP settings of 20–25 cm H_2O should be used. In some infants, this may need to be increased up to 30–40 cm H_2O for opening up alveoli.
- Initial PEEP should be set at 5 cm H_2O.
- *FiO_2 setting:* For the initial resuscitation of newborns greater than or equal to 35 weeks' gestation, set the blender to 21% oxygen. For the initial resuscitation of newborns less than 35 weeks' gestation, set the blender to 21–30% oxygen.
- *PPV is stopped:* When HR is >100 beats/min and baby has sustained spontaneous breaths.
- *Ventilation corrective steps:* When PPV is ineffective, one needs to take ventilation corrective steps **(Table 2)**.

The assistant needs to tap out the HR and also say out if HR is improving or getting worse. HR is counted for 6 seconds and multiplied by 10 to give an approximate HR. After prolonged PPV, consider inserting an orogastric (OG) 8 F feeding tube and 20 mL syringe measured by the distance between bridge of the nose to the earlobe to the point midway between xiphoid and umbilicus.

CHEST COMPRESSION

- *Indications for chest compressions:* When HR remains <60 beats/min despite 30 seconds of effective PPV.
- *Considerations during chest compressions:*
  - Application of electrocardiogram (ECG) leads if available.
  - Intubation if not done so far.
  - Increase oxygen concentration to 100% FiO_2.
  - Coordination with PPV.
  - Preparing for placement of umbilical venous (UV) line.
- *Methods of chest compression:* There are two methods—(1) thumb technique and (2) two-finger technique. In thumb technique, two thumbs are used to depress the sternum while hands encircle the torso and finger supports the spine. This is the preferred technique as it is superior in generating peak systolic and coronal perfusion pressure. Two-finger technique where the tips of the middle and index fingers are used to compress the sternum

perpendicularly. Pressure is applied to the lower third of the sternum and sternum is depressed to a depth of approximately one-third of antero-posterior (AP) chest diameter. The thumbs/tip of fingers should remain in contact with the chest during both compression and release.

- *Timing of chest compression:* Coordinated by counting loud "one and two and three and breathe and..." Each 2-second cycle of events comprises three compressions and one ventilation in 2 seconds [a total of 120 events—90 compression and 30 breaths (3:1) in 60 seconds; Ratio of 3:1]. Wait for 45–60 seconds and then assess HR again.
- *Indications to stop chest compression:* If HR is ≥60 beats/min, stop chest compressions and continue PPV with 40–60 breaths per minute.

INTUBATION

- *Indication for intubation:* Endotracheal intubation is considered when PPV with face mask is not resulting in clinical improvement or lasts more than few minutes, when chest compressions are needed and for reliable airway access in special situations such as need for surfactant, suspected congenital diaphragmatic hernia (CDH) or direct tracheal suction if the airway is obstructed with thick secretions.
- *Intubation procedure:* Determine size of endotracheal tube (ET), position the baby in sniffing position, ask for neck roll if needed, check light of the laryngoscope, hold the laryngoscope with left hand, use the stylet in tube if needed, insert tube to length of weight in kilograms + 6 or nasal-tragus length + 1, request/apply cricoid pressure if needed, and pass the tube into glottis beyond the markings on the tube. Stabilize ET tube against the hard palate and tape the tube.
- *Time to intubate:* Not more than 30 seconds for each trial.
- *Assessment of successful intratracheal intubation:* The operator watches tube pass through cords, symmetric adequate chest rise, bilateral breath sounds, increasing HR and improving saturations, mist in tube, change in colorimetric CO_2 detector from purple to yellow, and decreased or absent breath sounds over the stomach. Confirm with chest X-ray, if available, checking also for tube position and pneumothorax. Babies with poor cardiac output and extremely low birth weight (ELBW) babies may take time to show reliable color change. If epinephrine is given through ET tube it could falsely turn the color yellow.
- *Laryngeal mask airway (LMA):* May be used if PPV is ineffective and intubation is not feasible. Other indications include congenital anomalies involving mouth, lip, palate, tongue, neck, jaw, Pierre Robin sequence, and trisomy 21. Use size 1 for neonates. For insertion of LMA, position baby in sniffing, hold device like a pen and advance with the opening facing away from the operator. Inflate with 2–4 mL of air **(Fig. 5)**.

MEDICATION

Epinephrine

- *Indication:* When HR is <60 beats/min after 30 seconds of effective ventilation and another 60 seconds of coordinated chest compression and effective ventilation.
- *Dose:* Epinephrine 1:10,000 solution 0.1–0.3 mL/kg IV (given rapidly followed by a flush of 0.5–1 mL normal saline) and 0.5–1 mL/kg endotracheally. After epinephrine check HR in

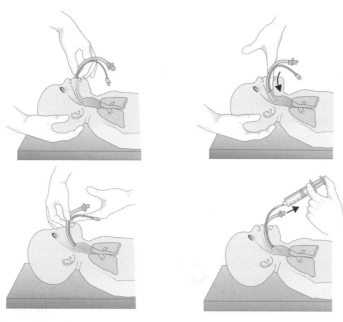

Fig. 5: Insertion of laryngeal mask airway.

1 minute and continue chest compressions and PPV with 100% oxygen. If HR is still less than 60 beats/min, repeat the dose of epinephrine every 3–5 minutes.

- *Volume expanders:* Volume expanders are indicated if the baby is not responding to the steps of resuscitation and has signs of shock or a history of acute blood loss. The recommended solution for treating hypovolemia is 0.9% NaCl (10 mL/kg normal saline). In case of severe fetal anemia one can use type-O Rh-negative blood (10 mL/kg). This can be given over 5–10 minutes and pausing to give the epinephrine flushes as needed if chest compressions are being done. Ringer's lactate is no longer recommended for treating hypovolemia.

SPECIAL SITUATIONS

If HR <60 beats/min in spite of effective ventilation, consider hypotension, pneumothorax, and other structural reasons like airway malformation, hydrops, abdominal ascites, CDH, pulmonary hypoplasia, chromosomal defects, metabolic acidosis, hypoxic-ischemic encephalopathy (HIE) or congenital heart disease (CHD).

- In prenatally diagnosed CDH, minimize face mask ventilation, perform early planned intubation, and use OG tube for gastric decompression.
- For pneumothorax/chylothorax/pleural effusion needle decompression at bedside if needed.
- For pulmonary hypoplasia and hydrops, higher PIPs need to be considered for adequate chest movement.
- For extreme prematurity, use of plastic bags, warm mattresses, and surfactant should be considered.

AFTER RESUSCITATION

- At the end of each resuscitation, it is important to debrief. Discuss briefly what went well during the resuscitation, was the leader effective and delegated tasks well, and was there good communication and team work, what was not done well, what could have been done better to improve. The goal is not to assign blame but to improve the process.
- *Reasons to stop resuscitation:* Resuscitation may be discontinued after 10 minutes of asystole, after maximal resuscitation effort.

KEY POINTS

➢ Birth asphyxia accounts for about 23% of the approximately 4 million neonatal deaths worldwide.
➢ Ventilation of the baby's lung is the most important and effective step in neonatal resuscitation.
➢ Frequent simulations and training of trained providers and instructors is key for continued improvement in morbidity and mortality in babies worldwide. It has been widely recognized that though theoretical knowledge is retained, skills deteriorate without practice.

SELF ASSESSMENT

1. **Baby is born limp and apneic. You place her under radiant warmer, position her airway, remove secretions, dry and stimulate her. If she remains still apneic, next step is to:**
   a. Provide positive pressure ventilation
   b. Provide free-flow oxygen
   c. Consider CPAP

2. **What should be size of endotracheal tube for a baby weighing <1,000 g?**
   a. 2.0 mm
   b. 2.5 mm
   c. 3.0 mm
   d. 3.5 mm

3. **Ratio of chest compression to ventilation is:**
   a. 1:3
   b. 3:1
   c. 5:2
   d. 2:5

4. **Which of the following devices provide PEEP during resuscitation (more than one may be true)?**
   a. Self-inflating bag
   b. T-piece resuscitator
   c. Flow-inflating bag

2
Chapter

Fluid and Electrolyte Management

Jogender Kumar, Venkataseshan Sundaram

INTRODUCTION

- An appropriate fluid and electrolyte management is an essential component of neonatal care primarily due to the constantly evolving fluid and electrolyte homeostasis from the fetal life throughout the infantile period and an abrupt transition to postnatal period.
- Inappropriate fluid management has been reported to be associated with chronic lung disease (CLD), patent ductus arteriosus (PDA), and necrotizing enterocolitis (NEC) in preterm neonates. Physiologically, total body water (TBW) comprises of extracellular fluid (ECF) and intracellular fluid (ICF), where ECF is the fluid within the intravascular and interstitial spaces and ICF is the fluid contained within individual cells. Early in fetal development, TBW comprises of about 90–95% of the total body weight. However, this proportion declines as gestation progresses, primarily due to decrease in ECF volume. During the first week of life, all healthy neonates experience a reduction in body weight.
- The major cause of this physiologic weight loss is a reduction in ECF, triggered by a rise in atrial natriuretic peptide (ANP) after birth. The initial transition passes through three less distinct phases—(1) pre-diuretic (1–2 days—low urine output (U.O.), normal to low serum sodium), (2) diuretic (2–4 days—increased urine output, normal to high serum sodium), and (3) a post-diuretic phase (4–5 days onward—stabilization of urine output at 2–5 mL/kg/hr). The diuretic phase is more pronounced in lower gestational age neonates with a urine output approaching 10 mL/kg/hr, which may potentially result in excessive weight loss and high sodium levels. The expected weight loss in the first week of life is 5–10% (1–2% per day) and 10–15% (2–3% per day) in term and preterm infants, respectively.

GOALS OF FLUID AND ELECTROLYTE MANAGEMENT

- Appropriate fluid management in a neonate comprises of maintenance fluid requirements per day, deficit replacement (if one such exists), and replacement of the ongoing losses.
- The maintenance requirement includes daily fluid and electrolyte requirement of the body, which in turn depends on the gestational and postnatal age, environmental factors, renal function and maturity, serum and urine electrolytes, and electrolyte composition of the fluid losses.
- In general, daily maintenance fluid requirement equals insensible water loss (IWL) + sensible water loss [urinary loss + stool loss (5–10 mL/kg) + growth requirements (10–15 mL/kg)]. A prototype of suggested daily fluid requirement can be found in **Table 1**.

Table 1: Fluid and electrolyte requirements in initial days of life.							
	Parenteral fluid in mL/kg/day *Days of life*						
Birth weight	*1*	*2*	*3*	*4*	*5*	*6*	*7*
≥1,500 g	60	75	90	105	120	135	150
<1,500 g	80	95	110	125	140	150	150
	Electrolyte requirement (mEq/kg) No electrolyte supplementation in the first 48 hours						
Sodium	1–3 (ELBW neonates may require up to 6–8 mEq/kg/day)						
Potassium	1–2 (start after onset of diuresis)						
Chloride	1–3						

(ELBW: extremely low birth weight)

TIPS FOR APPROPRIATE FLUID MANAGEMENT

- Administer electrolyte-free fluid in the first 48 hours of life to allow adequate physiological ECF volume loss to take place. This fluid would typically be a dextrose containing solution or parenteral nutrition as suitable with the concentration depending on the glucose requirement of the neonate.
- Watch for signs of hydration such as weight change, urine frequency, and adequacy of stool passage.
- In suspected cases of dehydration, serum sodium, urine-specific gravity, and serum osmolality may help to confirm or refute dehydration.

Deficit Replacement

General Calculations for Estimation of Fluid and Electrolyte Deficit

Fluid deficit volume
- The most precise method of assessing fluid deficit is weight loss.
- Fluid deficit (L) = Pre-illness weight – current weight (in kg).
- Percentage of dehydration = (Pre-illness weight – current weight)/pre-illness weight × 100.
- For every 1% dehydration = 10 mL/kg would be the arbitrary fluid deficit.

Solute deficit (isonatremic dehydration)
$$\text{Sodium deficit (mEq)} = \text{Fluid deficit (L)} \; 0.75 \times \text{ECF sodium (mEq/L)}$$

Excess electrolyte deficits (hyponatremic dehydration)
$$\text{Deficit} = (Na_{desired} - Na_{actual}) \, (mEq/L) \times \text{distribution factor (0.75)} \times \text{pre-illness weight (kg)}$$

Free water deficit
This is the amount of additional free water loss in hypernatremic dehydration.

Note: It requires 4 mL/kg of fluid to decrease serum Na^+ by 1 mEq/L. If serum Na^+ is >170 mEq/L, estimated requirement would be 3 mL/kg.

$$\text{FWD (mL)} = 4 \text{ mL/kg} \times \text{weight (kg)} \times [(\text{Present sodium concentration-desired sodium concentration})\text{meq/L}]$$

Solute fluid deficit
This is the amount of additional fluid volume loss beyond free water loss in a patient with hypernatremic dehydration.

SFD = Total fluid deficit – FWD

Solute sodium deficit

$$SSD = SFD (L) \times 0.75 \times normal\ ECF\ sodium,\ i.e.\ 145.$$

Note: 0.75 is the distribution factor of sodium and 0.25 of potassium in neonates.

Solute potassium deficit

$$SPD = SFD (L) \times 0.25 \times normal\ ICF\ potassium,\ i.e.\ 150.$$

Deficit Replacement Strategy

Replacement of fluid deficit has two components—(1) resuscitation of the intravascular compartment and (2) repletion of the deficit.

Initial resuscitation
Reserved for neonates who have clinical evidence of hemodynamic compromise such as tachycardia along with poor peripheral pulses and prolonged capillary refill time and/or hypotension, especially in the presence of blood loss or evidence of sepsis. Fluid of choice is isotonic saline [normal saline (NS)] at 10–20 mL/kg administered over 30–60 minutes. This initial resuscitation volume should be deducted from the total deficit replacement fluid.

Note: In preterm neonates, caution should be exercised while administering bolus fluid more rapid than the recommended rate of administration as rapid fluctuation in the cerebral blood flow may occur and may be associated with intraventricular hemorrhage.

Deficit repletion and maintenance: Following initial stabilization, the remaining deficit is replaced over the next 24–48 hours as shown in **Table 2**.

Replacement of ongoing losses
Renal losses: The total amount of urine output should be replaced volume or weight by volume, depending on the method of urine collection (nappy weighing/test tube/collection bags). Catheterization should be reserved for the circumstances where collection by the above methods is not feasible. In general, renal losses of greater than 4 mL/kg/hr should be

Table 2: Fluid replacement strategy in various conditions.			
Type of dehydration	*First 8 hours*	*Next 16 hours*	*Next 24 hours*
Isonatremic/hyponatremic			
• Fluid deficit volume • Na+ deficit (Add excess deficit in hyponatremia) • K+ deficit	Replace ½ of calculated deficit	Replace remaining ½ of calculated deficit	
Maintenance	1/3rd of maintenance fluid	2/3rd of maintenance fluid	
Hypernatremic			
Free water deficit	Replace ½ of the deficit over first 24 hours		Replace remaining ½ of over next 24 hours
• Solute fluid deficit volume • Solute Na+ deficit • Solute K+ deficit	Replace ½ of calculated deficit	Replace remaining ½ of calculated deficit	
Maintenance	To be given in addition to the above calculated deficit at an hourly rate		

Table 3: Approximate IWL in different birth weight categories.

Birth weight (g)	IWL (mL/kg/day)
750–1,000	82
1,001–1,250	56
1,251–1,500	46
>1,501	26

(IWL: insensible water loss)

Table 4: Choice of replacement fluid for ongoing losses.

Nature of losses	Type of fluid
Vomiting/nasogastric aspirates/polyuria	N/2 saline (0.45%) + 10 mEq/L KCl
Chest tube drainage/Third space losses	Normal saline (0.9% NS)
Diarrheal losses	N/5 saline (0.2%) in 5% dextrose + 20 mEq/L KCl

(KCl: potassium chloride)

replaced over the forthcoming 6 hours, even though extreme preterm neonates may often have physiological losses in this range, due to their immature renal concentrating ability.

Extrarenal loss/insensible water loss: Insensible water losses are primarily evaporative losses via the skin (two-thirds) and respiratory tract (one-third). IWL increases exponentially with decrease in weight and gestational age **(Table 3)**. As a rule of thumb, IWL equals (fluid intake – urine output) + weight change. IWL dramatically increases under a radiant warmer, when the skin is breached (due to probes and sensors) and in cases of high respiratory rate unaccompanied by respiratory humidification.

Strategies to prevent/reduce IWL:
- Avoid allowing the neonate to remain naked except while rewarming. Keep head and extremities adequately covered.
- Use of plastic bags and wraps during resuscitation helps in babies <32 weeks' gestation.
- Use transparent plastic sheets (food grade polythene sheets) to create a microenvironment while nursing under a radiant warmer (cling wrap).
- Humidify the ambient air up to 70–80% in extremely low birth weight neonates nursed in an incubator. However, avoid excessive humidification and rain out as well as prolonged durations of humidification to prevent fungal and bacterial colonization of the incubators.
- Respiratory gases used for noninvasive as well as invasive ventilatory support should preferably be warmed and humidified.
- Use of emollients (Topical application of coconut oil in very preterm and 750–1,500 g infants has been shown to reduce transepidermal water loss and improves skin maturity and integrity).

Gastrointestinal losses
Fluid losses from the gastrointestinal (GI) route are usually from the stomach (orogastric tube drainage), small intestine (vomiting and regurgitation, acute gastroenteritis), large intestine (enterocolitis), and surgical site drainage (small and/or large intestine losses). These losses would need assessment for quantity and a weight by volume replacement in an ongoing fashion. The type of fluid would depend on the type of losses.

The choice of replacement fluid should be as per the type of losses **(Table 4)**.

APPROACH TO DISORDERS OF SODIUM AND WATER BALANCE

Disorders of fluid and electrolyte imbalance can be grouped into disorders of tonicity (hypo/hypernatremia) or ECF volume.

The assessment and monitoring of fluid and electrolyte status will depend on maternal and neonatal history, physical examination and laboratory evaluation **(Table 5)**.

Isonatremic Disorders

Dehydration

Etiology
- It involves equal losses of Na and water.
- Losses through nasogastric, thoracostomy, or ventriculostomy drainage.
- Third space GI losses (Gastroschisis, omphalocele).

Diagnosis
- *Clinical:* Weight loss, decreased urine output, tachycardia, and hypotension.
- *Laboratory:* Metabolic acidosis, increased urine specific gravity, and increased blood urea nitrogen (BUN).

Management
See Table 3 and example 1.

Fluid Overload

Etiology
- Excessive isotonic fluid administration.
- Congestive cardiac failure.
- Sepsis.
- Neuromuscular paralysis.

Diagnosis
Weight gain, edema, pulmonary crepitations, and hepatomegaly.

Table 5: Assessment and monitoring of fluid and electrolyte status.		
History	*Physical examination*	*Laboratory evaluation*
• *Maternal:* NSAIDs, hydration status, oligohydramnios, oxytocin, antenatal steroids • *Neonatal:* Birth asphyxia, urinary stream and environmental factors (humidification, ventilation, warmers, and phototherapy)	• *Vital parameters* • *Skin and mucosa:* Edema, dryness, skin turgor (Sunken anterior fontanels and mucosal dryness are not reliable) • *Systemic:* Pulmonary crepts, cardiac gallop, and hepatomegaly indicate fluid overload • *Ancillary assessment:* Weight change, Intake, and output	• Serum and urine electrolytes • Plasma osmolarity • Urine specific gravity • Blood pH • Urea/creatinine • Fractional excretion of Na (FeNa)

(NSAIDs: nonsteroidal anti-inflammatory drugs)

Management
Restriction of sodium as well as water.

Example 1: A 15-day old term neonate, birth weight 3 kg, presents in the emergency department with lethargy and poor feeding from last 5 days. At admission, the baby had a weight of 2.7 kg and was hemodynamically stable. On evaluation, her serum sodium is 140 mEq/L. How will you chart fluids for this baby?

Step 1: Calculate replacement fluid
Fluid deficit volume (L) = Pre-illness weight − current weight (in kg) = 0.3 L = 300 mL

Sodium deficit (mEq) = Fluid deficit (L) × 0.75 × ECF Na = 0.3 × 0.75 × 145 = 32.6 mEq

Potassium deficit (mEq) = Fluid deficit (L) × 0.25 × ICF K = 0.3 × 0.25 × 150 = 11.25 mEq

Step 2: Calculate maintenance fluid
Fluid: 150 × 3 = 450 mL, Na = 3 × 3 = 9 mEq, K = 3 × 2 = 6 mEq

Step 3: Fluid schedule*

	First 8 hours	Next 16 hours
Deficit		
• Fluid deficit volume (mL)	150	150
• Na$^+$ deficit (mEq)	16.3	16.3
• K$^+$ deficit (mEq)	6	6
Maintenance		
• Fluid (mL)	150	300
• Na (mEq)	3	6
• K (mEq)	2	4
Total		
• Fluid (mL)	300	450
• Na (mEq)	19.3	22.3
• K (mEq)	8	10

*Add ongoing losses if any.

Hyponatremic Disorders (Etiologies given in Table 4)

The etiology of hyponatremia will depend on whether it is factitious, euvolemic, hypovolemic or hypovolemic **(Table 6)**.

Hypovolemic Hyponatremia

Diagnosis
Same as isonatremic dehydration.

Management
Reduce ongoing Na loss. Administer Na and water to replace deficits, also account for losses and maintenance.

Euvolemic Hyponatremia

Diagnosis of syndrome of inappropriate antidiuretic hormone
In the absence of volume-related stimulus to antidiuretic hormone (renal, adrenal or thyroid insufficiency, CCF or diuretic ingestion), the criteria lists in **Table 7** should be met.

Table 6: Causes of hyponatremia.

Factitious hyponatremia	Euvolemic hyponatremia	Hypovolemic hyponatremia	Hypervolemic hyponatremia
• Hyperlipidemia • Hyperproteinemia • Hyperglycemia	• Syndrome of inappropriate antidiuretic hormone secretion • Excessive IV fluids • Hypothyroidism	• Diuretic • Congenital adrenal hyperplasia • Renal tubular acidosis • Obstructive uropathy • Gastrointestinal losses • Skin losses • Necrotizing nterocolitis	• Congestive cardiac failure • Acute kidney injury • Neuromuscular blockade • Capillary leak due to Sepsis

(IV: intravenous)

Table 7: Criteria for diagnosis of syndrome of inappropriate antidiuretic hormone.

Parameter	Value
Urine osmolality (mOsm/kg)	>100 (usually > plasma)
Serum osmolality (mOsm/kg)	<280
Serum sodium (mEq/L)	<135
Urine sodium (mEq/L)	>30
Clinical	Oliguria, abnormal weight gain, and absence of edema

Management
- Fluid restriction alone (if serum Na >120 mEq/L).
- Three percent NaCl infusion (1–3 mL/kg)—if serum Na <120 mEq/L or neurologic signs of hyponatremia present.

Hypervolemic Hyponatremia

Diagnosis
Clinical: Weight gain, edema, decreased urine output.

Laboratory: Increased BUN and low fractional excretion of Na (FENa).

Management
Restrict sodium and water intake.

Correction of Sodium in Hyponatremia

Acute hyponatremia (<24 hours)
- Severe (<120 mEq/L) or symptomatic hyponatremia (seizures, neurologic symptoms) should be given a bolus of hypertonic saline (3% NaCl) to produce a rapid increase in serum sodium.
- Aim to correct to 120–125 mEq/L or until resolution of symptoms followed by the slow correction (over 16–24 hours) of the remaining deficit.
- Excess Na deficit (per kg) = Body weight × 0.75 × ($Na_{desired}$ – Na_{actual}).
- Each mL/kg of 3% NaCl increases the serum Na by approximately 1 mEq/L.
- A child with active symptoms often improves after receiving 4–6 mL/kg of 3% NaCl.

- *Inhaled nebulized beta-agonist (salbutamol, albuterol):*
    - ◆ Due to the immaturity of the β-receptor response in preterms, they might cause nonoliguric hyperkalemia.
    - ◆ Not recommended as primary therapy.
- *Correction of acidosis:*
    - ◆ Every 0.1 pH unit increase leads to a decrease of 0.6 mEq/L in serum potassium.
    - ◆ Sodium bicarbonate 1–2 mEq/kg over 5–10 minutes IV may be used.
    - ◆ Avoid rapid infusion to reduce the risk of intraventricular hemorrhage (IVH).
    - ◆ Respiratory alkalosis by hyperventilation in an intubated patient is an option but should be reserved for emergency conditions as there is a risk of hypoperfusion.

Step 4: Enhanced potassium excretion:
- Furosemide (1 mg/kg IV)
- Peritoneal dialysis
- Double volume exchange transfusion
- Cation exchange resins (Kayexalate):
    - ◆ Administered orally per gavage or per rectal.
    - ◆ Should not be given per oral in preterm neonates (increased risk of NEC).
    - ◆ Rectal administration (1 g/kg at 0.5 g/mL of NS) with a minimum retention time of 30 minutes decreases serum K levels by 1 mEq/L.

In clinical practice, the choice of therapy depends upon the clinical condition, ECG changes, and actual serum K level.

The algorithm for the management of hyperkalemia is described in **Flowchart 1**.

Flowchart 1: Algorithm for management of hyperkalemia.

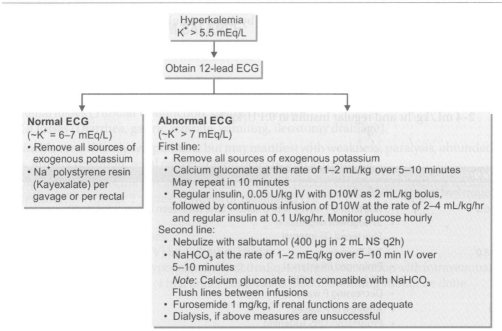

(ECG: electrocardiagram; IV: intravenous)

KEY POINTS

➢ An appropriate fluid and electrolyte management is an essential component of neonatal care.

➢ Fluid management in a neonate should take into account maintenance fluid requirements per day, deficit replacement (if one such exists) and replacement of the ongoing losses.

➢ Disorders of fluid and electrolyte imbalance can be disorders of tonicity (hypo/hypernatremia) or ECF volume. These should be managed cautiously to avoid overt overcorrection or undercorrection.

➢ Complications of hypernatremia include intracranial bleed, cerebral sinus venous thrombosis, renal vein thrombosis, seizures, demyelination, and cerebral edema.

➢ Hyperkalemia in neonates may be asymptomatic or may have a spectrum of signs including ventricular brady/tachyarrhythmia and hemodynamic instability.

SELF ASSESSMENT

1. **Conventionally, hyperkalemia is defined as a serum potassium:**
   a. >5.0 mEq/L
   b. >5.5 mEq/L
   c. >6.0 mEq/L
   d. >6.5 mEq/L

2. **All of the following are true about correction of acute hyponatremia except:**
   a. Severe (<120 mEq/L) or symptomatic hyponatremia (seizures, neurologic symptoms) should be given a bolus of hypertonic saline (3% NaCl) to produce a rapid increase in serum sodium.
   b. Aim to correct to 120–125 mEq/L or until resolution of symptoms followed by the slow correction (over 16–24 hrs) of the remaining deficit.
   c. Excess Na deficit (per kg) = Body weight × 0.75 × ($Na_{desired}$ – Na_{actual}).
   d. Each mL/kg of 3% NaCl increases the serum Na by approximately 3 mEq/L.

FURTHER READING

1. Bell EF, Acarregui MJ. Restricted versus liberal water intake for preventing morbidity and mortality in preterm infants. Cochrane Database Syst Rev. 2008;(1):CD000503.
2. Eichenwald EC, Hansen AR, Martin C, Stark AR. Cloherty and Stark's Manual of Neonatal Care, 8th edition. Philadelphia: Lippincott Williams & Wilkins (LWW); 2017.
3. Kliegman RM, Stanton B, St. Geme J, Schor NF. Nelson Textbook of Pediatrics, 20th edition. Philadelphia, PA: Elsevier/Saunders; 2016.
4. Toro-Ramos T, Paley C, Pi-Sunyer FX, et al. Body composition during fetal development and infancy through the age of 5 years. Eur J Clin Nutr. 2015;69(12):1279-89.

Disorders of Glucose, Calcium, and Magnesium

Chapter 3

Shiv Sajan Saini, Jogender Kumar

GLUCOSE METABOLISM

Glucose is the primary metabolic fuel in the fetal as well as postnatal life. In utero, there is continuous supply of glucose from the mother to the fetus. However, immediately after cord clamping, the newborn has to depend on his/her own endogenous glucose production for survival. After birth, blood glucose levels decrease to as low as 25–30 mg/dL in first 1–2 hours of life. With the onset of counter-regulatory metabolic responses, primarily glycogenolysis and gluconeogenesis, the blood glucose level increases to more than 45 mg/dL by 3–4 hours of life. Beyond 48 hours of life, glucose levels are generally above 60 mg/dL. Hypoglycemia as well as hyperglycemia are the common metabolic problems encountered in neonates.

HYPOGLYCEMIA

Definition

The definition of hypoglycemia remains a controversial issue in neonatology. Pediatric Endocrine Society states that "hypoglycemia cannot be defined as a specific plasma glucose concentration". However, the society recommends to maintain plasma glucose >50 mg/dL in the first 48 hours and >60 mg/dL beyond 48 hours. American Academy of Pediatrics (AAP) guidelines recommend maintaining plasma glucose levels >47 mg/dL in late preterm and term neonates beyond 24 hours of age and intervene in a symptomatic neonate at plasma glucose <40 mg/dL. National Neonatology Forum of India (NNF) recommends intervention at blood glucose <40 mg/dL (plasma glucose <45 mg/dL). Thus, most of the guidelines/protocols agree on the concept of operational threshold for intervention, if blood glucose falls below 40 mg/dL (~plasma glucose 45 mg/dL).

Incidence

The reported incidence of hypoglycemia among at-risk neonates such as small for gestational age (SGA), infants of diabetic mothers (IDM), large for gestational age (LGA) and late preterm infants has been reported to vary from 45% to 55%.

Clinical Features

Most of the hypoglycemic episodes in neonates are asymptomatic. The clinical presentation of hypoglycemia in neonate is usually nonspecific and includes lethargy, poor feeding, hypotonia, irritability, tremors, jitteriness, poor primitive reflexes, sometimes exaggerated Moro's reflex, high-pitched cry, seizures, apnea, and cyanosis.

Classification

Neonatal hypoglycemia can be classified as transient (first few hours to days of life, most common form) and persistent hypoglycemia (continues to stay beyond 7 days of life).

Transient Hypoglycemia

Etiology
Related to decreased energy stores, increased utilization of energy due to sickness or transient metabolic disturbances.

Decreased production/stores:
- Prematurity
- Small for gestational age/intrauterine growth restriction (IUGR)
- Delayed introduction of feeding
- Inadequate substrate intake.

Increased utilization:
- Asphyxia
- Hypothermia
- Sepsis
- Shock
- Respiratory distress
- Polycythemia
- Mother or neonate on beta-blockers (e.g. labetalol or propranolol).

Hyperinsulinemic hypoglycemia:
- *Transient hyperinsulinism:* IDM, LGA, erythroblastosis fetalis, etc.
- *Secondary to other conditions:* Birth asphyxia, syndromes such as Beckwith-Wiedemann syndrome, congenital disorders of glycosylation, mothers on tocolytic therapy with beta-sympathomimetic agents, infusion of high concentration of glucose through a malpositioned umbilical venous, sudden stoppage of high glucose infusion, and following exchange transfusion.

Monitoring/screening for hypoglycemia
All symptomatic neonates should be immediately screened for blood glucose. Serial monitoring of blood glucose should be done in asymptomatic at-risk neonates **(Table 1)**.

Frequency of monitoring
Neonates who are at risk of hypoglycemia but are asymptomatic should be first screened at 2 hours after birth. Glucose monitoring should be continued 4–6 hourly thereafter until feedings are well established and glucose values have normalized (generally 48 hours of life).

Table 1: Indications for routine blood glucose screening.

Neonatal conditions	Maternal conditions
• Premature and late preterm infants (<37 weeks) • Low-birth weight infants • Small or large for gestational age neonates • Sick neonates (including but not limited to sepsis, birth asphyxia, polycythemia, suspected inborn errors of metabolism) • Receiving intravenous fluids • Congenital heart diseases (TGA) • Total parenteral nutrition • Blood exchange transfusion • Rh hemolytic disease	• Insulin-dependent diabetic mothers • Gestational diabetic mothers • Obese mothers • Maternal drug ingestion, e.g. beta blockers, oral hypoglycemics, sympathomimetic • Mothers given large amounts of dextrose containing intravenous fluids during labor and delivery

(TGA: transposition of the great arteries)

Methods of blood/plasma glucose level estimation

■ *Point of care (POC) reagent strips* are most widely used tool for bedside screening of hypoglycemia. However, it is not very reliable at low plasma glucose levels. Therefore, low blood glucose values should be confirmed by laboratory analysis. However, due to risk of abnormal neurodevelopmental outcome associated with hypoglycemia, treatment must be initiated based on the results of reagent strips. The blood glucose value by glucometer is 10–15% lower than plasma glucose.

■ *Laboratory diagnosis*: This is the most accurate method [either glucose oxidase (calorimetric) method or glucose electrode method (as used in blood gas and electrolyte analyzer machine)]. The blood sample must be stored in fluoride/citrate vial and processed within the shortest possible turnover time. Delayed processing may lead to falsely low values (14–18 mg/dL/hr).

■ *Subcutaneous continuous glucose monitors (glucose oxidase based)*: The clinical use of these devices is currently not established in neonates.

Management

The management algorithm is shown in **Flowchart 1**. Intervention for hypoglycemia levels should be tailored to the clinical scenario and individualized for neonate in consideration. Unnecessary disruption of breast feeding and mother-infant relationship should be avoided. In Sugar Baby study 2013, it was seen that use of dextrose gel 40% in management of mild hypoglycemia in at risk infants decreased neonatal intensive case unit (NICU) admissions and decreased formula feeding rates at 2 weeks of age. While treating hypoglycemia with intravenous (IV) infusion, feeding should be allowed as it helps in better glycemic control. Glucose concentration >12.5% should not be infused via peripheral cannula and preferably given through either central line or peripherally inserted central catheter. If blood glucose remains <50 mg/dL despite glucose infusion rate (GIR) >12 mg/kg/min, refractory hypoglycemia should be considered.

Refractory Hypoglycemia

Defined if the infant remains hypoglycemic despite receiving GIR >12 mg/kg/min.

Flowchart 1: Algorithm for management of hypoglycemia.

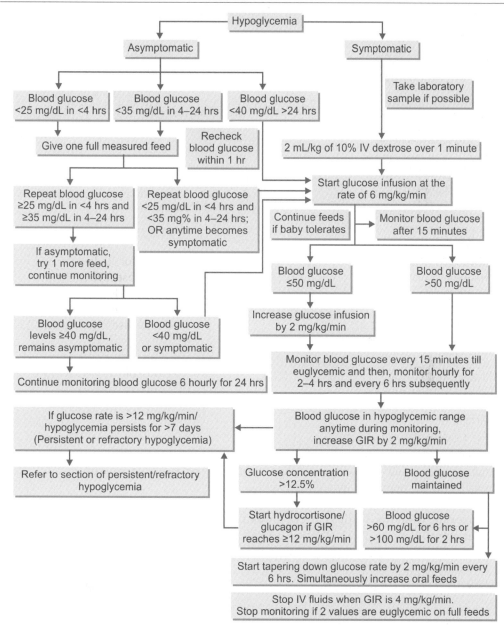

(GIR: glucose infusion rate; IV: intravenous)

Persistent/prolonged hypoglycemia
- Defined if the need for glucose infusion persists for >7 days.
- Persistent/refractory hypoglycemic baby must be evaluated by specialist for following endocrine or metabolic disturbances **(Table 2)**.

Table 2: Etiological workup for evaluation of persistent/refractory hypoglycemia.

Etiology	Investigations to be sent
Hormone deficiencies: • Congenital hypopituitarism • Adrenal insufficiency • Isolated growth hormone deficiency	*First line investigations:* • Insulin • Cortisol • Thyroid profile • Urine for ketone and reducing substances
Hormone excess (hyperinsulinemic state): • Beckwith-Wiedemann syndrome • Hereditary defects of pancreatic islet cells	*Second line investigations:* • Growth hormone levels • ACTH
Hereditary defects in carbohydrate metabolism: • Galactosemia • Glycogen storage disease • Fructose intolerance • Glycogen synthase deficiency • Fructose-1,6-diphosphatase deficiency • Ketogenic defects	• 17-OH-progesterone • Blood ammonia • Blood lactate levels • Galactose 1 phosphate uridyl transferase levels • Urine aminoacidogram • TMS • Free fatty acid levels
Hereditary defects in amino acid metabolism: • Maple syrup urine disease • Propionic acidemia • Methylmalonic acidemia • Tyrosinemia	
Fatty acid oxidation defects: • Acyl-CoA dehydrogenase—medium-, long-chain deficiency • 3-OH-3-methylglutaryl-CoA-lyase deficiency • *Mitochondrial disorders*	

(ACTH: adrenocorticotropic hormone; TMS: tandem mass spectroscopy)

Management of persistent/refractory hypoglycemia

Certain drugs should be used depending upon etiology/available workup in addition to increasing GIR for persistent hypoglycemia:

- Hydrocortisone: 5 mg/kg/dose IV BD
- Diazoxide: 10–25 mg/kg/day in three divided doses
- Glucagon: 0.1 mg/kg SC/IM/IV (max 0.3 mg)—maximum of three doses
- Octreotide: 2–10 µg/kg/day SC, 2–3 times/day.

Congenital Hyperinsulinism

It is the most common cause of persistent hypoglycemia. Its major causes involve defects in *ABCC8* and *KCNJ11* genes, which encode sulfonylurea receptors-1 (SUR1) and killer cell inhibitory receptors (Kir-6.2) of the pancreatic β-cell ATP-sensitive K1 channel, respectively.

When to suspect?

- Persistent hypoglycemia.
- Requirement of high glucose infusion rate (>10 mg/kg/min).
- Absence of ketonemia or acidosis in presence of hypoglycemia.

Diagnostic criteria (in critical blood sample with plasma glucose <45 mg/dL)

- Hyperinsulinemia (plasma insulin >2 µU/mL) and/or
- Plasma free fatty acids <1.5 mmol/L
- Plasma beta-hydroxybutyrate <2 mmol/L
- Positive glycemic response to injection glucagon with increase in blood sugar by ≥30 mg/dL.

Long-term Outcome and Follow-up

Factors on which long-term outcome of hypoglycemia is dependent include severity of hypoglycemia, its duration, cerebral utilization of glucose, and availability of alternative fuels such as ketone or lactate and associated comorbidities. The neonates who experience symptomatic hypoglycemia are at risk of seizures, hypotonia, microcephaly, visual/hearing impairment, and delayed neurodevelopment. Even the neonates with asymptomatic hypoglycemia are at risk of abnormal neurodevelopment. Therefore, these infants should be evaluated for vision at one-month corrected age. Follow-up should be continued at 3, 6, 9, 12, and 18 months corrected age for growth, neurodevelopment, vision and hearing. MRI at 4–6 weeks is a good modality to assess hypoglycemic brain injury and should be considered on follow-up.

HYPERGLYCEMIA

Definition

Hyperglycemia is defined as whole blood glucose level >125 mg/dL or plasma glucose >145 mg/dL. The presentation of neonatal hyperglycemia is nonspecific. The clinical presentation is usually secondary to hyperosmolarity and osmotic diuresis.

Etiology/Risk Factors

- Extremely low birth weight neonates (ELBW)
- Sick neonates (Sepsis, asphyxia, hypothermia)
- Neonates undergoing painful procedures
- Drugs (Glucocorticoids, caffeine, phenytoin, diazoxide, etc.)
- Lipid infusion
- Iatrogenic (excessive exogenous glucose infusion)
- Neonatal diabetes mellitus
- Immature development of glucose transporters.

Treatment

Prevention and early detection are keys to management of neonatal hyperglycemia. In addition, it is important to carefully titrate GIR and frequently monitor blood sugar and urine glucose. Management steps are:

- Monitor at-risk or symptomatic infants for blood glucose levels.
- Extremely low-birth weight neonates should be initiated on GIR of 4–6 mg/kg/min. Fluid balance and glucose levels should be closely monitored. If they develop hyperglycemia on 10% glucose, concentration should be decreased but hypotonic fluids with dextrose concentration <5% should be avoided.

- Feeding should be promoted wherever indicated as it promotes insulin secretion.
- Parenteral nutrition (amino acids) stabilizes glucose levels and should be used as soon as possible, wherever indicated.
- However if the glucose values exceed 250 mg/dL despite decreasing glucose delivery or if osmotic diuresis is present in setting of hyperglycemia, exogenous insulin therapy should be initiated as follows:
  - The usual rate of infusion is 0.05–0.2 units/kg/hr (usual starting dose is 0.05 units/kg/hr).
  - Blood sugar should be checked every 30 minutes until stabilized.
  - If blood sugar remains >180 mg/dL, infusion should be titrated in increments of 0.01 units/kg/hr.
  - In case of hypoglycemia while on insulin infusion, discontinue insulin infusion and administer IV bolus of 10%D at the rate of 2 mL/kg and start GIR infusion at 6 mg/kg/min. Titrate blood glucose level closely monitoring every 30 minutes.
  - Monitor for hypokalemia and rebound hyperglycemia.
- *Oral sulfonylureas* have been used in the long-term management of infants with Kir6.2 and SUR1 defects.

KEY POINTS

- ➤ Hypoglycemia is a common metabolic problem encountered in neonates.
- ➤ Most of the guidelines/protocols agree on the concept of operational threshold for intervention, if blood glucose falls below 40 mg/dL (~plasma glucose 45 mg/dL).
- ➤ Neonates who are at risk of hypoglycemia but are asymptomatic should be first screened at 2 hours after birth. Glucose monitoring should be continued 4–6 hourly thereafter until feedings are well established and glucose values have normalized (generally 48 hours of life).
- ➤ Hypoglycemia should be managed with oral feeds or dextrose gel or IV fluids depending on the severity of hypoglycemia and presence/absence of symptoms.
- ➤ Refractory or prolonged hypoglycemia may point toward an underlying endocrine or metabolic problem.
- ➤ Drugs such as diazoxide or octreotide may be required in cases of refractory or persistent hypoglycemia especially in the setting of hyperinsulinism.

SELF ASSESSMENT

1. **All of the following are diagnostic criteria (in critical blood sample with plasma glucose <45 mg/dL) for hyperinsulinism except:**
   a. Hyperinsulinemia (plasma insulin >2 µU/mL)
   b. Plasma-free fatty acids <1.5 mmol/L
   c. Plasma beta-hydroxybutyrate >2 mmol/L
   d. Glycemic response to inj. glucagon ≥30 mg/dL
2. **All of the following are correct approaches to manage hyperglycemia except:**
   a. Feeding should be promoted wherever indicated as it promotes insulin secretion.
   b. Amino acid stabilizes glucose levels and should be used as soon as possible, wherever indicated.

   c. However, if the glucose values exceed 250 mg/dL despite decreasing glucose delivery or if osmotic diuresis is present in setting of hyperglycemia, exogenous insulin therapy should be initiated.

   d. Lipid stabilizes glucose levels and should be increased in parenteral nutrition as soon as possible, wherever indicated.

CALCIUM METABOLISM

Calcium is an essential element of our body. Calcium levels are regulated by the interplay of parathyroid hormone (PTH), calcitonin, and vitamin D3. During the last trimester, there is active transport of calcium from mother to fetus even in the absence of a fetomaternal calcium gradient. Serum calcium (SCa) in the fetus is 10–11 mg/dL at term (1–2 mg/dL higher than mother). SCa levels start falling immediately after birth and reaches nadir in the first 12–24 hours after birth due to decreased PTH level, end organ unresponsiveness to PTH, abnormal vitamin D metabolism, hyperphosphatemia, hypomagnesemia, and hypercalcitoninemia. Gradually there is a rise in PTH level leading to increase in SCa. Adult levels of SCa are achieved by 2 weeks of age. During this transition phase, especially first 48 hours, the risk of early onset hypocalcemia is increased.

HYPOCALCEMIA

Half of serum calcium is bound and half is unbound or ionized (**Table 3**).

Types

Early-onset neonatal hypocalcemia (ENH): Hypocalcemia occurring within first 3 days of life (usually within 48 hours).

Late-onset neonatal hypocalcemia (LNH): Hypocalcemia occurring 4th day onward.

Etiology

The etiology of hypocalcemia is described in **Table 4**.

Clinical Features

Most of the ENH are asymptomatic in contrast to the LNH. Symptoms are:

- *Neuromuscular irritability*: Jitteriness, myoclonic jerks, exaggerated startle, seizures, tetany, and extensor hypertonia.
- *Cardiac:* Tachycardia, prolonged QT interval, decreased cardiac contractility, and congestive cardiac failure.
- *Nonspecific:* Apnea, laryngospasm with inspiratory stridor, wheezes due to bronchospasm, vomiting due to pylorospasm, circumoral cyanosis, tachypnea, edema, etc.

Table 3: Cut off values of serum calcium in term and preterm infants.		
	Total serum calcium level	Ionized calcium level
Preterm <1,500 g	<7 mg/dL (1.75 mmol/L)	<4 mg/dL
Term and preterm >1,500 g	<8 mg/dL (2 mmol/L)	<4.4 mg/dL

Table 4: Etiology of hypocalcemia.

Early-onset hypocalcemia	Late-onset hypocalcemia

• Prematurity
• Infant of diabetic mother
• Preeclampsia
• Perinatal stress/asphyxia
• Maternal hyperparathyroidism
• Maternal intake of anticonvulsants (phenobarbitone, phenytoin)
• Iatrogenic (alkaline pH, citrate blood products, diuretics, etc.)
	• Increased phosphate load:
	  – Dietary (cow milk, formula milk)
	  – Decreased excretion (renal insufficiency)
	• Vitamin D deficiency
	• Hypomagnesemia
	• Maternal vitamin D deficiency
	• Malabsorption
	• Hepatobiliary disease
	• Transient PTH resistance
	• Hungry bones syndrome
	• Metabolic alkalosis
	• Transient hypoparathyroidism
	• Congenital hypoparathyroidism (primary and secondary)
	• Iatrogenic (citrated blood products, lipid infusion, alkali therapy, loop diuretics, glucocorticoids, and phosphate supplementation)

(PTH: parathyroid hormone)

Diagnosis

Laboratory: Blood calcium levels can be assessed by measuring total or ionized serum calcium. Ionized calcium is the preferred method as it is biologically available form of calcium.

ECG: QoTc >0.22 seconds or QTc >0.45 seconds.

Management

Early-onset Neonatal Hypocalcemia

Prevention
Extremely low birth weight neonates and sick neonates can be screened by measuring ionized calcium at 12, 24, and 48 hours. Ionized calcium should also be evaluated in symptomatic neonates compatible with hypocalcemia and suspected congenital heart diseases.

Treatment
Treatment depends upon symptomatology as shown in **Flowchart 2**.

Late-onset Neonatal Hypocalcemia

Laboratory tests for diagnosis of late-onset hypocalcemia is given in **Table 5**. Treatment is specific to the etiology **(Table 6)** and may need lifelong therapy depending upon etiology.

Outcome

Prognosis is excellent in ENH as most of them resolve within 48–72 hours without any significant sequelae. In LNH, prognosis depends upon the etiology. LNH secondary to exogenous excessive intake of phosphate and magnesium deficiency responds well, whereas

Flowchart 2: Treatment of hypocalcemia.

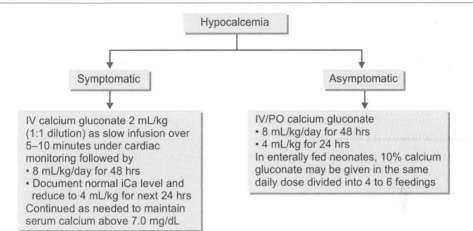

(IV: intravenous; PO: per oral; iCa: ionized calcium)

Table 5: Laboratory tests for diagnosis of late-onset hypocalcemia.	
First tier	*Second tier*
• Serum calcium • Serum phosphate • Serum alkaline phosphatase • Liver function tests • Renal function tests • Arterial/capillary blood pH • X-ray chest/wrist	• Serum magnesium • Serum PTH • Urine calcium creatinine ratio • Maternal calcium, phosphate, and ALP • Absence of thymic shadow on chest X-ray might suggest DiGeorge sequence

(ALP: alkaline phosphatase; PTH: parathyroid hormone)

Table 6: Treatment of late-onset neonatal hypocalcemia.	
Etiology	*Treatment*
Hypomagnesemia	• 0.2 mL/kg of 50% $MgSO_4$, IM × 2 doses, 12 hours apart followed by • 0.2 mL/kg/day of 50% $MgSO_4$; PO × 3 days until the serum Mg concentration is >1.5 mg/dL
Hypoparathyroidism	• Oral calcium (50 mg/kg/day in 3 divided doses) • 0.25 to 1 mcg/day calcitriol • Keep product of calcium and PO_4 < 55 mg^2/dL^2
Hyperphosphatemia	• Encourage exclusive breast-feeding. • Use low phosphate containing formula. • Low dose calcium can be given for 1–2 weeks. • Avoid phosphate binding products.
Vitamin D deficiency	• Vitamin D_3 supplementation 2,000 IU/Day for at least 3 months

(PO: per oral; IM: intramuscular)

those caused by hypoparathyroidism requires continued therapy with calcium and vitamin D metabolites and may last several weeks to months, or may be permanent.

HYPERCALCEMIA

Definition

Total serum calcium (TCa) >11 mg/dL and/or ionized calcium (iCa) >5 mg/dL (1.45 mmol/L).

Etiology

- Iatrogenic: Total parenteral nutrition (TPN), intravenous fluid (IVF)
- Decreased renal calcium clearance
- Hyperparathyroidism
- Hyperthyroidism
- Hypophosphatasia
- Hypervitaminosis D
- Idiopathic neonatal hypercalcemia
- Subcutaneous fat necrosis
- Associated with skeletal dysplasias, tumors, acute adrenal insufficiency, hypervitaminosis A, and thyrotoxicosis.

Clinical Features

It may be asymptomatic or symptomatic (poor feeding, vomiting, poor linear growth, constipation, polyuria, hypotonia, encephalopathy, nephrocalcinosis, hypertension, seizures, etc.). Persistent hypercalcemia may be associated with extraskeletal calcifications. Chronic moderate hypercalcemia may just present with failure to thrive.

Treatment

Acute Management

Acute management is reserved for symptomatic/severe hypercalcemia (TCa > 14 mg/dL or iCa > 1.8 mmol/L).

The medical management is directed to increase urinary calcium excretion. Calcium and vitamin D supplementation should be discontinued. Volume expansion is given with isotonic saline at twice the maintenance followed by furosemide (1 mg/kg intravenously) to be given over 6–8 hours. If hypercalcemia is severe and is accompanied with hypophosphatemia, 30–50 mg/kg/day of oral (preferable) or intravenous phosphorus can be given in addition. The goal of phosphate is to maintain serum phosphate levels between 3 mg/dL and 5 mg/dL. Serum calcium usually takes 24–48 hours to normalize. In resistant cases, glucocorticoids (prednisone, 2 mg/kg per day) can be added. Other therapies of hypercalcemia include calcitonin, bisphosphonate, dialysis, and total parathyroidectomy with autologous reimplantation.

Chronic Phase

- Dietary restriction
- Cellulose phosphate binders (limited experience).

DISORDERS OF MAGNESIUM METABOLISM

Magnesium is the second most abundant intracellular cation and plays an important role in metabolism, protein synthesis, membrane integrity, and neuromuscular activity. The plasma magnesium concentration is elevated in neonates (0.8 ± 0.16 mmol/L or 2.0 ± 0.4 mg/dL) as compared to adults.

HYPOMAGNESEMIA

Hypomagnesemia is defined if the serum magnesium concentrations are <0.66 mmol/L (1.6 mg/dL).

Etiology

Hypomagnesemia occurs secondary to decreased magnesium supply (e.g. maternal magnesium deficiency, intrauterine growth restriction, maternal diabetes, and malabsorption) or magnesium loss [e.g. double volume exchange transfusion (DVET) with citrated blood; decreased renal tubular reabsorption; maternal hyperparathyroidism; drugs such as loop diuretics, aminoglycosides and amphotericin B; polyuric phase of acute tubular necrosis, sometimes may be seen in neonates undergoing therapeutic hypothermia].

Clinical Features

Same as hypocalcemia and mostly coexists with late onset hypocalcemia. Hypocalcemia may give clue to hypomagnesemia.

Treatment

Treatment is directed to treatment of concurrent hypocalcemia. In severe hypomagnesemia, 0.05–0.1 mL/kg of 50% $MgSO_4$ solution IV over 1–2 hours can be given under cardiac monitoring. The dose can be repeated after 12–24 hours. Generally the condition improves with one or two doses, but may require longer magnesium supplements.

HYPERMAGNESEMIA

Hypermagnesemia is defined when serum magnesium concentration exceeds 1.15 mmol/L (2.8 mg/dL).

Etiology

Hypermagnesemia occurs due to increased magnesium supply secondary to maternal treatment with magnesium sulfate, secondary to neonatal magnesium therapy (e.g. asphyxia, pulmonary hypertension, antacids, and enema) or parenteral nutrition.

Clinical Features

Most neonates are asymptomatic. Symptoms include apnea, respiratory depression, lethargy, hypotonia, hyporeflexia, poor suck, decreased gastrointestinal (GI) motility, and urinary retention.

Treatment

Supportive measures may be required to ensure hydration. Feeds may be deferred till returns of bowel movement. Usually term neonates secrete magnesium effectively; however, preterm neonates may have compromised magnesium secretion. Calcium gluconate 2 mL/kg may be used in acute cases. Loop diuretic, exchange transfusion, and dialysis may be rarely needed.

KEY POINTS

➢ Calcium levels are regulated by the interplay of PTH, calcitonin, and vitamin D3.
➢ Prematurity, SGA, perinatal stress, infants of diabetic mother are common risk factors for early onset hypocalcemia.
➢ Intravenous calcium therapy should be preferably reserved for management of symptomatic hypocalcemia.
➢ Most common cause of late onset hypocalcemia in neonates is vitamin D deficiency.
➢ Hypomagnesemia [serum magnesium concentration <0.66 mmol/L (1.6 mg/dL)] often coexists with hypocalcemia and should be managed concurrently.

SELF ASSESSMENT

1. **Late onset hypocalcemia may be caused by all except:**
    a. Maternal vitamin D deficiency.
    b. Malabsorption or hepatobiliary disease.
    c. Metabolic acidosis
    d. Congenital hypoparathyroidism (primary and secondary).

2. **All of the following are true except:**
    a. Hypomagnesemia is defined if the serum magnesium concentration are <0.66 mmol/L (1.6 mg/dL).
    b. Magnesium is the second most abundant intracellular cation.
    c. Magnesium plays an important role in metabolism, protein synthesis, membrane integrity, and neuromuscular activity.
    d. The plasma magnesium concentration is low in neonates (0.8 ± 0.16 mmol/L, or 2.0 ± 0.4 mg/dL) as compared to adults.

FURTHER READING

1. Adamkin DH. Neonatal hypoglycemia. Curr Opin Pediatr. 2016;28(2):150-5.

Parenteral Nutrition

Anumodan Gupta, Sachin Kumar Dubey, Umesh Vaidya

INTRODUCTION

- Optimum nutrition is essential for survival, physical growth, mental development, productivity, health, and well-being across the entire life span.
- Parenteral nutrition (PN) or intravenous (IV) nutrition is an important part of critical care. Nutritional support prevents a catabolic state that is associated with critical illness and hastens recovery.
- Parenteral nutrition thus supports nutritional needs till adequate enteral nutrition is established.

GOALS OF PARENTERAL NUTRITION

Provision of:
- Adequate calories for energy expenditure and growth.
- Adequate carbohydrates with lipids and protein intake for a balanced ratio.
- Essential nutrients including minerals, electrolytes, vitamins, and trace elements.

INDICATIONS

Common indications in neonates are shown in **Table 1**. PN should be started at the earliest. PN can be stopped once enteral nutrition provides 75% of calorie needs.

Table 1: Indications of parenteral nutrition.	
Prematurity <28 weeks and/or <1,000 g	Prematurity <32 weeks and/or <1,500 g who are unable to achieve full enteral feeds by day 3
Prematurity >32 weeks and/or >1,500 g who are unable to achieve at least 50% enteral feeds by day 5	Necrotizing enterocolitis (stages II and III)
Surgical neonates (exomphalos, intestinal surgeries, gastroschisis)	Short bowel syndrome
All neonatal and infant catabolic states (weight loss, poor muscle mass) where enteral feeding is limited or not possible	

STEPS IN STARTING PARENTERAL NUTRITION

- Identify patient.
- Assess nutritional needs. Energy requirements for growth for preterm and term neonates on PN are 110–120 kcal/kg/day and 90–110 kcal/kg/day, respectively. It should be ensured that minimum 30 kcal/kg/day is provided for every g/kg of protein. This is calculated as a calorie-nitrogen ratio (CNR).
- Calculate PN.
- Prepare PN.
- Administer PN.

Components and dispensing for parenteral nutrition calculations: Purpose of PN is to provide the neonate macronutrients **(Table 2)** as well as micronutrients.

MICRONUTRIENTS

- *Vitamins:* Start on day 1 of PN. As per European Society for Paediatric Gastroenterology, Hepatology and Nutrition (ESPGHAN) recommendations, vitamins are added to the lipid emulsion during compounding. In India, pediatric multivitamin infusion (MVI) is not

Table 2: Macronutrients.		
Carbohydrates	*Lipids*	*Proteins*
Dextrose as a part of PN is on the lines of routine intravenous fluids (60% calorie intake)	• Lipids are energy dense and isoosmolar. They provide 30% (range 25–40%) of the caloric intake on PN • Apart from calories, lipids provide essential fatty acids (EFA—linoleic and linolenic acids) and/or DHA which are necessary for cell metabolism and particularly brain and retinal development	Early and adequate proteins lead to better nitrogen retention, better postnatal growth, better head growth and lesser incidence of bronchopulmonary dysplasia (provides 10% of energy)
Starts on day 1	Starts on day 1	Starts on day 1
Dose calculated on the basis of glucose infusion rate (GIR)	Minimum dose of 1 g/kg/day (desirable up to 3 g/kg/day)	Preterm: Minimum of 2 g/kg/day on day 1 (desirable 2.5 to 3 g/kg/day). Amino acids are graded up on consecutive days to a maximum of 3.5 g/kg/day)
	Tolerance of lipids: Serum triglyceride estimation (maintain below 200 mg/dL). In the past, there were concerns regarding the use of lipids in neonatal jaundice, sepsis and thrombocytopenia. Recent studies have shown lipids to be safe in these conditions if proper dosage and administration guidelines are followed. Dose of 1 g/kg/day are sufficient to prevent EFA deficiency	The calorie-nitrogen ratio (CNR) ensures adequate calories for the amount of proteins being given. It is calculated as follows: Calorie-nitrogen ratio = Non-protein calories (Dextrose + Lipids) 0.16 × proteins (g)

(DHA: docosahexaenoic acid; EFA: essential fatty acid; PN: parenteral nutrition)

Table 3: Doses of minerals used in PN.	
Sodium	0–3 mEq/kg/day (0 on day 1 and then 2–3 mEq/kg/day)
Potassium	0–2 mEq/kg/day (0 on day 1 and then 2–3 mEq/kg/day)
Chloride	0–5 mEq/kg/day (0 on day 1 and then 4–5 mEq/kg/day)
Calcium	42–120 mg/kg/day (preterm), 32 mg/kg/day (term)
Phosphorus	28–64 mg/kg/day (preterm), 14 mg/kg/day (term)
Magnesium	5 mg/kg/day

(PN: parenteral nutrition)

available and adult MVI is used as a substitute. Being water-soluble, adult MVI cannot be mixed in lipid solution and has to be mixed in dextrose, electrolyte containing solution. Limitations—higher vitamin A content (undesirable), no vitamin K, and is alcohol based. It also has benzoic acid as a stabilizer, which is not suitable for neonatal use.

- *Minerals:* Minerals are required in doses as described in **Table 3**.
- *Trace elements:* If the neonate needs to be on total parenteral nutrition (TPN) for more than 15 days, trace elements are started after 10 days of life. Presently T-pres/Celcel 5 (Trace element injection 5) is used in TPN solution which includes zinc, copper, chromium, manganese, and selenium.

CALCULATION OF PARENTERAL NUTRITION NEEDS (TABLE 4)

Nutritional requirements of premature babies have to be calculated very accurately to facilitate growth and to avoid complications.

Manual calculation is difficult, time consuming, needs training and validation before execution of order. Prescription errors up to 27.9% have been reported.

The process of writing repetitive tasks and tedious calculations thus leading to errors can be prevented by use of a dedicated software, thus improving the safety of PN administration.

Software Calculations

There are softwares for PN calculations which are accurate, validated, and reduce errors of calculation and compounding. It is used to keep track of patient's nutritional status on a serial basis. At neonatal intensive care unit (NICU) of KEM Hospital, Pune, we have developed user-friendly software named "Kimaya NICU software", which is in regular use.

COMPOUNDING OF TOTAL PARENTERAL NUTRITION (TABLE 5)

Compounding means preparing the PN solutions for administration once the calculations are done. There are two methods of compounding (manual and automated). Manual compounding implies preparation of PN solution by the nutritionist/nurse/doctor under a system called Laminar Flow system. Dextrose, amino acids, electrolytes, vitamins, and trace elements are compounded in one bottle, whereas the lipids are administered separately through a syringe.

Table 4: Total parenteral nutrition (TPN) calculation sheet.

Name: _____

Registration number: _____ Date: _____

Day of life: _____ Birth weight _____

Weight for calculation: _____
1. **Total fluid** (mL/kg) = _____ mL × wt =
2. **Lipids** = ___ g/kg = ___ g = ___ × 5 mL of 20% lipid solution = ___ mL ___ Rate = ___ mL/hr infusion over 24 hrs
3. **Additives** = (a + b + c + d) mL as below:
   a. Antibiotics ___ mL
   b. Feeds ___ mL
   c. Hep-lock solution ___ mL
   d. Others ___ mL
4. (Net fluid will contain amino acids + dextrose + electrolytes), etc.
   Net fluid remaining = Total fluids – (lipids + additives) = ___ mL ___ Rate = ___ mL/hr infusion over 24 hrs
   A. Amino acids = ___ g/kg = ___ g = ___ × 10 mL of 10% amino acid solution
   B. Na = ___ mEq/kg = ___ mEq = ___ × 2 mL of 3% NaCl = ___ mL
   C. K = ___ mEq/kg = ___ mEq = ___ × 0.5 mL of KCL = ___ mL
   D. Ca gluconate = ___ mL/kg = ___ mL
   E. MVI = ___ mL
   F. Remaining volume for **Dextrose** (Dex volume) = Net fluid volume – (A + B + C + D + E) = _____ mL

$$\text{Dextrose concentration required} = \frac{\text{Weight} \times \text{Glucose infusion rate} \times 144}{\text{Dextrose volume}} = \_\_\_\_\_\%$$

To calculate required dextrose concentration, we can use 50% and 5% dextrose

$$\text{Volume of low conc solution} = \frac{\text{High conc} - \text{desired conc}}{\text{High conc} - \text{low conc}} \times \text{Dextrose volume}$$

i. $$\text{Here volume of 5\% D} = \frac{50 - \text{desired conc}}{50 - 5} \times \text{Dextrose volume} = \_\_\_\_\_\text{ mL}$$

ii. Volume of 50% D = Dextrose volume – volume of 5% D = _____ mL

TPN calculation sheet example 2 kg neonate needing 150 mL/kg fluid
Weight for calculation _____
1. **Total fluid** (mL/kg) = 150 mL × wt = 300 mL
2. **Lipids** = 2 g/kg = 4 g = 4 × 5 mL of 20% lipid solution = 20 mL   Rate = 0.8 mL/hr infusion over 24 hrs
3. **Additives** = (e + f + g + h) mL as below
   e. Antibiotic = 5 mL
   f. Feed = 25 mL
   g. Hep-lock solution = 10 mL
   h. Others = 0 mL
4. (Net fluid will contain amino acids + dextrose + electrolytes), etc.
   Net fluid remaining = Total fluids – (lipids + additives) = 300 – (20 + 40) mL = 240 mL Rate = 10 mL/hr infusion over 24 hrs
   G. Amino acids = 3 g/kg = 6 g = 6 × 10 mL of 10% amino acid solution = 60 mL
   H. Na = 3 mEq/kg = 6 mEq = 6 × 2 mL of 3% NaCl = 12 mL
   I. K = 2 mEq/kg = 4 mEq = 4 × 0.5 mL of KCL = 2 mL
   J. Ca gluconate = 8 mL/kg = 16 mL
   K. MVI = 1 mL
   L. Remaining volume for **Dextrose** (Dex volume)
      = Net fluid volume – (A + B + C + D + E) = 240 – (60 + 12 + 2 + 16 + 1) = 240 – 91 = 149 mL

Contd…

Contd…

- Dextrose concentration required $= \dfrac{\text{Weight} \times \text{Glucose infusion rate} \times 144}{\text{Dextrose volume}} = \dfrac{2 \times 6 \times 144}{149} = 11.6\%$

  To calculate required dextrose concentration, we can use 50% and 5% dextrose

  Volume of low conc solution $= \dfrac{\text{High conc} - \text{desired conc}}{\text{High conc} - \text{low conc}} \times$ Dextrose volume

  iii. Here volume of 5% D $= \dfrac{50 - 11.6}{50 - 5} \times 149 = \dfrac{38.4}{45} \times 149 = 127$ mL

  iv. Volume of 50% D = Dextrose volume − volume of 5% D = 149 − 127 = 22 mL

(MVI: multivitamin infusion; KCL: potassium chloride)

Table 5: Compounding of parenteral nutrition.

Bottle	Syringe
Dextrose	Lipids
Amino acids	
Electrolytes—sodium, potassium, calcium, magnesium, chloride	
Minerals—zinc, manganese, copper, chromium, selenium	
Vitamins	

COMPATIBILITY AND STABILITY

The PN formulation is a complex mixture containing different chemical components that may cause problems with stability and compatibility.

Factors on which stability of the nutrients primarily depends on are:

- Amino acid constitution and pH of the solution
- *pH of the formulation*: Maintaining a final pH of 5.0 or above
- *Dextrose concentration*: Keeping the final dextrose concentration at 3.3% or greater
- Concentration of the electrolytes
- Order of mixing
- *Ca:PO₄ ratio*: Calcium and phosphorus are common essential electrolytes in PN solutions. If mixed in too high a concentration, calcium and phosphorus may form an insoluble precipitate of calcium phosphate. Pulmonary emboli secondary to calcium phosphate precipitates have been reported to be fatal.
- *Osmolarity*: The osmolarity of the final PN formulation dictates the administration route. Osmolarity is primarily dependent on the dextrose, amino acid, and electrolyte content.

Photoprotection of Parenteral Nutrition

Peroxide formation in PN is now considered as an important issue that needs attention. Sources of peroxide in PN are many, viz. amino acids (tryptophan, tyrosine, methionine, cysteine, and phenylalanine), multivitamins (riboflavin), trace elements, lipid emulsion (polyunsaturated fatty acid), and additives used for stabilization of PN.

Effects: Hypertriglyceridemia and impairs glucose uptake in muscle and fat; disrupts cell membrane integrity; mediates tissue injury; and changes quality of PN and causes loss of potency of PN by reducing levels of some vitamins and amino acids.

QUALITY CONTROL OF PARENTERAL NUTRITION PREPARATION

- Visual check for precipitation or particulate matters.
- *Biological integrity of the product:* On periodic basis, random samples of 5–10 mL are aseptically drawn from prepared TPN solutions. They are sent to microbiology laboratories for sterility testing.
- *High-efficiency particulate air (HEPA) filter hood environmental samples:* Periodically swabs for culture must be taken from working surface of the HEPA hood.
- *High-efficiency particulate air filter hood certification:* HEPA filter hoods must be tested for its efficiency once every 6 months.

SETTING UP

- Total parenteral nutrition solutions must be administered using an IV-infusion set with filter.
- Never add anything to a TPN solution. Never piggy back a TPN solution with any other preparations due to physical, chemical, and biological incompatibility.
- Use of Y connectors or triple lumen connectors for administrating amino acid solution and lipid together from same line. Alternatively, some units infuse amino acid-dextrose-electrolyte solution and lipids through separate infusion lines at different sites.
- Infusion sets need to be changed daily. Bacterial filters are changed every 3 days.

ROUTES AND TECHNIQUES OF PARENTERAL NUTRITION ADMINISTRATION

Total parenteral nutrition can be administered through peripheral or central lines (umbilical or central venous route). Use of peripheral line is safer when PN is needed for less than 10 days.

Percutaneous inserted central catheter (PICC) is inserted to avoid phlebitis when:

- Concentrations of >12.5% glucose are needed.
- Osmolarity of solution is >900 mOsm/L.
- Prolonged period of TPN is anticipated.

The position of the tip of the catheter needs to be in a large vessel preferably the superior or inferior vena cava outside the heart with position confirmed by X-ray prior to use. Single lumen central lines are preferred over multiple lumen catheters due to less risk of sepsis. PN lines should be handled minimally and with all aseptic techniques.

KEY POINTS

- Parenteral nutrition can be provided by peripheral or central route.
- Both amino acids and lipids should be started on day 1 of life.
- Starting dose of amino acids and lipids is 1 g/kg/day. Lipids need to be increased daily keeping check on triglyceride concentrations.
- Parenteral nutrition calculation software is a good alternative to manual calculation.

SELF ASSESSMENT

1. **Maximum osmolality which can be tolerated while giving parenteral nutrition through peripheral route is**
   a. 800 mOsm/L
   b. 1,200 mOsm/L
   c. 900 mOsm/L

2. **Trace elements need to be added to parenteral nutrition if it is given for more than:**
   a. 5 days
   b. 10 days
   c. 15 days

3. **How many calories are needed per gram of protein for best accretion of protein?**
   a. 20 calories
   b. 30 calories
   c. 40 calories

FURTHER READING

1. Bhave SA, Vaidya UV. Parenteral nutrition in developing countries: problems and perspectives. In: Gupte S (Ed). Recent Advances in Pediatrics. Vol. 4. New Delhi: Jaypee Brothers Medical Publishers (P) Ltd; 1993. pp. 106-21.
2. Blackmer AB, Partipilo ML. Three-in-one parenteral nutrition in neonates and pediatric patients: risks and benefits. Nutr Clin Pract. 2015;30(3):337-43.
3. Brown CL, Garrison NA, Hutchison AA. Error reduction when prescribing neonatal parenteral nutrition. Am J Perinatol. 2007;24(7):417-27.
4. Chaudhari S, Vaidya UV. Total parenteral nutrition in India. Indian J Pediatr. 1988;55(6):935-40.
5. Chessex P, Harrison A, Khashu M, et al. In preterm neonates, is the risk of developing bronchopulmonary dysplasia influenced by the failure to protect total parenteral nutrition from exposure to ambient light? J Pediatr. 2007;151(2):213-4.
6. Deshpande G, Maheshwari R. Intravenous lipids in neonates. In: Patole S (Ed). Nutrition for the Preterm Neonate: A Clinical Perspective. New York: Springer Publication; 2014. pp. 215-32.
7. Havranek T, Armbrecht E, Scavo LM. Compassionate use of Omegaven in preterm neonates with parenteral nutrition associated direct hyperbilirubinemia. J Pediatr Neonatal Care. 2014;1(1):00004.
8. Raimbault M, Thibault M, Lebel D, et al. Automated compounding of parenteral nutrition for pediatric patients: characterization of workload and costs. J Pediatr Pharmacol Ther. 2012;17(4): 389-94.
9. Tagare A, Vaidya U. Clinical nutrition guidelines: neonatal parenteral nutrition. 2010.
10. Tagare A, Vaidya U. Parenteral nutrition: Current guidelines. J Neonatol. 2007;21(3):186-8.
11. Vaidya UV, Hegde VM, Bhave SA, et al. Reduction in parenteral nutrition related complications in the newborn. Indian Pediatr. 1991;28(5):477-84.
12. Ziegler EE, Carlson SJ. Early nutrition of very low birth weight infants. J Matern Fetal Neonatal Med. 2009;22(3):191-7.

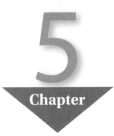

5
Chapter

Enteral Nutrition in Preterm Neonate

Pankaj Garg, Ajoy Kumar Garg

INTRODUCTION

Preterm survivors are at a higher risk of growth failure and developmental disabilities compared to their healthy term counterparts. With improved survival of preterm neonates, optimizing nutrition has become an essential component in management of sick infants.

IMPORTANCE OF NUTRITION

- To avoid postnatal growth failure
- Prevent necrotizing enterocolitis and other feed-related morbidities
- To improve neurodevelopmental outcomes.

Current nutrition guidelines suggest achievement of postnatal growth rates approximating the intrauterine growth of a normal fetus of the same postmenstrual age **(Table 1)**.

However, this goal is often difficult to achieve because of the physiologic limitations associated with prematurity. Extrauterine growth restriction remains a clinical complication of prematurity with rates ranging from 30% to 97%.

BENEFITS OF ENTERAL NUTRITION

- Trophic benefits of nutrient stimulation to the gut
- More physiological
- Avoid prolonged use of parenteral nutrition and associated complications.

Table 1: Recommended growth for preterm very low birth weight babies.	
AAP guidelines	
Weight gain	18–20 g/kg/d
OFC gain	0.9–1.0 cm/week
Length gain	0.9–1.0 cm/week

(AAP: American Academy of Pediatrics; OFC: occipito-frontal circumference)

NUTRITION REQUIREMENTS

The requirements for fully enterally-fed preterm very low birth weight (VLBW) infants is described in (**Table 2**).

Options for Enteral Nutrition

- Mother's own milk—first choice
- Pasteurized donor human milk
- Preterm formula.

BENEFITS OF HUMAN MILK

- Reduction in necrotizing enterocolitis (NEC), late onset sepsis, bronchopulmonary dysplasia (BPD), and retinopathy of prematurity (ROP).
- Lesser gastric residuals and early advancement of feeds.
- Improved neurodevelopmental outcomes.

FORTIFICATION OF HUMAN MILK

Need

In preterm neonates, unfortified human milk (mother's own milk or donor) does not meet the recommended energy and protein requirements. They need to be fortified with human milk

Table 2: Requirements for fully enterally-fed preterm very low birth weight infants.		
Nutrients	*ESPGHAN (2010)/kg/day*	*Koletzko et al. (2014)/kg/day*
Fluids (mL)	135–200	135–200
Energy (kcal)	110–135	110–130
Protein (g)	4.0–4.5 (<1 kg) 3.5–4.0 (1–1.8 kg)	3.5–4.5
Lipids (g)	4.8–6.6 (<40% MCT)	4.8–6.6
DHA (mg)	12–30	55–60
Carbohydrate (g)	11.6–13.2	11.6–13.2
Calcium (mg)	120–140	120–200
Phosphate (mg)	60–90	60–140
Magnesium (mg)	8–15	8–15
Iron (mg)	2–3	2–3
Zinc (mg)	1.1–2.0	1.4–2.5
Copper (µg)	100–132	100–230
Selenium (µg)	5–10	5–10
Vitamin A (µg)	400–1,000	400–1,100
Vitamin D (IU)	800–1,000/day	(400–1,000 per day from milk + supplement)

(DHA: docosahexaenoic acid; ESPGHAN: European Society for Paediatric Gastroenterology Hepatology and Nutrition; MCT: medium change triglyceride)

Table 3: Nutritional content of EBM, EBM fortified with HMF, and preterm formula.

		At full feeds of 180 mL/kg/day		
	Recommended intakes (kg/day) (ESPGHAN 2010)	Unfortified EBM (kg/day)	EBM fortified with fortifier (4 g/100 mL) (kg/day)	Preterm formula (kg/day)
Energy (kcal)	110–135	120	143.6	144
Protein (g)	(<1,000) 4–4.5 (1,000–1,800) 3.5–4	1.98	3.8	3.6
Fat (g)	4.8–6.6	8.46	8.74	7.9
Vitamin A (IU)	1,500–3,300	400	1,800	837
Vitamin D (IU)	800–1,000	45	964	167
Calcium (mg)	120–140	40	156.2	185
Phosphorus (mg)	60–90	23	78	93
Iron (mg)	2–3	0.162	2.2	2.5

(EBM: expressed breast milk; ESPGHAN: European Society for Paediatric Gastroenterology Hepatology and Nutrition; HMF: human milk fortifier)

Table 4: Guidelines for human milk fortification.

Whom to start?	Preterm <32 weeks and/or birth weight <1,800 g
When to start?	Baby is on feeds 100 mL/kg/day
How long?	Postmenstrual age—40 weeks or baby is on direct breast feeds

fortifier (bovine-based or human milk-based) to meet calorie and protein demands of these babies **(Table 3)**.

The guidelines for human milk fortification is described in **Table 4**. If there is non-availability of human milk (mother's own milk or donor milk) then preterm formula should be used. Infants on preterm formula should be supplemented with vitamin A and D.

Human Milk Fortification: Evidence (Cochrane)

- Improve short-term growth.
- Increased nitrogen retention.
- No long-term neurodevelopmental benefits.

Types of Fortification

- Standardized (most commonly used and practical in our scenario)
- Individualized
- Targeted [blood urea nitrogen (BUN)-based].

OTHER SUPPLEMENTATION IN VERY LOW BIRTH WEIGHT BABIES

Calcium and Phosphorus

Calcium absorption depends on calcium, vitamin D, phosphorus intakes, and nitrogen retention. Calcium intake of 120–140 mg/kg/day ensures retention of 60–90 mg/kg/day as absorption is 55–60%. Considering a nitrogen retention ranging from 350 mg/kg/day to 450 mg/kg/day and calcium retention from 60 mg/kg/day to 90 mg/kg/day, the adequate phosphorus intake represents 60–90 mg/kg/day of a highly absorbable phosphate source (90%) with a calcium to phosphorus ratio between 1.5 and 2.0. The American Academy of Pediatrics (AAP) Committee on Nutrition issued guidelines that laboratory monitoring of VLBW infants should begin at 4–5 weeks after birth. Serum phosphorus concentration below 4 mg/dL should be followed up carefully. Serum alkaline phosphatase levels greater than 800 IU/L or clinical concern for fractures should lead to a radiographic workup for rickets.

Vitamin D

Vitamin D is essential for various physiological processes such as neuromuscular function and bone mineralization. Vitamin supplementation should be able to reach target value of circulating 25(OH)D to at least 75 nmol (30 ng/mL). A vitamin D intake of 800–1,000 IU/day (and not per kilogram) during the first months of life is recommended in both breast-fed and formula-fed preterm babies.

Iron

Iron is essential for brain development and iron deficiency anemia may result in poor neurodevelopment in infants. On the other hand, excessive iron supplementation may lead to increased risk of infection, poor growth, and interfere with absorption or metabolism of other minerals. Excessive iron may increase the risk of retinopathy of prematurity by formation of free oxygen radicals. Thus, iron deficiency as well as iron overload is detrimental. Due to association of increased oral intake of iron with possible adverse effects, an intake of 2–3 mg/kg/day is recommended. Prophylactic enteral iron supplementation (given as a separate iron supplement, in preterm formula or in fortified human milk fed infants) should be started at 2–6 weeks of age (2–4 weeks in extremely low birth weight infants). Laboratory monitoring pertaining to nutritional supplementation of preterm infants is described in (**Table 5**).

Nutritional supplementation at discharge:
At time of discharge, VLBW babies need to be supplemented depending upon the type of feed (**Tables 6 and 7**).

Table 5: Laboratory monitoring pertaining to nutritional supplementation of preterm infants.		
	Timing	*Targets*
Serum calcium, phosphorus, alkaline phosphatase	Start at 4 weeks of life Frequency—fortnightly till discharge	Alkaline phosphatase should be less than 800 IU
Hemoglobin, reticulocyte count	Start at 4 weeks of life Frequency—fortnightly till discharge	Do ferritin before starting iron

Table 6: Nutritional supplementation in very low birth weight babies till 40 weeks postmenstrual age.

Nutrient	Direct breast feeding	EBM fortified with human fortifier (4 g/100 mL)	Preterm formula
Calcium and phosphorus	Add calcium (140–160 mg/kg/day) and phosphorus (70–80 mg/kg/day) once baby is on full feeds	Not needed	Not needed
Vitamin A	Add multivitamin (MV) drops 1 mL once a day	Add MV drops 1 mL once a day	MV drops 0.5 mL/day
Vitamin D	Vitamin D drops 400 IU/day (rest from ostocalcium)	Vitamin D drops 400 U/day	Vitamin D drops 800 IU/day
Iron	Start iron at 2–3 mg/kg/day at 2–4 weeks of life	Start iron at 2–3 mg/kg/day at 2–4 weeks of life	Start iron at 2–3 mg/kg/day at 2–4 weeks of life

(EBM: expressed breast milk)

Table 7: Nutritional supplementation from 40 weeks onward.

Nutrients	Dose	Till
Vitamin D	800 U/day	1 year
Iron	2–3 mg/kg/day	1 year

Table 8: Evidences to support for aggressive enteral nutrition without increasing the risk of necrotizing enterocolitis (NEC).

Cochrane review	Primary comparisons	Population	Result
Morgan et al. (2013)	Trophic feeding <4 days of age for at least 7 days vs. enteral fasting	9 trials 754 very low birth weight or very preterm	No difference in days to full feeds (MD –1.05, 95% CI –2.61 to 0.51), risk of NEC (RR 1.07, 95% CI 0.67 to 1.70)
Morgan et al. (2014)	Delayed (>4 days) progressive feeding vs. early (<4 days) feeding	9 trials, 1,106 infants, few <28 weeks or <1,000 g	Decreased length of stay for the early feeding group (MD 2.11 days, 95% CI 0.31 to 3.9, P = .02). No difference in risk of NEC (RR 0.93, 95% CI 0.64 to 1.34), mortality (RR 1.18, 95% CI 0.75 to 1.88)
Oddie et al. 2017	Slow (<24 mL/kg per day) vs. faster	10 trials, 3,753 infants	Higher incidence of invasive infection in the slow advancement group (RR 1.46, 95% CI 1.03 to 2.06, P = .03). No difference in NEC (RR 1.02, 95% CI 0.64 to 1.62) mortality (RR 1.18, 95% CI 0.90 to 1.53)

(RR: relative risk, CI: confidence interval; MD: mean difference)

INITIATION AND ADVANCEMENT OF ENTERAL FEEDINGS

Present practice favors early start of enteral feed at least minimal enteral feeding, also referred to as trophic feeding or gastrointestinal (GI) priming, as lack of enteral feeding has been shown to delay gut maturation in preterm infants and results in negative effects **(Table 8)**.

SUGGESTED FEEDING REGIMEN BASED ON ABOVE EVIDENCE

Feeding protocol may vary from unit to unit. Systematic feeding regimen is an evidence-based intervention shown to reduce NEC. Advancement of feed should be based on clinical and abdominal examination. Feed intolerance can manifest as abdominal distension or increased abdominal girth >2 cm from baseline, increased gastric residual >50% of prefeed, and hemorrhagic or bilious vomiting. In these cases, infants should be closely monitored and worked up for sepsis, NEC, and electrolyte imbalance.

Birth weight	Initiation volume	Advancement
<1,000 g	15–20 mL/kg/day	15–20 mL/kg/day
1,000–1,500 g	30 mL/kg/day	30 mL/kg/day

Protocol for feeding small for gestational age (SGA) babies with/without history of absent/reversed end diastolic umbilical flows (AREDF) is as under:

- If examination of abdomen is normal, feeding can be initiated after 24 hours of life and advanced by making small increments in volume.
- Especially in preterm SGA < 29 weeks with AREDF, increments should be very slow in first 10 days.
- Human milk remains milk of choice.

MODES OF FEEDING

Different modes of feeding have been described in **Table 9**.

ISSUES PERTINENT TO ENTERAL NUTRITION IN VERY LOW BIRTH WEIGHT BABIES

Nasogastric versus Orogastric Feeding

Feeding can be given by nasogastric or orogastric route. Nasogastric route is easy to secure but may increase work of breathing owing to neonates being obligate nasal breathers. On the

Table 9: Mode of feeding.		
Gestational age	Feeding skills	Feeding methods
<28 weeks	• No sucking efforts • Poor gut motility	• Parenteral nutrition • Initiate minimal enteral feeding (EBM) if no risk for NEC, i.e. absent or reversed end diastolic feeds and hemodynamically stable
29–31 weeks	• Sucking burst develops • No coordination between suck, swallow, and breathing	Gavage feeding—nasogastric or orogastric feed, continuous or intermittent, progressive feed
32–34 weeks	• Mature sucking begins • Better coordination between swallowing and breathing	Feed by spoon, paladai or cup feeding
>34 weeks	Mature sucking coordination between swallowing and breathing	Breast feeding if hemodynamically stable

(NEC: necrotizing enterocolitis; EBM: expressed breast milk)

other hand, frequent movement of the orally placed tube may result in mucosal trauma. In addition, it can increase the risk of apnea and bradycardia due to vagal stimulation. Evidence is insufficient to suggest use of one over another.

Continuous versus Bolus Feeding

Bolus and continuous feedings are both suitable feeding strategies for preterm infants, both presenting clinical benefits as well as disadvantages. Bolus feeding is more physiological and promotes cyclical releases of hormones. Continuous feeding decreases energy expenditure, stimulates duodenal motor function, and does not have adverse effects on pulmonary function. A Cochrane review including seven trials, involving 511 infants, found no differences in time to achievement of full enteral feeds by either feeding methods. A trend toward earlier discharge was observed in infants less than 1,000 g birth weight fed by the continuous tube feeding method compared to intermittent nasogastric tube feeding method (mean difference –11 days; 95% confidence interval –21.8 to 0.2).

Growth Monitoring—Which Growth Curves to be Used?

Growth of all preterm babies should be plotted on Intergrowth 21 charts or Fenton 2013 growth charts till 50 weeks of postmenstrual age and subsequently on WHO growth standard charts.

CONCLUSION

To achieve the goals of nutrition for preterm infants, aggressive and adequate enteral nutrition is needed. In recent years, focus has shifted from the overall energy intake to the optimal protein intake and P/E ratio. A high overall energy intake may result in increased accretion of adipose tissue, whereas high protein intake may have beneficial effects on the quality of growth and long term neurodevelopmental outcomes. Fortified human milk (own followed by donor) is milk of choice for preterm babies. Preterm formula should be used whenever there is decreased supply of human milk due to some reasons. Systematic feeding regimen (having unit protocol for feeding) leads to decrease NEC in these babies.

KEY POINTS

➤ Early and aggressive nutrition leads to better neurodevelopmental outcomes.
➤ Enteral nutrition should be introduced as early as possible preferably on day 1 if baby is hemodynamically stable.
➤ Human milk (own mother's followed by donor) is feeding of choice in preterm babies.
➤ Human milk needs fortification to meet nutritional needs of premature babies.

SELF ASSESSMENT

1. **A very low birth weight baby is receiving expressed breast milk fortified with human milk fortifier. He needs to be given calcium and phosphorus supplementation in addition to it.**
   a. True
   b. False

2. **Dose and timing of iron supplementation in extremely low birth weight babies are:**
   a. 2–3 mg/kg/day and 4–8 weeks of life
   b. 1–2 mg/kg/day and 2–4 weeks of life
   c. 2–3 mg/kg/day and 2–4 weeks of life
   d. 1–2 mg/kg/day and 4–8 weeks of life

3. **At what age should we start screening VLBW babies for osteopenia of prematurity?**
   a. 2 weeks
   b. 4 weeks
   c. 6 weeks
   d. 8 weeks

FURTHER READING

1. Agostoni C, Buonocore G, Carnielli VP, et al.; ESPGHAN Committee on Nutrition. Enteral nutrient supply for preterm infants: commentary from the European Society of Paediatric Gastroenterology, Hepatology and Nutrition Committee on Nutrition. J Pediatr Gastroenterol Nutr. 2010;50(1):85-91.
2. American Academy of Pediatrics (AAP). Nutritional needs of preterm infants. In: Kleinman RE (Ed). Pediatric Nutrition Handbook, 6th edition. Elk Grove Village, IL: American Academy of Pediatrics; 2009. pp. 79-112.
3. American Academy of Pediatrics (AAP). Nutritional needs of preterm infants. In: Kleinman RE (Ed). Pediatric Nutrition Handbook, 5th edition. Elk Grove Village, IL: American Academy of Pediatrics; 2004.
4. Arslanoglu S, Corpeleijn W, Moro G, et al.; ESPGHAN Committee on Nutrition. Donor human milk for preterm infants: current evidence and research directions. J Pediatr Gastroenterol Nutr. 2013;57(4):535-42.
5. Koletzko B, Poindexter B, Uauy R. Recommended nutrient intake levels for stable, fully enterally fed very low birth weight infants. World Rev Nutr Diet. 2014;110:297-9.
6. Kumar P, Jain N, Thakre R, et al. Evidence Based Clinical Practice Guidelines. New Delhi: National Neonatology Forum of India; 2010.
7. Patole S. Strategies for prevention of feed intolerance in preterm neonates: a systematic review. J Matern Fetal Neonatal Med. 2005;18(1):67-76.
8. Ziegler EE. Meeting the nutritional needs of the low-birth-weight infant. Ann Nutr Metab. 2011;58(Suppl 1):8-18.

Respiratory Distress Syndrome

Amrit Jeevan, Nandkishor S Kabra

INTRODUCTION

Respiratory distress syndrome (RDS, previously called as hyaline membrane disease) is due to pulmonary surfactant deficiency. It is characterized by low pulmonary compliance. It is the leading cause of respiratory distress in preterm infants. The onset of respiratory distress occurs at or soon after birth.

INCIDENCE

Gestational age	Percentage
<28 weeks	60–80%
28–32 weeks	25–50%
32–36 weeks	15–30%
>37 weeks	1–3%

RISK FACTORS

- Prematurity—single most important risk factor
- Maternal diabetes
- Perinatal asphyxia
- Rh isoimmunization
- Male sex
- History of RDS in siblings
- Lack of antenatal steroids

SURFACTANT

- Surfactants are surface-active chemicals which lower the surface tension and prevent the collapse of alveoli at the end of expiration.
- The composition of surfactant is 90% lipids and 10% proteins (approximately).
- Dipalmitoylphosphatidylcholine (DPPC), also known as lecithin, is the predominant phospholipid in surfactant. It has a hydrophilic head and hydrophobic tail which makes it a surface-active agent.

- Dipalmitoylphosphatidylcholine is in the form of a gel at body temperature, however, presence of some unsaturated phospholipids and cholesterol is responsible for its fluid state.
- Phosphatidylglycerol is also considered as an indicator of lung maturity; it acts with the hydrophobic surfactant proteins to enhance its biophysical activity.
- The approximate surfactant pool size in term and preterm infants is 100 mg/kg and 4–5 mg/kg, respectively at birth.

PATHOGENESIS

- In surfactant-deficient lungs, there is epithelial cell necrosis within half an hour of birth.
- Necrosed alveolar cells detach from basement membrane and formation of hyaline membrane starts. In addition, there is interstitial edema.
- By 24 hours, there is extensive generalized hyaline membrane formation which lines the bronchioles up to respiratory bronchiole and alveolar ducts.
- After 24 hours, inflammatory cells appear within airway lumen which are mostly macrophages and polymorphs.
- Ingestion of membrane by macrophages takes place over next 2–3 days as the membrane separates.
- Epithelial regeneration is detectable after 48 hours beneath the separating membranes.
- Gradual formation of lamellar bodies and surfactants.
- Some of the reparative cells are thick, hampering gas exchange.
- By day 7, all the hyaline membranes disappear in an uncomplicated patient **(Flowchart 1)**.

CLINICAL FEATURES

- Triad of tachypnea, expiratory grunt, and inspiratory retractions especially in a premature infant
- Increased work of breathing
- Flaring of alae nasi
- Chest retractions
- Cyanosis
- Pallor
- Lethargy
- Apnea

Silverman-Anderson score can be used for objectively scoring the severity of respiratory distress in preterm infants.

SILVERMAN-ANDERSON SCORE

Feature	Score 0	Score 1	Score 2
Upper chest movement with respect to abdomen	Synchronized breathing	Lag on inspiration	See-saw respiration
Lower chest retractions	None	Minimal	Marked
Xiphoid retractions	None	Minimal	Marked
Nasal flaring	None	Minimal	Marked
Expiratory grunt	None	Audible wheeze by stethoscope	Audible wheeze

Flowchart 1: Pathophysiology of respiratory distress syndrome (RDS).

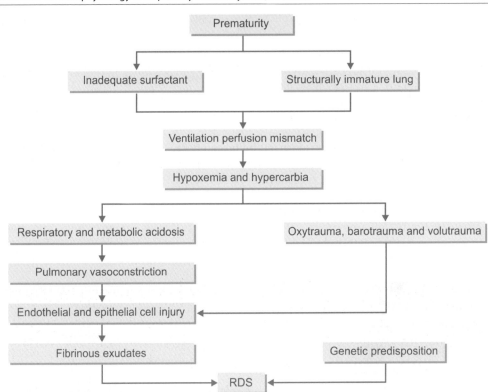

Source: Image reproduced with permission from Medscape Drugs and Diseases; Medscape. (2015). Respiratory Distress Syndrome. [online] Available from: https://emedicine.medscape.com/article/976034-overview [Last accessed on September, 2019].

SA score 1–3: Mild RDS, oxygen supplementation

SA score 4–6: Moderate RDS, noninvasive ventilation, consider surfactant

SA score >6: Severe RDS, mechanical ventilation, surfactant.

NATURAL COURSE OF THE ILLNESS

- The onset of respiratory distress is usually within first few hours after birth and in severe cases, it may occur immediately after delivery during first few breaths.
- Usually the respiratory distress is progressive and may worsen in the first 24–72 hours after birth and then improves gradually over a few days. In severe cases or if not supported well, the course may be relentlessly progressive. Left to right shunt through the ductus during recovery phase may lead to congestive heart failure. Complications of assisted ventilation may lead to air leak syndromes and bronchopulmonary dysplasia (BPD). Disseminated intravascular coagulation may lead to massive pulmonary bleed.

DIAGNOSTIC EVALUATION

- Arterial or capillary blood gas may reveal respiratory/mixed acidosis, hypoxemia, and hypercarbia.
- Blood glucose needs to be monitored as in any sick infant.
- Complete blood count and blood culture should be done especially in preterm infants at risk of infection such as presence of maternal chorioamnionitis, prolonged leaking/preterm premature rupture of membranes (PPROM), or other risk factors.
- *Anteroposterior (AP) and lateral chest radiograph*: Chest X-ray in RDS is essentially a low volume lung. It helps in grading the severity of RDS and also in ruling out other possible causes of respiratory distress like congenital pneumonia, transient tachypnea of newborn, pneumothorax, congenital lung malformations, and cardiac causes of respiratory distress.
- Echocardiogram (if clinically indicated).

X-ray Grading of RDS (Figs. 1A to D)

- *Grade I:* Symmetrical reticulogranular pattern, decrease in transparency of the lung, no certain difference to normal findings.

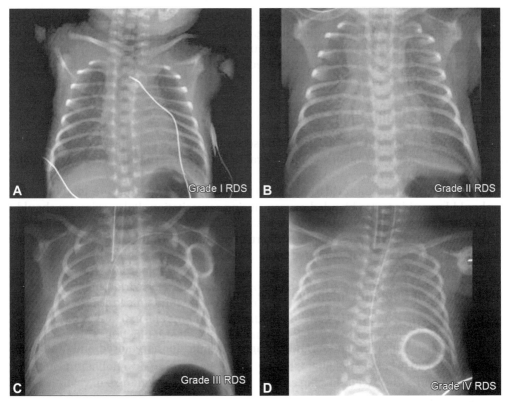

Figs. 1A to D: Grading of respiratory distress syndrome (RDS).
Courtesy: Dr Roalnd Talanow kinderradiologie-online.de

RESPIRATORY SUPPORT AND SURFACTANT

- Exogenous surfactants should be given as early as possible in the course of RDS. Natural surfactants are preferred over synthetic.
- A second and sometimes a third dose of surfactant should be administered if there is evidence of ongoing RDS such as persistent oxygen requirement and need for mechanical ventilation.
- More mature infants can often be extubated to noninvasive support (CPAP) immediately following surfactant. In infants who need mechanical ventilation, the goal should be to ventilate for the shortest possible time and all efforts should be made to prevent hyperoxia, hypocarbia, and volutrauma.
- Infants should be maintained on CPAP or nasal intermittent positive pressure ventilation (NIPPV) in preference to ventilation if possible.

RECOMMENDATIONS TO IMPROVE OUTCOME IN RDS

- Preventing preterm births
- Antenatal steroids:
  - ◆ Decrease RDS most consistently between 28 weeks and 34 weeks of gestational age (RR–0.65; 95% CI 0.47–0.75); number needed to treat to benefit (NNTB) 12.
  - ◆ *<27 weeks*: No reduction in RDS.
  - ◆ *<32 weeks*: Antenatal steroids and surfactant therapy act synergistically in reducing severity of RDS, decrease mortality and air leak when compared to either intervention alone or no intervention.
- Delivery room CPAP
- Early rescue surfactant
- Noninvasive ventilation
- Volume targeted ventilation
- Early extubation
- Avoiding reintubation.

PROGNOSIS

Increased use of antenatal steroids, delivery room CPAP, surfactant replacement therapy, and other supportive care has resulted in decrease in neonatal mortality to the tune of <5% in babies weighing 1,000–1,500 g and to <10% in babies weighing 750–999 g in advanced neonatal centers in India.

KEY POINTS

- ➤ Surfactant deficiency disorder is the most common cause of respiratory distress in preterm infants.
- ➤ Early CPAP should be considered in all preterm infants with RDS.
- ➤ Surfactant replacement should be done in infants with CPAP failure.
- ➤ Increased use of antenatal steroids, delivery room CPAP, surfactant replacement therapy and other supportive care has resulted in decrease in neonatal mortality.

SELF ASSESSMENT

1. **Which of the following statement is false?**
   a. Surfactants are surface-active materials that lower surface tension.
   b. Pulmonary surfactant is composed of approximately 90% lipids and 10% proteins.
   c. The main phospholipid in surfactant is phosphatidylinositol.
   d. Term infants have a surfactant storage pool of approximately 100 mg/kg, while in preterm infants the estimated pool size of 4–5 mg/kg at birth.
2. **Which of the following statement is false?**
   a. Early rescue surfactant therapy in infants with established RDS reduces the risk of mortality, air leak, BPD and BPD/death as compared to late rescue therapy.
   b. Infants below 28 weeks should be given prophylactic surfactant.
   c. Initiation of CPAP from birth with early selective surfactant administration for babies showing signs of RDS is recommended.
   d. Both animal derived and newer synthetic surfactants (having SP-B like activity) decrease acute respiratory morbidity and mortality in preterm infants with RDS.

FURTHER READING

1. Polin RA, Carlo WA; Committee on Fetus and Newborn; American Academy of Pediatrics. Surfactant replacement therapy for preterm and term neonates with respiratory distress. Pediatrics. 2014;133(1):156-63.
2. Sweet DG, Carnielli V, Greisen G, et al. European Consensus Guidelines on the Management of Respiratory Distress Syndrome - 2016 Update. Neonatology. 2017;111(2):107-25.

Meconium Aspiration Syndrome, Persistent Pulmonary Hypertension, and Air Leak

B Vishnu Bhat, B Adhisivam, Nishad Plakkal

MECONIUM ASPIRATION SYNDROME

INTRODUCTION

- Meconium is the first intestinal discharge from newborns, a viscous, dark-green substance composed of intestinal epithelial cells, lanugo, mucus, and intestinal secretions like bile.
- Fetal hypoxic stress may stimulate colonic activity, resulting in the passage of meconium. It may also stimulate fetal gasping movements that result in meconium aspiration.
- Meconium aspiration syndrome (MAS) reflects a spectrum of disorders in infants born with meconium-stained amniotic fluid (MSAF), ranging from mild tachypnea to severe respiratory distress.
- Since meconium is rarely found in the amniotic fluid prior to 34 weeks gestation, meconium aspiration primarily affects infants born at term and post-term.
- Factors that promote the passage in utero include placental insufficiency, maternal hypertension, preeclampsia, oligohydramnios, infection, acidosis, and maternal drug abuse, especially use of tobacco and cocaine.

INCIDENCE

- Nearly 10–15% of births are complicated by meconium passage before birth.
- Among the total births complicated by meconium passage, 10–12% of neonates develop MAS.
- It accounts for 10% of all causes of respiratory failure in neonates with mortality of 15–20% in developing countries.

PATHOPHYSIOLOGY

The pathophysiology of MAS is described in **Flowchart 1**.

Flowchart 1: Pathophysiology of meconium aspiration syndrome.

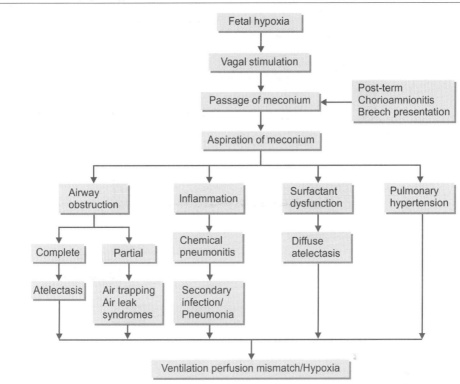

CLINICAL FEATURES

- History of MSAF.
- Affected infants are frequently small for gestational age (SGA) or postmature.
- Respiratory distress with marked tachypnea, cyanosis, intercostal and subcostal retractions, abdominal breathing, grunting, and nasal flaring.
- The vernix, umbilical cord, and nails may be meconium-stained.
- Neurologic and/or respiratory depression at birth typically due to hypoxia or shock.
- Chest is hyperinflated and crepts and rhonchi are noted bilaterally.
- Radiologic findings are initially coarse nodular opacities, followed by hyperinflation, and alternating diffuse patchy densities with areas of expansion **(Fig. 1)**. Consolidation, collapse, pneumothorax, and air leaks may be noted **(Fig. 2)**.

SEVERITY (WISWELL CLASSIFICATION)

Grade	Clinical features
Mild	Neonate requires less than 40% oxygen for less than 48 hours
Moderate	Neonate requires more than 40% oxygen for more than 48 hours with no air leak syndromes
Severe	Neonate requires assisted ventilation for more than 48 hours

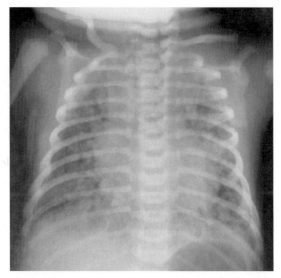

Fig. 1: Chest X-ray showing bilateral coarse infiltrates in a neonate with meconium aspiration syndrome.

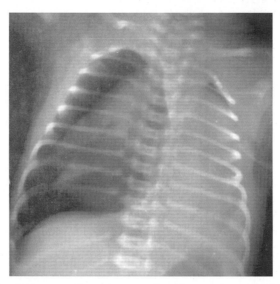

Fig. 2: Chest X-ray showing right pneumothorax in a neonate with meconium aspiration syndrome.

DIFFERENTIAL DIAGNOSIS

- Transient tachypnea of the newborn
- Sepsis or pneumonia
- Persistent pulmonary hypertension of the newborn
- Miscellaneous—pulmonary edema or pneumothorax
- Lung malformations.

MANAGEMENT

Delivery Room Management

- Routine intrapartum oropharyngeal suction and immediate postnatal suction in vigorous babies were abandoned in the Neonatal Resuscitation Program (NRP) 2005 guidelines.
- The 2015 updated guidelines from the American Heart Association (AHA), American Academy of Pediatrics (AAP), and International Liaison Committee on Resuscitation (ILCOR) do not recommend routine endotracheal suction for nonvigorous infants with MSAF.
- The primary reason that endotracheal suction is not able to reduce the risk of MAS significantly could be because both meconium passage and aspiration occur in utero and the tracheal suctioning is unlikely to benefit as meconium already is in the distal lung at the time of birth.
- The care of these infants should be guided by the same general principles for further intervention including endotracheal intubation, which are based on inadequate respiratory effort (gasping, labored breathing, or poor oxygenation) or heart rate (<100 beats/min).

A. Investigations:
- Chest radiograph
- Arterial blood gas
- Blood glucose, calcium, and electrolytes periodically or as indicated
- Septic screen if risk factors for sepsis are present

B. Supportive care:
- Maintain thermoneutral environment
- Oxygen therapy/assisted ventilation, continuous positive airway pressure (CPAP), positive pressure ventilation, high frequency ventilation as required. Synchronized intermittent mandatory ventilation or assist/control with adequate sedation is preferred. The aim of mechanical ventilation should be to improve oxygenation and simultaneously minimize barotrauma
- Maintain/correct blood sugar and calcium levels
- Correction of metabolic acidosis
- Maintain adequate perfusion—inotropic support if needed
- Monitor vitals and SPO_2 (91–95%)
- Minimize tactile and other stimulations

C. Others:
- Routine antibiotic is not required except in cases where infection is suspected
- Surfactant therapy and inhaled nitric oxide (iNO) if indicated. As secondary surfactant deficiency is expected with MAS, surfactant administration may reduce the severity of respiratory illness and decrease the number of infants with progressive respiratory failure requiring support with extracorporeal membrane oxygenation (ECMO). The Canadian Pediatric Society recommends exogenous surfactant for all intubated infants with MAS requiring FiO_2 ≥50%.
- Management of persistent pulmonary hypertension (PPHN)
- Treatment of other complications like pneumothorax, convulsions, etc.

COMPLICATIONS

Short-term	Long-term
• Air leak syndromes	• Increased incidence of respiratory infections in the first year of life
• Atelectasis	• Increased risk of reactive airway disease in the first 6 months of life
• Pneumonia	• Chronic lung disease
• Persistent pulmonary hypertension	• Neurologic deficits, including central nervous system (CNS) damage, seizures, mental retardation, and cerebral palsy depending on associated asphyxia

PERSISTENT PULMONARY HYPERTENSION

INTRODUCTION

Persistent pulmonary hypertension (PPHN) is associated with significant mortality and morbidity in the NICU and is characterized by increased pressure in the main pulmonary artery, i.e. pulmonary hypertension (PHT) leading to right to left shunt and causing hypoxemia in the neonate. PPHN usually refers only to the acute forms of pulmonary hypertension commonly seen in the first few days of life. A more chronic form of PHT associated with bronchopulmonary dysplasia (BPD) is increasingly being recognized. PPHN is classically associated with conditions like MAS and congenital diaphragmatic hernia (CDH), but can be due to a wide variety of causes. It can occur in term as well as preterm infants.

INCIDENCE

- 1–2 per 1,000 live births in the West
- Likely higher incidence in India
- Mortality rate > 10–20%.

ETIOLOGY

Categories of PPHN	Examples of conditions
Congenital abnormalities with increased pulmonary vascular resistance (PVR)	• Congenital diaphragmatic hernia (CDH) • Pulmonary hypoplasia • Alveolar capillary dysplasia with malalignment of pulmonary veins
Pulmonary disease leading to increased PVR	• Meconium aspiration syndrome (MAS) • Respiratory distress syndrome (RDS) • Transient tachypnea of newborn (TTN) • Pneumonia
Extrapulmonary conditions associated with elevated PVR	• Perinatal asphyxia • Sepsis • Polycythemia • Down syndrome • Drug-induced (e.g. maternal intake of selective serotonin reuptake inhibitors or nonsteroidal anti-inflammatory drugs)
Idiopathic	• When no definite cause is identified

PATHOGENESIS

Some of the important mediator pathways involved in pulmonary vasoreactivity and the site of action of some drugs are illustrated in **Figure 3**.

- Prostacyclin (PGI_2) is synthesized from arachidonic acid in the endothelial cell, through reactions catalyzed by cyclooxygenase (COX) and prostacyclin synthase (PGIS). PGI_2 then stimulates adenylate cyclase through prostacyclin receptors (IP) in the vascular smooth muscle cell, leading to the synthesis of cyclic adenosine monophosphate (cAMP) from adenosine triphosphate (ATP). cAMP decreases calcium levels in the cytoplasm and the vascular smooth muscle relaxes. Exogenously administered prostacyclin (acting through

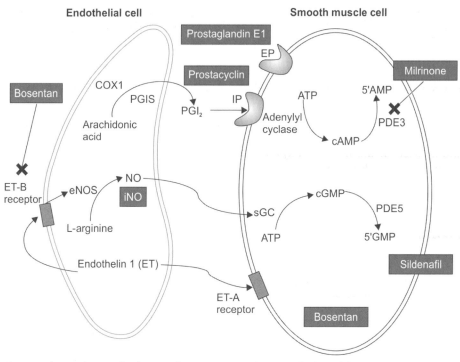

Fig. 3: Key vascular mediators of pulmonary hypertension and action of selected drugs.
(ATP: adenosine triphosphate; cAMP: cyclic adenosine monophosphate; cGMP: cyclic guanosine monophosphate; COX1: cyclooxygenase-1; eNOS: endothelial nitric oxide synthase; iNO: inhaled nitric oxide; NO: nitric oxide; PGIS: prostacyclin synthase; PGI$_2$: prostacyclin; PDE: phosphodiesterase; sGC: soluble guanylate cyclase; IP: prostacyclin)

IP receptors) and prostaglandin E1 (acting through EP receptors) both result in pulmonary vasodilation. Milrinone is an inhibitor of phosphodiesterase 3A (PDE3), which degrades cAMP.

- Endothelin-1 (ET) is a potent vasoconstrictor and mediates its effects through ET-A receptors on the smooth muscle cell. ET-B receptors on endothelial cells stimulate nitric oxide (NO) synthesis. Bosentan is an ET antagonist at both ET-A and ET-B receptors.
- NO synthesis is catalyzed by endothelial nitric oxide synthase (eNOS). Through soluble guanylate cyclase (sGC), NO stimulates the production of cyclic GMP (cGMP), which also decreases cytosolic calcium levels and relaxes vascular smooth muscle. Sildenafil, a PDE5 inhibitor, prevents the breakdown of cGMP.

CLINICAL FEATURES

- *Hypoxemia*—hallmark of PPHN, but can also be due to underlying pulmonary disease.
- Labile oxygenation, with wide swings is associated with a variety of stimuli:
  - Stimuli include touch, loud noises or pain
  - Lability reflects the variability in pulmonary vascular resistance (PVR).
- Difference in preductal (right upper limb) and postductal (lower limb) SpO$_2$ > 5–10%.

♦ Seen with right-to-left shunting of deoxygenated blood across the patent ductus arteriosus (PDA)

♦ No pre-post ductal difference if shunt is at atrial level or PDA is closed.

INVESTIGATIONS

Echocardiography:
- Tricuspid regurgitation (TR)
- Bulging of the interventricular septum to the left side
- Right-to-left or bidirectional shunt at the PDA/patent foramen ovale (PFO)
- TR jet velocity helps to estimate the pulmonary arterial pressure

X-rays:
- Features of underlying disease (like MAS or CDH)
- Prominent right cardiac border

Blood gas:
- Hypoxemia is the hallmark
- Hypercarbia can be a major problem in CDH, pulmonary hypoplasia, MAS, etc.
- Oxygenation index (OI) is helpful in assessing severity and response to therapy
- OI is calculated as follows:

$$OI = \text{Mean airway pressure (MAP)} \times 100 \times \frac{FiO_2}{PaO_2}$$

  - *OI ≤15*: Mild PPHN
  - *OI 15 to ≤25*: Moderate PPHN
  - *OI 25 to ≤40*: Severe PPHN
  - *OI >40*: Very severe PPHN (evaluate for ECMO)
- Inhaled nitric oxide is typically considered if the OI is >20–25.

Laboratory parameters:
- Normal calcium and electrolyte levels are targeted.
- Biomarkers and blood culture if infectious etiology is suspected.

DIFFERENTIAL DIAGNOSIS

▪ Key consideration is to rule out congenital heart disease masquerading as PPHN.

▪ Total anomalous pulmonary venous return with obstruction and left sided obstructive lesions (like hypoplastic left heart syndrome and critical coarctation of aorta) can be associated with pulmonary venous hypertension and hypoxemia, mimicking PPHN.

▪ An experienced echocardiographer should be able to differentiate these conditions from PPHN.

▪ Conditions like alveolar capillary dysplasia are rare and easily missed without a high index of suspicion.

TREATMENT

The primary goal is to improve tissue oxygenation. This is usually attained by increased oxygen administration, enhancing pulmonary vasodilation and improving cardiac function, in addition to general measures and treatment of the underlying condition.

General measures:
- Minimize the stimuli that can worsen PPHN
- Care in a quiet environment
- Use eye shields and ear muffs
- Fentanyl is the preferred drug for analgesia
- Paralyzing agents are rarely used
- Most may require parenteral nutrition

Oxygenation:
- Oxygen is a potent pulmonary vasodilator
- Hyperoxia is not beneficial
- Preductal SpO_2 target of 91–95% is adequate (85–95% in CDH)
- *Tissue oxygenation*—assess indirectly using pulse oximetry, blood gas, lactate level
- Near infrared spectroscopy (tissue oxygenation) is not routine

Ventilation:
- Target CO_2 at normal level or slightly high (40–50 mm Hg)
- Up to 65 mm Hg can be tolerated in CDH if pH is >7.2
- Limit tidal volume and peak pressure to minimize lung injury
- Surfactant therapy in cases with underlying RDS or MAS but not routinely
- Surfactant therapy is not useful in CDH

Circulatory management:
- Maintaining a normal systemic BP helps reduce right-to-left shunt
- Target mean BP close to upper limit of normal (45–55 mm Hg) in term infants
- Intravenous fluids for maintenance
- Packed cells to maintain the hematocrit >40%
- No definite evidence to support use of one inotrope over another
- In practice, one may start with dobutamine and then add dopamine if required

Pulmonary vasodilators:
- Inhaled nitric oxide:
  - Selective pulmonary vasodilator
  - Can reduce the need for ECMO in infants with severe PPHN
  - May not reduce mortality in Western settings
  - No evidence of benefit in infants with CDH
  - Started at a dose of 20 ppm
- *Sildenafil*:
  - Especially useful in settings where iNO is not available
  - *IV sildenafil:* A loading dose of 400 µg/kg infused over 3 hours, followed by a maintenance infusion of 1.6 mg/kg/day
  - Oral sildenafil is less expensive and was shown to reduce mortality in resource-limited settings. Starting dose is 250–500 µg/kg once every 6 hours and increase, as required, to not more than 2 mg/kg once every 4 hours
- *Milrinone*:
  - Useful to reduce PVR
  - Improves myocardial function
  - Avoid in hypotensive infants
  - *Dose:* 50–75 µg/kg/hr over 30–60 minutes and then a continuous IV infusion of 30–45 µg/kg/hr. Loading dose may cause hypotension
- *Low-dose arginine vasopressin*:
  - Reduces PVR
  - Increases systemic BP
  - Reduces right-to-left shunt
  - Experience is limited
  - *Dose:* 0.02 units/kg/hr; increase as required to not more than 0.1 units/kg/hr
- *Bosentan*:
  - Role in PPHN is not clear and evidence is conflicting
- IV prostaglandin or inhaled prostacyclin
  - Considered in patients who do not respond adequately to iNO

FOLLOW-UP

Infants with severe PPHN are at high risk of abnormal neurodevelopmental outcomes and should be followed up to a year of age or longer. Hearing testing is done before hospital discharge and on follow-up.

AIR LEAK

INTRODUCTION

- Pneumothorax, pneumomediastinum, pulmonary interstitial emphysema, and pneumopericardium are more common.
- Pneumoperitoneum and subcutaneous emphysema are rare.
- Incidence is higher among preterm infants especially those with pulmonary disease.
- Risk factors include underlying lung disease (MAS, pulmonary hypoplasia) and mechanical ventilation.

PNEUMOTHORAX

- A common complication of MAS.
- Pneumothorax should be suspected in any newborn with sudden onset of respiratory distress especially in a mechanically ventilated neonate with unexplained deterioration in oxygenation, ventilation, or cardiovascular status.
- Small pneumothorax may be asymptomatic. However, signs of respiratory distress such as tachypnea, grunting, pallor, and cyanosis are usually present.
- Physical examination may reveal chest asymmetry with hyperinflation of the affected side, decreased breath sounds on the affected side, and shift of cardiac impulse away from the affected side.
- Chest X-ray is the preferred investigation. However, transillumination and ultrasonography may also be useful.
- Radiological features of common air leak syndromes are described below:

Air leak	Chest X-ray findings
Pneumothorax	• Air in the pleural cavity (the area appears hyperlucent with absent pulmonary markings) • Collapse of the affected lung • Displacement of the mediastinum and heart shadow to opposite side • Bulging intercostal spaces • Downward displacement of the diaphragm on the affected side
Pneumomediastinum	• Halo around the heart border • Lateral view may show retrosternal translucency • The mediastinal air can elevate the thymus away from the pericardium, resulting in a "spinnaker sail" appearance
Pulmonary interstitial emphysema	• Hyperinflation and small cysts (localized or diffuse) • Linear radiolucencies variable in length and do not branch • Extreme cases—large bullae may appear

MANAGEMENT

- Oxygen supplementation should be provided to maintain adequate saturation.
- Fluid balance, nutrition, and cardiovascular support should be managed appropriately.
- Adopting a ventilatory strategy aimed at achieving acceptable gas exchange with the least amount of mean airway pressure possible to prevent further barotrauma and volutrauma.
- Infants without respiratory distress may be observed closely without specific treatment.
- In case of symptomatic or tension pneumothorax, emergency needle thoracocentesis should be done followed by intercostal tube drainage.

KEY POINTS

- Meconium-stained amniotic fluid occurs in 10–15% of births; out of these 10% develop MAS; out of these 15–20% die.
- Usually complicates term and near-term neonates.
- NRP 2015 does not recommend routine endotracheal suctioning of nonvigorous neonates born through MSAF.
- It requires supportive treatment and in some cases surfactant therapy and iNO and/or ECMO.
- PPHN is the most common cause of mortality in MAS.
- PPHN is manifested by severe, labile hypoxemia, and evidence of R>L shunting at PDA/PFO level.
- Oxygenation index is a good indicator of clinical severity in these cases.
- Apart from supportive care, iNO and drugs have a significant role to play in the management.
- Air leak syndrome, especially pneumothorax, is a common complication of MAS.
- Transillumination is a simple bedside test for air leak; though X-ray chest remains diagnostic.
- In case of symptomatic or tension pneumothorax, emergency needle thoracocentesis should be done followed by intercostal tube drainage.

SELF ASSESSMENT

1. **Which of the following statements is false regarding meconium aspiration syndrome?**
   a. Routine intrapartum suctioning and immediate postnatal suction in babies is not recommended.
   b. Usually affects SGA or postmature infants.
   c. According to Wiswell classification, neonates requiring less than 40% oxygen for less than 48 hours are classified as moderate disease.
   d. Antibiotics are not routinely recommended.

2. **Which of the following statements is false regarding management of PPHN?**
   a. Preductal saturation should be 95–98%.
   b. Target CO_2 should be at normal level or slightly high (40–50 mm Hg).
   c. Surfactant therapy in cases with underlying RDS but not routinely.
   d. Inhaled nitric oxide is started at a dose of 20 ppm.

FURTHER READING

1. Abman SH, Baker C, Gien J, et al. The Robyn Barst Memorial Lecture: Differences between the fetal, newborn, and adult pulmonary circulations: relevance for age-specific therapies (2013 Grover Conference series). Pulm Circ. 2014;4(3):424-40.
2. Abman SH, Hansmann G, Archer SL, et al.; American Heart Association Council on Cardiopulmonary, Critical Care, Perioperative and Resuscitation; Council on Clinical Cardiology; Council on Cardiovascular Disease in the Young; Council on Cardiovascular Radiology and Intervention; Council on Cardiovascular Surgery and Anesthesia; and the American Thoracic Society. Pediatric Pulmonary Hypertension: Guidelines From the American Heart Association and American Thoracic Society. Circulation. 2015;132(21):2037-99.
3. Chettri S, Adhisivam B, Bhat BV. Endotracheal suction for nonvigorous neonates born through meconium stained amniotic fluid: a randomized controlled trial. J Pediatr. 2015;166(5):1208-13.e1.
4. Chettri S, Bhat BV, Adhisivam B. Current concepts in the management of meconium aspiration syndrome. Indian J Pediatr. 2016;83(10):1125-30.
5. Jain A, McNamara PJ. Persistent pulmonary hypertension of the newborn: Advances in diagnosis and treatment. Semin Fetal Neonatal Med. 2015;20(4):262-71.
6. Nangia S, Thukral A, Chawla D. Tracheal suction at birth in non-vigorous neonates born through meconium-stained amniotic fluid. Cochrane Database Syst Rev. 2017;(5):CD012671.

8 Chapter

Invasive Ventilation in Neonates

Arti Maria, Tapas Bandyopadhyay

INTRODUCTION

- Spontaneous breathing is negative pressure ventilation wherein air is actively drawn into the lungs as a result of exaggeration of physiological negative intrathoracic pressure during inspiration and then expired out due to passive recoil of the chest wall and lungs. This is in contrast to the mechanical ventilation that drives in air through a ventilator.
- The term invasive ventilation conveys a form of mechanical ventilation wherein an endotracheal tube is placed to serve as an interface between the ventilator and the baby's lungs to get the pressures delivered to achieve the desired gas exchange.
- The concept of gas exchange implies elimination of CO_2 (ventilation) in exchange of oxygen (oxygenation) and continues throughout the respiratory cycle. The gas exchange through the expiration is maintained by virtue of the functional residual capacity of the lungs.

INDICATIONS OF VENTILATION

Clinical	Laboratory
Weak, absent and/or poor respiratory effort: • Apnea	pH <7.2 and not improving, PCO_2 >65 on days 0–3, >70 beyond day 3, PaO_2 <50 mm Hg
Severe respiratory distress: • Downes'/Silverman score ≥7 • Failure of continuous positive airway pressure (CPAP)	
Miscellaneous: • Cardiovascular collapse—shock, cardiopulmonary resuscitation, preoperative	

WHAT IS A VENTILATOR?

It is easiest to understand any ventilator as being a T-piece device with the baby being interposed in the middle of a continuous flow of gases running across from one end (inspiratory limb) to the other end (expiratory limb) of the circuit following the path of least resistance. However, as and when the flow on expiratory side is interrupted by complete closure of the positive end expiratory pressure (PEEP) valve, the baby gets a breath (inspiration).

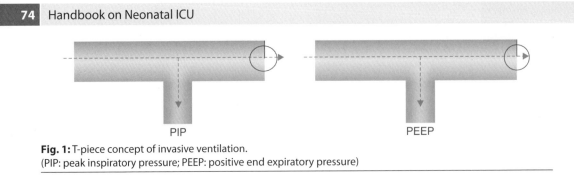

Fig. 1: T-piece concept of invasive ventilation.
(PIP: peak inspiratory pressure; PEEP: positive end expiratory pressure)

The duration for which the valve remains closed determines the inspiratory time, the periodicity with which this event occurs, determines the ventilator rate (frequency) and the degree of closure determines the peak inspiratory pressure **(Fig. 1)**. During expiration, the PEEP valve is partially closed producing "positive end expiratory pressure".

SOME BASIC CONCEPTS

Control Variables (Which are Controlled by the Ventilator to Generate Inspiration)

- Pressure (airway pressure is controlled) ⎫
- Volume (tidal volume is controlled) ⎬ Most common
  ⎭

Differences between volume controlled ventilation (VCV) and pressure controlled ventilation (PCV)		
Features	VCV	PCV
Control variable	Volume	Pressure
Trigger	Patient or machine	Patient or machine
Limit	Flow	Pressure
Cycle	Volume or flow	Time or flow
Delivered tidal volume	Constant	Variable
Delivered peak pressure	Variable	Constant
Inspiratory flow waveform	Square	Ramp descending

Phase Variable (Which Changes the Phase of Respiratory Cycle)

- Trigger (which causes the breath to begin)—time, patient (pressure or flow)
- Limit (which regulates the gas flow during breath)—pressure, volume, and flow
- Cycling (which causes the breath to end)—time, pressure, flow, and volume.

Ventilatory Parameters

- *Oxygenation:* It depends upon mean airway pressure (MAP) and fraction of inspired oxygen (FiO_2). MAP is the average area under the curve of the pressure waveform **(Fig. 2)**.
- *Ventilation:* It depends upon minute ventilation (MV).

$$MV = \text{respiratory rate} \times \text{tidal volume}$$

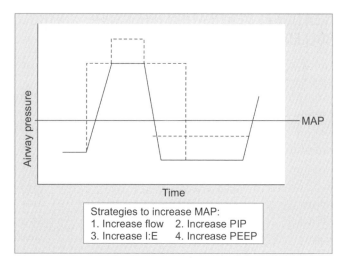

Strategies to increase MAP:
1. Increase flow   2. Increase PIP
3. Increase I:E   4. Increase PEEP

Fig. 2: Strategies to increase mean airway pressure (MAP).
(PIP: peak inspiratory pressure; PEEP: positive end expiratory pressure; I:E: inspiratory and expiratory time)

Ventilatory parameters and their description, range, and side effects

Parameter	Effect	Typical range	Target	Side effects
PIP (peak inspiratory pressure)	↑PaO_2 and ↓$PaCO_2$	12–25 cm H_2O	Just visible chest rise	Barotrauma
PEEP (positive end expiratory pressure)	↑PaO_2	4–8 cm H_2O	Optimum PEEP— adequate lung inflation on chest X-ray	Too high—gas trapping, decreases cardiac output Too low— derecruitment
Rate	↓$PaCO_2$	Term: 40–45 Preterm: 50–60	$PaCO_2$ in target range	Higher rates— compromise inspiratory time (Ti), expiratory time (Te), and ratio between inspiratory and expiratory time
Inspiratory time or I:E	Increase Ti: ↑PaO_2 Increase I:E: ↓$PaCO_2$	0.3–0.5 s	3–5 times of time constant (compliance × resistance)	Changes have modest effect on gas exchange
FiO_2 (fraction of inspired oxygen)	↑PaO_2	21–100%	SpO_2 between 90% and 95%	FiO_2 >0.6–0.7 increases the risk of oxytrauma
Flow rate	↑PaO_2	6–10 L/min	To attain sinusoidal waveform	↓ airflow—air hunger and ↑work of breathing ↑airflow—turbulence, auto PEEP and ↓ gas exchange

MODES OF CONVENTIONAL VENTILATION (PRESSURE CONTROLLED/ VOLUME CONTROLLED)

- *Intermittent mandatory ventilation*: Ventilator delivers mandatory breaths at fixed time intervals, irrespective of baby's spontaneous breathing efforts.
- *Patient-triggered ventilation*: Delivery of a mechanical breath in response to signal ("trigger") from the baby. This is further classified into synchronized intermittent mandatory ventilation (SIMV), assist control ventilation (A/C), and pressure support ventilation (PSV).

Classification of patient-triggered ventilation and their description:

Variables (Depend on)	SIMV	A/C	PSV
Rate	Ventilator	Baby	Baby
Inspiratory time	Ventilator	Ventilator	Baby
PIP	Ventilator	Ventilator	Ventilator
PEEP	Ventilator	Ventilator	Ventilator
Advantage	• Good inspiratory synchrony • Augments spontaneous breath	• All breaths above trigger level—supported • Good inspiratory synchrony	• Improves cycling as well as trigger • Inspiratory and expiratory synchrony
Disadvantage	• Asynchrony—expiratory all breaths, inspiratory few breaths • ↑Work of breathing if spontaneous breaths are unsupported	• Asynchrony—expiratory all breaths • Not useful for conditions with high spontaneous rates (generates auto-PEEP)	• Not useful for babies with apnea • Ventilators use back up rate for apnea patients; then it functions as IMV

(IMV: intermittent mandatory ventilation; SIMV: synchronized intermittent mandatory ventilation; A/C: assist control ventilation; PSV: pressure support ventilation)

DISEASE SPECIFIC VENTILATION AND INITIAL SETTINGS IN COMMON CLINICAL SCENARIOS

Disease condition	Normal lung	Respiratory distress syndrome	Meconium aspiration syndrome	Pneumonia
Pathophysiology				
Compliance	N	↓	↓/N	↓
Resistance	N/↑ (because of ET)	N/↑	↑	N/↑
Functional residual capacity	N	↓	↓/↑	↓
Time constant	N	↓	↑	↓
Initial settings				
PIP (cm H$_2$O)	12	15–16	14–15	15–16
PEEP (cm H$_2$O)	4	5	4–6	5
Rate (per minute)	30	50–55	40–45	50–55: Preterm 40–45: Term
Inspiratory time(s)	0.4	0.3–0.35	0.38–0.40	0.35–0.40
FiO$_2$%	0.21	0.5 or as required	As required	As required

(ET: endotracheal tube; PEEP: positive end expiratory pressure; PIP: peak inspiratory pressure)

Settings may need to be modified according to the progression/improvement in the disease status.

TARGETS FOR OPTIMAL VENTILATION

Clinical (Most important)		Blood gas	Radiological
• Baby should be breathing comfortably • Just visible chest rise • Absent or minimal retractions • Equal air entry	• Color—pink, capillary filling time—<3 s, normal blood pressure, adequate urine output • Saturation: 90–95%	• pH—7.35–7.45 • pCO$_2$—40–50 mm Hg • pO$_2$—50–80 mm Hg • BE—± 5 • Bicarbonate—20–24 mEq/L	• In anteroposterior view, the lung expansion should be up to sixth to eighth posterior ends of the ribs • Endotracheal tube (ET) should be at the level of T2 vertebrae • No role of serial chest radiograph in the absence of clinical indication

Subsequent monitoring of respiratory distress can be done using Downes' or Silvermans' score every 2–3 hours.

GUIDE FOR SUBSEQUENT ADJUSTMENT OF VENTILATOR SETTINGS TARGETING NORMAL BLOOD GAS PARAMETER

PaO$_2$ (mm Hg)	PaCO$_2$ (mm Hg)	Intervention	Remarks
↓	N	• ↑ FiO$_2$ • ↑ PEEP	Optimize PEEP as per lung inflation
↓	↑	• ↑ PIP • Optimize PEEP as per lung inflation	Consider ↑ FiO$_2$ appropriate for PEEP
↓	↓	• ↑ FiO$_2$	Persistent pulmonary hypertension (PPHN) may present with purely oxygenation difficulty; do not hyperventilate
N	↑	• ↑ Ventilator rates	Exclude endotracheal tube block
N	↓	• ↓ PIP • ↓ Ventilator rates	Consider ↓ rates if PaO$_2$ is low normal
↑	↓	• ↓ PIP	Decrease the settings
↑	↑	• ↓ PEEP	Optimize PEEP as per lung inflation
↑	N	• ↓ FiO$_2$ • ↓PEEP	Optimize PEEP as per lung inflation

PRINCIPLES OF SUPPORTIVE CARE AND BEDSIDE BEST PRACTICES FOR VENTILATED BABY

- Optimize ventilation and minimize duration and complications.
- Maintain neutral thermal environment and provide adequate nutrition.
- Prevention of infection.

Bedside best practices for ventilated baby	
Practice	Action
Humidification of inspiratory gases	Warmed to 37°C and fully saturated [100% relative humidity (RH) or 44 mg/L of vapor] when they reach the airway
Endotracheal suctioning	• Strict asepsis with stepwise protocol • Suctioning should be done only if there are visible secretions/desaturations and/or decreased breath sounds • Closed "inline" suctioning decreases respiratory contamination and pulmonary infections • Routine normal saline irrigation prior to the suctioning should not be done
Prevention of ventilator associated pneumonia	• Elevation of head end of bed to 30° • Strict asepsis during handling and performing procedure • Avoid breaking into respiratory circuit • Oral suction must follow and not precede ET suction or else separate ET and oral suctioning tubing • Sterile water in humidification systems • Periodic drainage of condensate from breathing circuits • Keeping the ET tube and Y-piece at 90° to each other • Daily assessment for extubation readiness
Positioning and physiotherapy	• Change position every 4–6 hours • Physiotherapy has a therapeutic role in presence of chest X-ray consistent with collapse • Should not be done in very preterm infants during the 1st week of life
Follow-up	• Long-term neurodevelopmental assessment • Neuroimaging • Retinopathy of prematurity (ROP) screening as indicated } Before discharge • Hearing assessment

ACUTE DETERIORATION OF A BABY ON VENTILATOR

It is recognized by sudden onset of desaturation and/or cyanosis and/or bradycardia and/or hypotension and/or cardiopulmonary arrest. Stepwise algorithm for recognition and management of such an event is shown in **Flowchart 1**.

These events can be prevented by regular clinical monitoring, setting appropriate alarms limits, responding to alarms, keeping emergency tray handy, and timely appropriate action.

WEANING AND EXTUBATION

The process of shifting the work of breathing from the ventilator back to the patient by gradually decreasing the level of support is called weaning.

Principles: Injurious parameters (PIP) should be weaned first; wean one parameter at a time; avoid changes in large magnitude; and assess the response to each of the changes as shown in **Flowchart 2**.

Extubation settings: At PIP—12-13 (15 in case of prolonged ventilation), PEEP—4-5, Rate—25-30, FiO_2—≤0.3 [very low birth weight babies are extubated to nasal continuous positive airway pressure (CPAP) of 5-6 cm H_2O].

Flowchart 1: Algorithm for acute deterioration of a baby on ventilator.

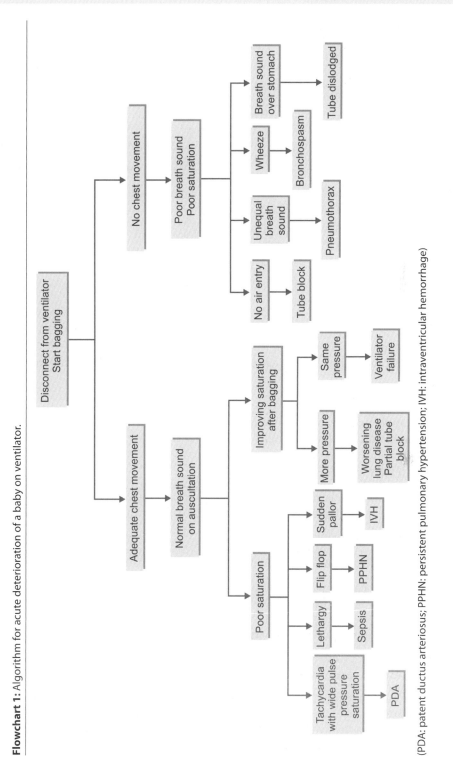

(PDA: patent ductus arteriosus; PPHN: persistent pulmonary hypertension; IVH: intraventricular hemorrhage)

Flowchart 2: Algorithm for stepwise weaning of babies on invasive ventilation.

```
              At first ↓PIP to 25
                     │
                     ▼
        Then alternately ↓PIP and FiO₂
                     │
                     ▼
          Till PIP 20; FiO₂ 0.6
```

Saturation; PaO₂ Maintained →	Decrease FiO₂; PEEP →	Extubation settings: • PIP–12–13 (15 in case of prolonged ventilation) • PEEP–4–5 • Rate–25–30 • FiO₂– ≤0.3
PaO₂; PaCO₂ Maintained →	Decrease PIP →	
Clinical parameters; PaCO₂ Maintained →	Decrease RR →	

(FiO₂: fraction of inspired oxygen; PIP: peak inspiratory pressure; PEEP: positive end expiratory pressure; RR: respiratory rate)

Peri-extubation Care

- Feeding is stopped 3–4 hours prior to extubation.
- In babies <1.5 kg, loading dose of caffeine can be used to improve the respiratory drive.

Post-extubation Care

- Humidification, nebulization, and frequent position change should be done.
- Meticulous monitoring for respiratory distress and vitals should be done.

HIGH FREQUENCY VENTILATION

Principle: It is a form of invasive ventilation that uses small tidal volumes, sometimes less than dead space, and very rapid rates (2–20 Hz or 120–1,200 cycles/min) to achieve gas exchange.

Salient features of high frequency oscillatory ventilation
• Very small tidal volumes
• Active expiration
• Oxygenation and ventilation can be controlled independently
• Increase in frequency leads to CO_2 retention and vice versa

Indications of high frequency ventilation in neonates	
Established	Other
• Air leak	• Persistent pulmonary hypertension (PPHN)
• As "rescue mode" in severe respiratory failure refractory to conventional ventilation [high PIP (22–24 in PT, 24–28 in term)]	• Meconium aspiration syndrome
• Pulmonary hypoplasia	• Congenital diaphragmatic hernia
• Adjunct to inhaled nitric oxide (iNO) in babies with PPHN	

(PT: preterm)

COMPLICATIONS OF INVASIVE VENTILATION

Upper airway	Lower airway	Extrapulmonary
• Palatal grooving, abnormality of dentition • Subglottic edema • Tracheal stenosis	• Chronic lung disease • Air leak • Pulmonary hemorrhage • Atelectasis • Ventilator-associated pneumonia	• Retinopathy of prematurity • Healthcare-associated sepsis • Intraventricular hemorrhage • Periventricular leukomalacia

KEY POINTS

➤ Mechanical ventilation is responsible for respiratory support of sick, preterm neonates with respiratory failure. Current thinking is in favour of noninvasive ventilation like CPAP and use of invasive mechanical ventilation has gone down over years.

➤ Pressure controlled, time limited ventilation is the most common ventilator strategy used.

➤ Flow synchronized ventilation is the only way to do inspiratory and expiratory synchrony.

➤ Invasive ventilation is associated with barotrauma, ventilator associated pneumonia, pulmonary hemorrhage, intracranial hemorrhage, and ventilator dependence.

➤ All ventilated neonates should be followed up for long-term neurodevelopment outcome.

SELF ASSESSMENT

1. **Which of the following is not a part of mean airway pressure?**
   a. PIP
   b. PEEP
   c. FiO_2
   d. Inspiratory time

2. **If a baby is not maintaining on ventilator, you disconnected the ventilator and started giving manual breaths and baby started improving. What is the diagnosis?**
   a. Pneumothorax
   b. Endotracheal tube dislodged
   c. PIP is low for the lung condition
   d. Intraventricular hemorrhage

FURTHER READING

1. Keszler M, Chartburn RL. Overview of assisted ventilation. In: Goldsmith JP, Karotkin EH, Keszler M, Suresh GK (Eds). Assisted Ventilation of the Neonate. 6th edition. Philadelphia: WB Saunders; 2017. pp. 140-52.

2. Pfister RH, Soll RF. Initial respiratory support of preterm infant: the role of CPAP, the INSURE method, and noninvasive ventilation. Clin Perinatol. 2012;39(3):459-81.

3. Sant'Anna GM, Keszler M. Weaning infants from mechanical ventilation. Clin Perinatol. 2012;39(3):543-62.

Noninvasive Ventilation in Neonates

Chapter

9

Abdul Razak, Karthik Nagesh N

DEFINITION

Noninvasive respiratory support (NRS) is defined as support provided to nasal airway of spontaneously breathing infant in absence of endotracheal tube.

TYPES (FLOWCHART 1)

- Nasal continuous positive airway pressure (NCPAP) includes continuous positive pressure provided by a device (ventilator or bubble CPAP or variable flow device) administered via nasal route through mask or binasal prongs or nasopharyngeal tube.
- Nasal intermittent positive pressure ventilation (NIPPV) includes positive pressure inflation on the top of CPAP provided by a ventilator (synchronous or nonsynchronous) administered via nasal route through mask or binasal prongs or nasopharyngeal tube. The peak pressures are higher and inspiratory times are lower compared to biphasic positive airway pressure (BIPAP).
- Biphasic positive airway pressure includes noninvasive support that cycles between two pressure levels provided by a variable flow device (synchronous or nonsynchronous way) administered via nasal route through mask or binasal prongs or nasopharyngeal tube. The peak pressures are lower and inspiratory times are higher compared to NIPPV.
- Heated humidified high flow nasal cannula (HHHFNC) includes heated and humidified gas flows greater than 1 L/min provided by a high-flow apparatus via nasal route through binasal prongs.
- Low-flow nasal cannula (LFNC) includes gas flows less than 1 L/min provided by a high-flow apparatus via nasal route through binasal prongs.
- Nasal high frequency oscillatory ventilation (NHFOV) includes continuous distending pressure with superimposed oscillations provided by ventilator administered via nasal route through mask or binasal prongs or nasopharyngeal tube.
- Noninvasive neurally adjusted ventilatory assist (NIV-NAVA) includes positive pressure inflation on the top of CPAP provided by a ventilator in a synchronous way determined by the electrical activity of diaphragm (detected by NAVA catheter placed in esophagus) administered via nasal route through mask or binasal prongs or nasopharyngeal tube.

Nasal CPAP is most commonly used mode of noninvasive support. HHHFNC has recently been used by many units with variable levels of success. Nasal invasive mechanical ventilation

Flowchart 1: Types of noninvasive respiratory support modes used in preterm infants.

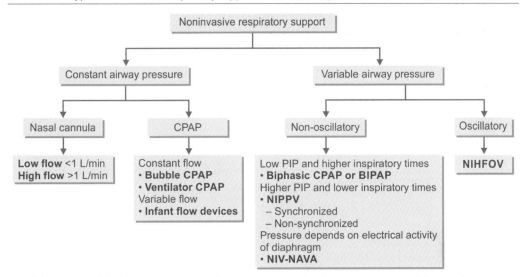

(BIPAP: biphasic positive airway pressure; CPAP: continuous positive airway pressure; NIV-NAVA: noninvasive neurally adjusted ventilatory assist; NIPPV: nasal intermittent positive pressure ventilation; NIHFOV: noninvasive high frequency oscillatory ventilation)

(IMV) and biphasic support is also being used. Nasal high frequency and NIV-NAVA are recent noninvasive strategies which are mainly in research phase and in this chapter, we shall restrict ourselves to CPAP, HHHFNC, and nasal IMV.

GOALS OF NONINVASIVE VENTILATION

- All devices provide some distending pressure, thereby increasing transpulmonary pressure and decreasing work of breathing.
- Recruiting collapsed alveoli thereby preserving gas exchange and minimizing work of breathing.
- Prevents lung injury by avoiding shear injury (atelectotrauma).
- Splints the upper airway and reduces obstructive apnea.
- By avoiding intubation, risk of airway trauma, inflammation, and infection are reduced.

  The mechanism by how the various noninvasive respiratory support modes work in neonatal population is as shown in **Table 1**.

NASAL CONTINUOUS POSITIVE AIRWAY PRESSURE

It has been most used form of noninvasive ventilation to support spontaneously breathing neonates with lung disease.

History

In 1971, Gregory et al. reported first successful application of CPAP through an endotracheal tube or a head box in a series of spontaneously breathing premature infants with respiratory

Table 1: Mechanism of various noninvasive respiratory modes.

	Oxygenation	Ventilation	Apnea of prematurity
NCPAP	Increasing functional residual capacity	• Increasing functional residual capacity • Reduces upper airway resistance	Maintains patency of airway by constant flow of gases
HFNC	Provides constant distending pressures (although variable)	• Washes out the anatomical dead space in the upper airway • Reduces upper airway resistance	Unclear but might work as NCPAP by providing constant flow of gases
NIPPV and BIPAP	Same as NCPAP	Same as NCPAP plus additional fixed rate of intermittent pressure on the top of baseline pressure helps clearing carbon dioxide	Same as NCPAP plus fixed rate of intermittent pressure on the top of baseline pressure helps infants with poor respiratory drive
NIV-NAVA	Same as NIPPV plus an additional advantage of synchronized pressure delivery proportional to the electrical activity of diaphragm improving patient-ventilator synchrony		
NHFOV	Same as NCPAP	Same as NCPAP but higher carbon dioxide clearance due to impact of oscillation	Same as NCPAP plus oscillation stimulates breathing (controversial)

(BIPAP: biphasic positive airway pressure; HFNC: high-flow nasal cannula; NCPAP: nasal continuous positive airway pressure; NHFOV: nasal high frequency oscillatory ventilation; NIPPV: nasal intermittent positive pressure ventilation; NIV-NAVA: noninvasive neurally adjusted ventilatory assist)

distress syndrome (RDS). In this era, mortality rates close to 60% were common in premature infants receiving IMV. CPAP was welcomed as a missing link between oxygen and mechanical ventilation.

Indications	Contraindications
• RDS • Transient tachypnea of neonate • Meconium aspiration syndrome • Pneumonia • Apnea of prematurity • Postoperative situations like surgical repair of congenital diaphragmatic hernia and congenital heart disease • Paralysis of hemidiaphragm • Bronchiolitis • Laryngo-, broncho- and tracheomalacia	• Shock and severe cardiovascular instability • Severe apneic episodes • Upper airway abnormalities like cleft palate, choanal atresia, tracheoesophageal fistula, and unrepaired diaphragmatic hernia • Respiratory failure (pH <7.25 and $PaCO_2$ > 60 mm Hg)

Physiologic Effects of Continuous Positive Airway Pressure

- Decreases tachypnea
- Decreases work of breathing
- Increases functional residual capacity and PaO_2

- Decreases transpulmonary shunting and improve lung compliance
- Stabilizes compliant chest wall of preterm baby
- Stabilizes upper airway
- Decreases thoracoabdominal asynchrony.

Methods of Generating Continuous Positive Airway Pressure

There are two types of CPAP:
1. *Continuous flow CPAP:* Continuous distending pressure (CDP) is generated at device. Bubble CPAP and ventilator-driven CPAP generate CDP by this method. In bubble CPAP, CDP is generated by depth of immersion of expiratory limb into bubbling chamber. In ventilators, CPAP is generated by closure of expiratory valve.
2. *Variable flow CPAP:* CPAP is generated at the prongs near patient end. Infant flow drivers use variable flow CPAP. They work on principle of Coanda effect in which air or fluid follows the curved surface of the wall.

Continuous flow CPAP (preferably bubble CPAP) is the most commonly used CPAP method.

Set-up of Bubble Continuous Positive Airway Pressure (Fig. 1)

- *Compressed source of air and oxygen:* It can be provided by means of compressed gas supply from cylinders or there can be centralized air and oxygen supply. In case of centralized supply, pressure should be monitored on daily basis.
- *Humidifier:* Dry and cool gas at high flows can damage the cilia leading to pneumonia and infections. So it needs to be warmed and humidified with a servo controlled humidifier to a temperature of 37°C.
- *Inspiratory limb:* Inspiratory limb is the limb of circuit joining the humidifier to nasal interface. There are two types of inspiratory limb—one contains heater wire and one does not contain heater wire. The one containing heater wire is preferred. Drawback of the one which does not contain heater wire is that there can be condensation in the inspiratory circuit and water can go to the baby.
- *Interface:* Various types of interfaces are available. Out of all the available interfaces, short binasal prongs are the best.
- *Expiratory limb:* Expiratory limb attaches from nasal interface and goes to bubbling chamber. The depth to which expiratory limb is immersed in the bubbling chamber determines the level of PEEP which child is getting.

Continuous Positive Airway Pressure Interfaces

Multiple devices have been used as interfaces to deliver CPAP **(Fig. 2)**.
- *Bilateral nasopharyngeal prongs:* They are long (length 40–90 mm) as compared to nasal prongs (9–14 mm). Long length leads to increase in resistance in airway thereby leading to increase in work of breathing.
- *Unilateral nasopharyngeal prong:* Conventionally nasal CPAP was delivered by endotracheal tube which is cut to approximately 5–6 cm length and placed through one nare. Drawback of this method is leakage through other nostril and increase in resistance because of length.

Complications of Continuous Positive Airway Pressure

- Nasal injury
- Malpositioned nasal prongs
- Inadvertent positive end expiratory pressure (PEEP) leading to hyperinflation of lungs and decreased perfusion
- Pneumothorax
- Gastrointestinal distension—usually benign, is called CPAP belly syndrome.

NASAL INTERMITTENT POSITIVE AIRWAY PRESSURE

Nasal IPPV combines the use of nasal CPAP with intermittent breaths. It can be provided by nasal prongs through any ventilator used in NICU. It can be used as primary mode to treat RDS or in apnea of prematurity or in postextubation state **(Table 3)**.

Evidence

Cochrane systematic reviews have shown NIPPV is more effective than NCPAP for reducing the need for intubation and invasive ventilation in preterm infants with RDS and postextubation.

Heated Humidified High Flow Nasal Cannula (Fig. 3)

This is one of the innovations, which has gained popularity in last few years despite limited evidence for its use.

Where it can be used?
- RDS
- Postextubation state
- Apnea of prematurity
- Weaning from nasal CPAP.

How does it work?
- Provides distending pressure
- Gas conditioning effects—decreases $PaCO_2$ by washing out nasopharyngeal dead space.
- It reduces inspiratory resistance thereby leading to decrease in resistive work of breathing.

Table 3: Settings of nasal intermittent positive airway pressure.		
Ventilator variable	*RDS*	*Postextubation*
Rate, breath/min	40	10–25
PIP, cm H_2O	2–4 >PIP on manual positive pressure ventilation	2–4 >PIP on mechanical ventilator
PEEP, cm H_2O	4–6	<5
Inspiratory time, sec	0.4–0.45	0.3–0.5
Flow rate, L/min	8–10	8–10

(PIP: peak inspiratory pressure; PEEP: positive end expiratory pressure; RDS: respiratory distress syndrome)
Adapted from Louise S Owen, Colin J Morley, Peter G Davis. Neonatal nasal intermittent positive pressure ventilation: what do we know in 2007? Arch Dis Child Fetal Neonatal Ed. 2007;92(5):F414–18.

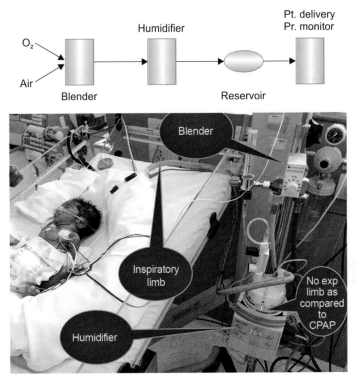

Fig. 3: Setup for heated humidified high-flow nasal cannula.
(CPAP: continuous positive airway pressure)

Difference in CPAP Prongs and High-flow Prongs

Whereas in CPAP, we advocate least or no leak, leak across nasal prong is mandatory in HHHFNC. The diameter of nasal prongs should be around 50% of internal nares diameter.

Benefits

- Ease of application
- Allows more access to face
- Easier for feeding and do Kangaroo mother care
- Less nasal trauma
- Ease of nursing care.

Practical Guidelines for HHFNC

- Start at 5–8 L/min depending upon weight of baby.
- Increase flow depending upon FiO_2 needs, work of breathing.
- If FiO_2 exceeds >50–60%, change to other modes (preferably CPAP before intubation).
- For weaning, wean FiO_2 first, and then flow.

- Once FiO_2 is <30%, decrease flow in decrements of 0.5–1 L/min q 12–24 hourly depending on clinical status.
- Take off if infant is stable for 24 hours on flow of 3–4 L/min.

KEY POINTS

➤ Bubble CPAP is most commonly used form of nasal CPAP.
➤ For primary RDS, nasal CPAP is treatment of choice.
➤ In postextubation state, HHHFNC is good alternative to nasal CPAP.
➤ Blender and humidifier are a must in setting up of any noninvasive ventilation.

SELF ASSESSMENT

1. **Preterm baby of 30 weeks is having RDS immediately after birth. His Downes' score is 6/10. Preferred mode of ventilator support in this baby is:**
   a. Oxygen by hood
   b. HHHFNC
   c. Bubble CPAP
   d. Intubation, surfactant and ventilation

2. **Which of following statements is true?**
   a. Baby on nasal CPAP is having abdominal distension, warrants withholding feed and increases risk of NEC
   b. X-ray with FRC of 4–6 ribs shows adequate lung expansion
   c. CPAP cannot be given in babies having meconium aspiration syndrome
   d. CPAP failure is defined as need for PEEP more than 8 cm H_2O and FiO_2 needs >50% with blood gas showing pH <7.25, $PaCO_2$ >60 mm and metabolic acidosis

FURTHER READING

1. Kotecha SJ, Adappa R, Gupta N, et al. Safety and efficacy of high-flow nasal cannula therapy in preterm infants: A meta-analysis. Pediatrics. 2015;136(3):542-53.
2. Lemyre B, Davis PG, De Paoli AG, et al. Nasal intermittent positive pressure ventilation (NIPPV) versus nasal continuous positive airway pressure (NCPAP) for preterm neonates after extubation. Cochrane Database Syst Rev. 2017;2:CD003212.
3. Lemyre B, Laughon M, Bose C, et al. Early nasal intermittent positive pressure ventilation (NIPPV) versus early nasal continuous positive airway pressure (NCPAP) for preterm infants. Cochrane Database Syst Rev. 2016;12:CD005384.
4. Morley CJ, Davis PG, Doyle LW, et al. Nasal CPAP or intubation at birth for very preterm infants. N Engl J Med. 2008;358(7):700-8.
5. Wilkinson D, Andersen C, O'Donnell CP, et al. High flow nasal cannula for respiratory support in preterm infants. Cochrane Database Syst Rev 2016;2:CD006405.

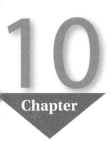

10

Chapter

Bronchopulmonary Dysplasia

Supreet Khurana, Praveen Kumar

INTRODUCTION

Bronchopulmonary dysplasia (BPD), also known as neonatal chronic lung disease, is one of the most common chronic respiratory morbidities of prematurity. "Classic or Old BPD" originally described by Northway was characterized by areas of significant atelectasis and fibrosis following severe respiratory distress syndrome (RDS) in presurfactant era in infants without antenatal steroid exposure and exposed to aggressive mechanical ventilation. In the current era, the most common form is "New BPD" seen in extremely preterm neonates due to their better survival with advances in neonatal care, and which has hallmark findings of arrest of alveolarization during early phase of lung development.

DEFINITION AND CLASSIFICATION

Neonates who need supplemental oxygen for a cumulative duration of ≥28 days (each day defined as need for >21% FiO_2 for >12 hours per day) satisfy the definition of BPD. Further classification of severity of BPD as given by National Institute of Child Health and Human Development (NICHD) in 2001 is based on gestational age along with need for supplemental oxygen and mechanical ventilation.

Gestational age (weeks)	Age at assessment	Mild	Moderate	Severe
<32 weeks	36 weeks postmenstrual age or discharge (whichever earlier)	Breathing room air	FiO_2 <30%	FiO_2 >30% and/or need for ventilation (either invasive or noninvasive)
≥32 weeks	56 days (8 weeks) postnatal age (PNA) or discharge (whichever earlier)			

Physiologic Definition of Bronchopulmonary Dysplasia

The need for supplemental oxygen is based on oxygen saturation (SpO_2) during a room air challenge performed at 36 weeks' postmenstrual age (PMA) (or 56 days for infants

≥32 weeks' PMA) or before hospital discharge. Persistent SpO_2 <90% is the cutoff below which supplemental O_2 should be considered.

Incidence

Incidence is inversely related to gestational age and birth weight.
- 35–50% in <28 weeks gestation as per western literature and 9–50% as per Indian literature.
- Neonates with birth weight <1,250 g account for 97% of cases.

RISK FACTORS

Inherent to patient:
- Prematurity
- Fetal growth restriction
- Male gender
- Caucasian race
- Higher correlation is seen in monozygotic twins
- Single nucleotide polymorphisms of endothelial nitric oxide synthase (eNOS) can increase risk of developing BPD.

Ventilation strategies:
- Aggressive mechanical ventilation using large tidal volumes causing volutrauma
- Surfactant deficiency both early as well late in the course of disease
- Oxygen toxicity due to even brief periods of hyperoxia leads to generation of free radical species that along with weak antioxidant defenses worsens lung injury
- Use of few high pressure inflation breaths at birth is known to cause significant barotrauma to preterm lungs and it is further established that presence of an endotracheal tube even for brief periods causes biotrauma.

Parenteral and enteral nutrition strategies:
- Neonates who receive excessive early intravenous fluids and/or do not show diuresis are predisposed to BPD
- Inadequate nutritional support for high calorie and protein needs along with vitamin deficiencies (especially vitamin A, D, and LCPUFA deficiency) in sick preterm neonates worsens lung injury and impedes repair.

Infections/Inflammation:
- Chorioamnionitis is found to be associated with BPD in many studies
- *Ureaplasma urealyticum* colonization of respiratory tract at 36 weeks PMA has been found to be significantly associated with increased risk of BPD
- Intrauterine *Chlamydia* infection has also been proposed as a risk factor.

Comorbid conditions:
- PDA and surgical ligation of PDA both are known predisposing factors.

(LCPUFA: long chain polyunsaturated fatty acids; BPD: bronchopulmonary dysplasia; PDA: patent ductus arteriosus; PMA: postmenstrual age)

PATHOGENESIS

"New BPD" encountered nowadays is characterized by arrest of alveolar septation during saccular phase of lung development in response to multitude of antenatal and postnatal factors enumerated above. It has pathognomic features of fewer and larger alveoli and abnormal pulmonary vasculogenesis that is in contrast to "Old BPD" which occurred due to structural injury during alveolar phase of lung development and had predominant features of inflammation and fibrosis.

CLINICAL FEATURES

Due to routine use of antenatal corticosteroids and judicious use of surfactant and gentle ventilation strategies, the usual clinical course observed is of a neonate with RDS having gradually improving ventilation with either abrupt deterioration or static course with inability to wean off from oxygen or ventilation. The respiratory findings may be a combination of findings of tachypnea, retractions, rales, prolonged expiration, expiratory wheeze, features of pulmonary arterial hypertension, and hypoxemia with some findings more predominant than others depending upon disease pathology.

INVESTIGATIONS

- *Chest X-ray:* With evolution of disease, lung findings change from clear lung fields to findings of diffuse haziness and coarse interstitial infiltrates **(Fig. 1)**. Lung volume may remain normal in early stage while with disease progression, areas of atelectasis with trapping appear and in those with severe disease there occurs streaky or cystic shadows accompanied with severe hyperinflation **(Fig. 2)**.
- *Arterial-blood gas:* Blood gases during early phases show hypercarbia with hypoxemia. A picture of respiratory acidosis compensated with metabolic alkalosis is seen after 2–3 weeks. Diuretic induced hyponatremia, hypokalemia, hypochloremia, and hypercalciuria with eventual nephrocalcinosis may occur.
- *Pulmonary function tests:* Decreased tidal volume, increased airway resistance, and decreased dynamic lung compliance with increasing ventilation/perfusion mismatch.
- *2D ECHO:* It is useful to look into alternate etiologies causing left to right shunts like PDA which can be a compounder for BPD. It is also a useful adjunct to assess severity of pulmonary arterial hypertension and right ventricular hypertrophy.
- *Biomarkers:* Though not used routinely but have been studied frequently for research purposes; so a brief overview of some of these is being provided in the table below.

(ECHO: echocardiography)

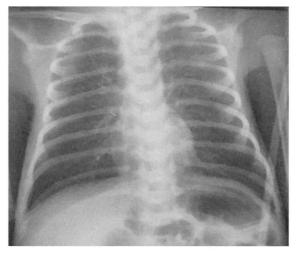

Fig. 1: Increased lung volume with diffuse haziness and interstitial opacities.

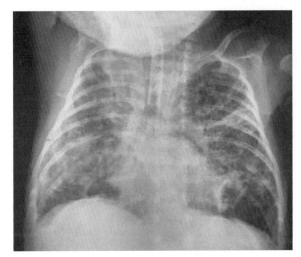

Fig. 2: Multiple areas of atelectasis and localized hyperinflation with fibrocystic changes.

Biomarkers	
Blood	*Characteristics*
Inflammatory markers	• Higher serum concentrations of IL-1β, IL-6, 8, 10, IFN-γ, and lower concentration of IL-17, RANTES, and TNF-β have been found to be associated with BPD/death in preterms
Angiogenic growth factors	• Low proangiogenic ANG-1 and high antiangiogenic endostatin in cord blood predict subsequent BPD • VEGF and PDGF BB significantly elevated on day 5 in neonates who developed BPD • High levels of PGF in cord blood predispose to BPD • Possibility of EMAP II in causation
Epithelial and fibrotic markers	• Elevated cord blood ratio of MMP-9:1 and KL-6 predict moderate-severe BPD • Conflicting evidence against levels of CCP (Clara cell proteins) in cord blood and serum
Tracheal aspirate/BAL	*Characteristics*
Inflammatory, fibrotic, and epithelial markers	• Increased IL-1β concentrations; IL-1β/IL-6 ratios increase risk for BPD • MCP-1, 2, 3 increased in neonates developing BPD • Neutrophil-gelatinase-associated lipocalin (NGAL) increased in infants developing BPD
Oxidant injury markers	• 3-chlorotyrosine and malondialdehyde correlate with BPD occurrence Higher levels of PUFA and plasmalogens are initially associated with a reduced risk of developing BPD, and their levels decrease with ventilation
Angiogenic growth factors	• Low levels of VEGF in tracheal aspirate fluid along with elevated soluble VEGF receptor 1 (VEGFR1) levels on day 1 of life, are biological markers for the BPD • Role of EMAP II is under investigation

Contd...

Contd...

Urine	Characteristics
Inflammatory and oxidative stress markers	• 8-hydroxydeoxyguanosine (8-OHdG) levels on day 7 independent risk factor for severe BPD • Leukotriene E4 levels on day 7 of life were higher than the values in classic BPD • High urinary concentrations of bombesin like peptide, associated with an increased BPD
Genomic biomarkers	Characteristics
GWAS (genome-wide association study)	• SPOCK2 as susceptibility gene, role not confirmed • Pathway analyzes confirmed involvement of CD44, phosphorus oxygen lyase activity, and indicated adenosine deaminase/miR-219 role
Respiratory microbiome	Characteristics
16S rRNA sequencing	• Reduced diversity of the microbiome may be an associated factor in the development of BPD

(ANG-1: angiopoietin 1; EMAP II: endothelial monocyte activating polypeptide II; PDGF BB: platelet derived growth factor BB; KL6: Krebs von den lungen 6; mir 219: microRNA-219; MMP9: matrix metallopeptidase 9; MCP 1, 2, 3: monocyte chemoattractant protein 1,2,3; PGF: proangiogenic growth factor; RANTES: regulated on activation, normal T cell expressed and secreted; TNF- β: tumor necrosis factor beta, VEGF: vascular endothelial growth factor, SPOCK2: SPARC/osteonectin, cwcv and kazal like domains proteoglycan 2)

DIFFERENTIAL DIAGNOSIS

Radiological findings of BPD can mimic certain diseases if the exact clinical course and ventilation history of neonate along with physical findings are not known. Some of the differentials include:

- Severe hyaline membrane disease (HMD)
- Congenital pulmonary lymphangiectasia
- Neonatal tuberculosis
- Cystic fibrosis.

MANAGEMENT

Management of established BPD is directed toward reducing further injury, providing optimal nutritional and developmental support for growth and recovery, and early detection, prevention, and treatment of associated complications. The following tables describe salient features of respiratory management, fluid administration and nutrition, diuretics, bronchodilators, corticosteroids, supportive care, and discharge planning.

Respiratory management:
- Gentle ventilation strategies using low tidal volumes (3–5 mL/kg), with optimal positive end expiratory pressure (PEEP) (5–7 cm H_2O). Volume targeted ventilation is preferred mode.
- Tolerating permissive hypercapnia $PaCO_2$ = 55–65 mm Hg (up to 70 mm Hg in patients with severe and chronic disease) with pH >7.25.
- Provide supplemental O_2 to maintain PaO_2 of 55–80 mm Hg avoiding both hypoxia and hyperoxia. Maintain target SpO_2 of 90–94%.
- Defer routine suctioning and perform calibrated suctioning up to premeasured endotracheal tube depth only when required.

Contd...

Contd…

- A planned weaning attempt to bring down pressure support followed by timely extubation to noninvasive ventilation is desirable. Continuous positive airway pressure (CPAP) and heated humidified high-flow nasal cannula (HHHFNC) are equivalent for post-extubation support, however, data for use in <28 weeks' neonates and those with evolving/established BPD is lacking. HHHFNC has the advantage of reduced nasal trauma and does not increase the risk of pneumothorax.
- Use of aseptic techniques while handling during invasive/noninvasive ventilation helps in avoiding nosocomial infections that can precipitate exacerbations and increase severity of BPD.

Fluid administration and nutrition:
- Minimal fluid restriction of 140–150 mL/kg per day, with target serum Na = 140–145 mEq/L and urine output = 1 mL/kg/hr is usually sufficient. In severely affected neonates with features of pulmonary edema/anasarca, fluid restriction to 110–120 mL/kg per day may be necessary.
- Providing energy of 120–150 kcal/kg/day and protein intake of 3.5–4 g/kg/day is needed for optimal growth of these neonates. In view of high energy requirement and fluid restricted states, fortification of feeds is often required.
- Routine monitoring and supplementation of calcium, phosphorus, and vitamin D depending upon osteopenia status of neonate is important.

Diuretics:
- In case of ventilator dependence with features of volume overload in form of pulmonary edema/excessive weight gain even after fluid restriction, diuretics can offer short-term benefits with no effect on long-term outcomes.
- Furosemide at IV doses of 1 mg/kg or oral 2 mg/kg/day can be used. Keeping a close watch and early management of electrolyte imbalances, hyponatremia and hypokalemia becomes mandatory.
- Thiazide diuretics—hydrochlorothiazide (2–4 mg/kg/day) or chlorothiazide (20–40 mg/kg/day) can be used to avoid furosemide induced toxicity.
- Combination of loop diuretics with spironolactone can help prevent electrolyte imbalances caused by furosemide and we prefer them if required for longer use.

Bronchodilators:
- Inhaled beta-2 agonists (e.g. salbutamol or levosalbutamol) may improve short-term function in case of acute exacerbation.
- Clinical response in form of improved SpO_2, decreased respiratory distress, and improved ventilation graphics can be observed.
- If beneficial, continue for a 48-hour period followed by weaning. If no response then discontinue use.
- Do not recommend for routine or chronic use because of lack of long-term efficacy and their adverse effects in form of tachycardia, hypertension, and arrhythmias.
- Nebulized ipratropium also has physiological advantage of improving pulmonary mechanics but studies for its efficacy are not available.

Corticosteroids:
- Though postnatal systemic corticosteroids (most studies have used dexamethasone) improve short-term pulmonary outcomes in neonates with established BPD, they are associated with serious short-term and long-term side effects.
- Therefore, risk–benefit ratio is not in favor of routine administration of postnatal steroids for either prevention or treatment of BPD.
- Though prophylactic hydrocortisone has shown promise of better survival without BPD, without an increase in adverse events, this approach unnecessarily exposes significant number of preterms to steroids and conclusive data are lacking to recommend this.

- Parental participation in decision making is essential with discussion about potential risks and benefits of use if steroid therapy is planned.
- Currently there is minimal evidence to support use of inhaled steroids for treatment of established BPD.

Contd…

Contd…

Supportive care:
- Developmentally supportive care and family integrated care must be provided to all neonates in view of higher incidence of neurodevelopmental abnormalities associated with BPD.
- Appropriate management of acute exacerbations and infectious episodes is crucial.
- Growth and developmental assessment should form part of routine management.
- Serial eye examinations for early detection and treatment of retinopathy of prematurity (ROP) are mandatory.
- Hearing evaluation by brainstem electric response audiometry (BERA) before 3 months corrected age must not be missed.

Discharge planning:
- Aim is to wean the supplemental oxygen and maintain stable respiratory status with adequate weight gain prior to discharge.
- However, some infants with prolonged oxygen dependency have to be discharged on home oxygen. Guidance with regard to oxygen delivery devices, pulse oximetry, and saturation targets, training for bag and mask ventilation, and liaising with pediatric specialist in proximity to patient's residence is essential.
- Appropriate training regarding cardiopulmonary resuscitation and suctioning along with advice for optimal nutrition and developmental stimulation, follow-up visual and hearing assessment must be given.
- Essential immunization pre- and post-discharge must be advised along with information for optional vaccination. Influenza and pneumococcal vaccination is recommended for BPD patients.
- Scheduled visits must be planned with multidisciplinary support.

COMPLICATIONS AND SEQUELAE

Acute	Subacute or late
• Acute exacerbations • Infections • Pulmonary air leaks • Electrolyte imbalance • Complications related to invasive and non-invasive ventilation—trauma to nasal septum, trachea, larynx, subglottic stenosis, vocal cord paresis • Early growth failure	• Pulmonary hypertension occurs in 1 out of 4–5 preterms with BPD, those with combined BPD and pulmonary arterial hypertension (PAH) have higher mortality • Systemic hypertension • Hearing loss • ROP • Nephrocalcinosis • Osteopenia • Gastroesophageal reflux • Growth failure • Asthma and recurrent respiratory illness requiring hospitalization • Neurological sequelae—higher rates of developmental delay and behavioral impairment • Mortality rate of 10–20% during infancy

PREVENTION

Intervention	Current status and evidence
Antenatal steroids	Decrease incidence and severity of RDS, however, did not decrease BPD incidence
Caffeine citrate	Strong recommendation for use of caffeine therapy and initiation of therapy soon after birth. As per systematic review, caffeine use is associated with reduction in BPD rates in preterm neonates and also has advantage if started early. We practice starting caffeine in preterm neonates born ≤32 weeks' gestation and having respiratory distress soon after birth requiring any form of respiratory support or having apneas

Contd…

Contd…

Intervention	Current status and evidence
Gentle ventilation and noninvasive ventilation	• Delivery room CPAP, early rescue surfactant by INSURE (INtubation SURfactant Extubation) or less invasive methods, avoiding intubation and positive pressure ventilation (PPV) • Gentle ventilation with permissive hypercapnia • Avoiding hyperoxia • Volume targeted ventilation • High frequency ventilation
Less invasive surfactant administration (LISA)	LISA technique reduced need for mechanical ventilation (MV) by 34%, BPD at 36 weeks by 27% and composite outcome of death/BPD at 36 weeks by 25%
Fluid restriction	Excessive fluid administration in first few days of life is associated with increased risk of left-to-right shunt across PDA and BPD. However, systematic review shows no effect of fluid restriction on BPD, mortality or duration of mechanical ventilation
Early selective surfactant	Given within first 30–60 minutes, reduces need for MV and O_2, however, did not decrease BPD incidence
Vitamin A	Weak recommendations for extremely low-birth weight (ELBW) neonates and difficulties of repeated IM injections
Postnatal steroids	• Routine use of early postnatal steroids is not recommended because of short-term and long-term side effects. A meta-regression analysis of trials has shown that only if the risk of BPD is >65%, postnatal steroids can potentially decrease the chance of death or cerebral palsy • As per recent meta-analysis, combination of early inhaled budesonide-surfactant in very low-birth weight (VLBW) neonates with RDS reduced BPD by 43% and composite outcome of death and BPD by 40%. However, a larger trial is needed for recommendations regarding its use • However, same effect on BPD has not been found with late inhalational steroids, i.e. ≥7 days
Azithromycin	Low quality evidence and not recommended for routine use
Investigational therapies	• Inhaled nitric oxide (iNO) • Surfactant and iNO combination • Antioxidants—melatonin, recombinant human Cu/Zn SOD, recombinant human CCP10, and catalase • Intratracheal mesenchymal stem cells (MSCs) transplantation—results of ongoing trials regarding safety and efficacy awaited • Docosahexaenoic acid (DHA)

KEY POINTS

➢ Bronchopulmonary dysplasia, also known as neonatal chronic lung disease, is one of the most common chronic respiratory morbidities of prematurity.

➢ Neonates who need supplemental oxygen for a cumulative duration of ≥28 days are said to have BPD.

➢ Risk factors include prematurity, poor ventilatory strategies, poor nutrition, and sepsis.

➢ "New BPD" encountered nowadays is characterized by arrest of alveolar septation during saccular phase of lung development in response to multitude of antenatal and postnatal factors.

➢ Management of established BPD is directed toward reducing further injury, providing optimal nutritional and developmental support for growth and recovery, and early detection, prevention, and treatment of associated complications.

SELF ASSESSMENT

1. **Which of the following is not a management strategy in management of BPD?**
   a. Gentle ventilation strategies using low tidal volumes (3–5 mL/kg), with optimal PEEP (5–7 cm H_2O). Volume targeted ventilation is preferred mode
   b. Tolerating permissive hypercapnia $PaCO_2$ = 55–65 mm Hg (up to 70 mm Hg in patients with severe and chronic disease) with pH >7.25
   c. Provide supplemental O_2 to maintain PaO_2 of 55–80 mm Hg avoiding both hypoxia and hyperoxia. Maintain target SpO_2 of 90–94%
   d. Routine endotracheal suctioning

2. **Which of the following is not an evidence-based strategy to prevent BPD?**
   a. Antenatal steroids
   b. Caffeine therapy
   c. Vitamin A supplementation
   d. LISA

FURTHER READING

1. Bancalari E, Claure N, Sosenko IR. Bronchopulmonary dysplasia: Changes in pathogenesis, epidemiology and definition. Semin Neonatol. 2003;8(1):63-71.
2. Jensen E, Foglia E, Schmidt B. Evidence-based pharmacologic therapies for prevention of bronchopulmonary dysplasia: Application of the grading of recommendations assessment, development, and evaluation methodology. Clin Perinatol. 2015;42(4):755-79.

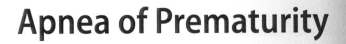

11

Chapter

Apnea of Prematurity

Swarna Rekha Bhat

INTRODUCTION

Apnea of prematurity is one of the most common problems encountered by sick preterm neonates. It could be primarily as a result of an immature nervous system or it could occur secondary to other neonatal problems such as sepsis, pneumonia, respiratory distress, etc.

DEFINITION AND CLASSIFICATION

Apnea or apneic episodes may be defined as cessation of respiration for a duration of 20 seconds with or without bradycardia and/or cyanosis or cessation of respiration for shorter periods with bradycardia and/or cyanosis. Apneic episodes may be classified as follows:

Type (incidence among all apneic episodes)	Pathology
Central (40%)	Cessation of respiration secondary to central nervous system (CNS) immaturity
Obstructive (10%)	Secondary to obstruction to airflow
Mixed (50%)	Combination of both

It can also be classified based on etiology as:

		Timing
Apnea of prematurity (AOP)	Occurring in preterm neonates primarily due to immature nervous system	2–7 days of postnatal life
Apnea occurring in preterm neonates	Occurs due to an underlying problem	Anytime during the first 28 days
Apnea occurring in term neonates	These are usually not apneic episodes but may be a manifestation of seizure activity or respiratory depression secondary to a CNS insult	

Periodic Breathing

Periodic breathing is a physiologic phenomenon occurring in preterm neonates and is characterized by brief periods of cessation of respiration, usually less than 10 seconds and not associated with cyanosis and bradycardia.

INCIDENCE

Apnea of prematurity is more common among neonates less than 35 weeks. Incidence among neonates <35 weeks will be around 10–20% and nearly 60–80% among neonates <28 weeks. Apnea of prematurity usually resolves around 37–40 weeks gestation.

PATHOGENESIS

Apnea of prematurity occurs as a result of physiologic immaturity of respiratory control by the central nervous system and decreased sensitivity of chemoreceptors.

Central apnea occurs due to:
- Respiratory irregularity is most frequently seen during rapid eye movement (REM) sleep and REM sleep is the predominant pattern in preterm neonates.
- Decrease in central chemosensitivity.
- Respiratory depression secondary to hypoxia.
- Decreased ventilator response to hypercapnia and hypoxia.
- Upregulation of inhibitory neurotransmitters like gamma-aminobutyric acid (GABA) and adenosine.
- Decrease in carotid body chemoreceptor sensitivity.

Obstructive apnea occurs due to:
- Upper airway block.
- Decreased laryngeal and pharyngeal reflexes, which help clearing airways and keeping upper airway open.

There may be a genetic predisposition as evidenced by:
- Presence of polymorphisms in A2A adenosine receptor gene in neonates with apnea of prematurity.
- *PHOX2B* gene mutation is seen in neonates with congenital central hypoventilation syndrome.

RISK FACTORS/SECONDARY CAUSES

In preterm neonates, the etiology is because of prematurity. However, both in term and preterm neonates, other risk factors can trigger episodes of apnea; these are listed in **Table 1**.

CLINICAL FEATURES

In a neonate who is not being monitored, apneic episodes manifest as cessation of respiration with or without cyanosis. If the apneic episode lasts for more than 30–45 seconds, there may be pallor (due to hypoxia), hypotonia, and eventually the neonate may become unresponsive.

In a neonate who is being monitored with a saturation monitor or apnea monitor, there may be bradycardia and desaturations.

INVESTIGATIONS

Investigations that are mentioned in **Table 1** may have to be done based on clinical suspicion. Baseline investigations would include blood sugar, serum electrolytes, hematocrit, blood counts, C-reactive protein (CRP), and blood culture.

Table 1: Risk factors and investigations.

Risk factors		Investigations
Temperature instability	Hypothermia Hyperthermia	
Metabolic	Hypoglycemia/hyperglycemia Hyponatremia/hypernatremia Hypocalcemia/hypercalcemia Hypomagnesemia Metabolic acidosis	Metabolic workup (Blood sugar, electrolytes, calcium, and magnesium blood gases)
Central nervous system	Perinatal asphyxia Intracranial bleed Seizures	Neuroimaging, EEG
Respiratory	Respiratory distress syndrome Pneumonia Pulmonary hemorrhage Airway obstruction	Chest X-ray, blood gases
Cardiovascular	Patent ductus arteriosus Hypotension/shock Cardiac failure	ECHO
Gastrointestinal	Gastroesophageal reflux Necrotizing enterocolitis	Abdominal X-ray, sepsis workup
Hematologic	Anemia Polycythemia	Hematocrit
Infections	Septicemia Meningitis	Sepsis screen, blood culture, CSF examination
Miscellaneous	Inborn errors of metabolism Improper posture resulting in airway obstruction	IEM workup

(ECHO: echocardiography; EEG: electroencephalogram; IEM: inborn errors of metabolism; CSF: cerebrospinal fluid)

MANAGEMENT

Monitoring

All neonates <35 weeks should be monitored in the first 7 days.

All sick preterm neonates should be monitored for longer periods.

Monitoring in preterm neonates, who have had apneic episodes, should continue for at least 5–7 days apnea-free period.

Method of Monitoring

Apnea monitors should be used if available. These will detect only central apneas. Most centers do not use apnea monitors because of their high false alarms.

Pulse oximeters and multisystem monitors will help pick up apneas if there is desaturation and bradycardia.

Recently Vergales et al. have demonstrated that computer-assisted detection of apneic episodes, utilizing data from monitors, is more effective than manual recording by nursing personnel.

TREATMENT

Immediate measures include:
- Stimulating the neonate
- Correcting any obvious problem (temperature instability, posture, and airway secretions)
- Administering oxygen if there is desaturation
- Positive pressure ventilation with bag and mask if apneic episode does not respond to stimulation.

Correct underlying problems:
- Antibiotics for sepsis
- Packed cell transfusion to maintain hematocrit >25
- Correction of metabolic abnormalities.

VENTILATION

Invasive ventilation is required only if the neonate does not have spontaneous respiration after initial measures.

Noninvasive ventilation is the treatment of choice. These include:
- Continuous positive airway pressure (CPAP)
- Nasal intermittent positive pressure ventilation (NIPPV)
- Heated humidified high flow nasal oxygen (HHHFNO)
- CPAP is the most frequent modality used.

Mode of Action

- Splints upper airway
- Increases oxygenation and functional residual capacity (FRC)
- Stimulates stretch receptors, which in turn stimulate breathing.
  Continuous positive airway pressure is started at 4–6 cm H_2O pressure, with FiO_2 as required to maintain saturations between 90% and 95%.
  It can be discontinued once there are no more episodes of apnea/desaturations for a period of 24–48 hours.

PHARMACOTHERAPY

Drugs used include:
- Aminophylline (not used because of adverse effects, narrow therapeutic index, and need to monitor drug levels).
- Caffeine **(Table 2)**.
- Doxapram (not used anymore because of adverse effects particularly related to benzyl alcohol, which is used as a preservative).

Table 2: Dose of caffeine.			
	Dose	*Base*	*Serum level*
Loading dose	20 mg/kg IV or PO	10 mg/kg	
Maintenance dose	5–8 mg/kg PO	2.5–5 mg/kg	5–20 µg/mL

Caffeine

Caffeine citrate is the drug of choice.

Mechanism of Action

- Respiratory stimulant
- Increases minute ventilation
- Improves CO_2 sensitivity
- Decreases hypoxic respiratory depression
- Increases diaphragmatic activity
- Decreases periodic breathing
- Acts as a bronchodilator.

Duration

Continue medications till 33–34 weeks or an apnea-free period of at least 5–7 days whichever is earlier [American Academy of Pediatrics (AAP) guidelines]. For babies <28 weeks gestation, a longer apnea-free period is recommended.

Adverse Effects

Adverse effects include tachycardia, feed intolerance, and mild diuretic effect. There are no long-term side effects of caffeine use, in fact caffeine for apnea of prematurity (CAP) trial by Schmidt et al. demonstrated better neurodevelopmental outcome at 18 months to 21 months, 5 years, and 11 years.

PREVENTION

Apneic episodes can be prevented by preventing prematurity and the risk factors such as hypoglycemia, anemia, etc.

The CAP trial by Schmidt et al. has demonstrated that using caffeine prophylactically for 10 days postnatal period in neonates with birth weight between 500 g and 1,250 g reduces incidence of bronchopulmonary dysplasia and improves survival without disability. Other retrospective studies have demonstrated both short-term and long-term benefits—decrease in apneic episodes, patent ductus arteriosus (PDA), bronchopulmonary dysplasia (BPD), and mortality. However, current evidence is insufficient to routinely recommend use of prophylactic caffeine therapy in preterm and very low birth weight (VLBW) neonates.

Long-term effects due to repeated episodes of hypoxia can be prevented by monitoring all at-risk neonates.

PROGNOSIS

Unrecognized episodes of apnea can be fatal. Repeated episodes can result in long-term neurodevelopmental sequelae and retinopathy of prematurity. Immediate and long-term prognosis is linked to the other associated problems.

KEY POINTS

➤ Apnea of prematurity primarily affects neonates <35 weeks of gestation warranting routine monitoring in these neonates.
➤ It is most commonly of mixed type.
➤ It could be primary because of lung maturity or secondary to sepsis, seizure, respiratory depression, genetic reasons, etc.
➤ Caffeine citrate is most commonly used pharmacotherapy with very less side effects and possible long-term neurodevelopment advantages.
➤ Mechanical ventilation (preferably noninvasive) may be required for refractory cases.

SELF ASSESSMENT

1. **Which of the following statements is false about apnea of prematurity?**
   a. Is defined by any cessation of breathing if associated with bradycardia and cyanosis/desaturations
   b. Usually occurs any time in first 28 days of life
   c. Incidence is around 80% in <28 weeks gestation
   d. Usually resolves by 37–40 weeks of gestation

2. **Which of the following statements is false about caffeine therapy?**
   a. In current day neonatology practice, it is the drug of choice for apnea of prematurity
   b. All neonates <35 weeks should be started on caffeine therapy on D1 of life and continued for 10 days at least
   c. Continue caffeine till 33–34 weeks or an apnea-free period of at least 5–7 days whichever is earlier
   d. Long-term trials have shown neurodevelopmental advantage to those preterm neonates who received caffeine therapy

FURTHER READING

1. Abdel-Hady H, Nasef N, Shabaan AE, et al. Caffeine therapy in preterm infants. World J Clin Pediatr. 2015;4(4):81-93.
2. Eichenwald EC; AAP Committee on Fetus and Newborn. Apnea of prematurity. Pediatrics. 2016;137(1):e20153757.
3. Schmidt B, Roberts RS, Davis P, et al.; Caffeine for Apnea of Prematurity Trial Group. Caffeine therapy for apnea of prematurity, N Engl J Med. 2006;354(20):2112-21.
4. Schmidt B, Roberts RS, Davis P, et al. Long-term effects of caffeine therapy for apnea of prematurity. N Engl J Med. 2007;357(19):1893-902.
5. Vergales BD, Paget-Brown AO, Lee H, et al. Accurate automated apnea analysis in preterm infants. Am J Perinatol. 2014;31(2):157-62.

12

Chapter

Approach to Suspected Congenital Heart Disease

Ranjan Kumar Pejaver, Maneesha PH, Susanta Kumar Badatya

INTRODUCTION

Approximately one-third of all major congenital anomalies are constituted by congenital heart disease (CHD) which have prevalence rates ranging from 9.3 per 1,000 live births in Asia, 8.2 per 1,000 live births in Europe to 8.2 per 1,000 live births in North America. Incidence and prevalence of CHD vary worldwide possibly due to differences in genetic and environmental factors.

The recurrence risk with a prior sibling who has a cardiovascular anomaly is between 1% and 4%. Improvement in diagnostic modalities and success of available treatment options has increased the survival of these children.

A proper approach and effective screening protocols are important to suspect, diagnose, and treat these potentially morbid conditions.

ETIOLOGY

Congenital heart diseases are proposed to be the result of multifactorial interactions between genetic predisposition and environmental factors. Both chromosomal disorders (Down's syndrome, 22q11 deletion syndrome, Trisomy 18, Trisomy 13) and single gene defects (Noonan's syndrome, Williams's syndrome) have been found in children with CHD. In addition to hereditary and genetic factors, teratogens have also been implicated in its causation. Teratogens may be drugs like valproate, lithium, paroxetine or infections (e.g. rubella) or metabolic conditions like diabetes mellitus and phenylketonuria.

CLASSIFICATION

Based upon levels of arterial oxygen saturation, newborns with heart diseases are classified as acyanotic and cyanotic heart diseases, former being more common. **Table 1** illustrates the categorization of CHDs by their pathophysiology.

CLINICAL PRESENTATION

As the CHD includes a wide number of anatomical and physiological cardiac abnormalities, clinical presentation may also vary. Manifestation can be grouped into four common modes of presentation:
1. Asymptomatic baby with murmur
2. Cyanosis

Table 1: Classification of congenital heart disease.

Type	Basic pathology	Examples
Cyanotic heart disease	Decreased pulmonary blood flow	Tetralogy of Fallot Tricuspid atresia
	Increased pulmonary blood flow	Transposition of great vessels (with VSD) Total anomalous pulmonary venous return
Acyanotic heart disease	Shunt lesions (left to right)	Ventricular septal defect Atrial septal defect Patent ductus arteriosus
	Obstructive lesions	Coarctation of aorta Aortic stenosis Pulmonary valve stenosis

(VSD: ventricular septal defect)

3. Circulatory collapse
4. Congestive cardiac failure.

Asymptomatic Baby with Murmur

On routine examination, as much as 80% of pediatric population can have a heart murmur. Not all murmurs are due to heart disease and not all newborns without a murmur are free of CHD. Timing of appearance of murmurs also depends upon the nature of lesion and pulmonary pressure. Small to moderate left to right shunts usually present with a murmur around age of 3–4 weeks when pulmonary pressures fall. Murmurs detected at birth or within 6 weeks of examinations should be sent for early pediatric cardiological evaluation.

Cyanosis

Cyanosis can be presenting feature in both cardiac and noncardiac causes and pulse oximetry will help in identifying central cyanosis. X-ray and clinical examination can point toward respiratory cause of cyanosis. Most common heart defects causing cyanosis in infancy include tetralogy of Fallot (TOF), pulmonary atresia, severe pulmonary stenosis, truncus arteriosus, transposition of great arteries and total anomalous pulmonary venous connection. Timing of presentation may range from birth itself to few days to few postnatal weeks depending on the presence of heart lesion and ductal closure.

Circulatory Collapse

Duct dependent systemic circulation such as coarctation of aorta, hypoplastic left heart syndrome, interrupted aortic arch, and critical aortic valve stenosis present as shock when duct closes decreasing perfusion to the whole or lower part of body. This manifests with insidious onset of poor feeding, lethargy, hypothermia, and blue episodes usually after 1–3 weeks of normalcy. CHD should be kept as a differential diagnosis in addition to inborn error of metabolism or late onset sepsis. Four limb BP and differential saturation can give important clue in these conditions.

Congestive Cardiac Failure

Neonates with cyanotic heart disease with high pulmonary flow, severe valvular regurgitant lesions, and significant shunt lesions like ventricular septal defect (VSD) and rhythm dysfunctions can cause ventricular dysfunction. The cardiac failure state presents as difficulty in feeding, increased duration to feed (>30 min), pallor, excessive sweating during feeding, respiratory distress, irritability during feeding, and failure to thrive.

Physical Examination

Clinical examination may show signs of impaired myocardial function and compromised tissue perfusion, signs of pulmonary congestion, and signs of systemic venous congestion as mentioned in **Table 2**.

Table 2: Approach to suspected cardiac disease.	
History	
Antenatal history	• Metabolic disorders (e.g. diabetes, phenylketonuria) • Exposure to teratogens (e.g. lithium, SSRI, anticonvulsants) • Exposure to prostaglandin synthetase inhibitors (e.g. ibuprofen, salicylic acid) • Rubella infection/TORCH infection • Autoimmune disease in the mother (e.g. systemic lupus erythematosus, Sjögren's syndrome) • Familial inherited disorders (e.g. Marfan and Noonan syndromes) • An obstetric ultrasound screening, findings of a prior fetal echocardiogram
Postnatal history	• Mode and difficulty of delivery, Apgar score • Time of onset of symptoms—shock, cyanosis, respiratory difficulty • Extracardiac abnormality
Family history	• History of consanguinity in parents • Early neonatal deaths • Family history or sibling with congenital heart disease
Clinical examination	
General examination	• Heart rate, rhythm, pulse volume—femoral pulse, edema • Four limb BP • Preductal and postductal saturation difference • Vascular collapse/shock—pale, mottled skin, cold extremities, prolonged capillary refill time (>3 s), increased skin—core temperature difference (>2°C)
Cardiovascular system examination	Signs of systemic venous congestion: Hepatomegaly (>3 cm or more) Signs of impaired myocardial function: • Gallop rhythm • Heart murmur • Cardiomegaly (clinical and radiographic) Signs of pulmonary congestion: • Tachypnea (respiratory rate of >60/min) • Subcostal or intercostal recession • Crepitations

Contd...

Contd...

Investigations	
Cardiac tests	Pulse oximetry screening Hyperoxia test, chest X-ray Electrocardiogram, echocardiography, and cardiac catheterization
Associated tests	Karyotype, USG cranium/MRI brain, USG KUB

(KUB: kidneys, ureters, bladder; MRI: magnetic resonance imaging; SSRI: selective serotonin reuptake inhibitor; USG: ultrasonography)

DIFFERENTIAL DIAGNOSIS

Aforementioned variable clinical presentation mimics many noncardiac conditions, which should be kept as a possibility while evaluating a suspected case of CHD.

- *Central cyanosis:*
  - *Respiratory disorders*—respiratory distress syndrome (RDS), pneumonia, pneumothorax, persistent pulmonary hypertension of the newborn (PPHN), and methemoglobinemia.
  - *Neurologic disorders*—central apnea and neuromuscular dysfunction.
- *Circulatory collapse:* Septic shock and inborn errors of metabolism.

INVESTIGATIONS

Whenever CHD is in differential diagnosis, investigations must be done to rule out and confirm diagnosis of CHD.

Screening Tests

Optimal care will ideally be feasible when CHD is detected antenatally or in neonatal period before it manifests clinically. This is possible by fetal echocardiography in antenatal period and universal pulse oximetry screening (POS) postnatally.

Fetal Echocardiography

Antenatal detection of major congenital heart defects like coarctation of aorta, transposition of great arteries, and hypoplastic left heart syndrome have significant impact on postnatal management and survival. Based on the type, the severity of heart defect and its prognosis, antenatal counseling could be done regarding management options, such as medical termination of pregnancy, planned delivery in a tertiary cardiac center.

Despite advancements in imaging, lesions like coarctation of aorta, interrupted aortic arch, aortic stenosis, and total anomalous pulmonary venous return (TAPVR) could well be missed by fetal screening. But a pooled sensitivity of 68.1% and a specificity of 99.9% seem to be reasonable for fetal echocardiography as a screening test.

Fetal echocardiography is indicated in presence of risk factors:

- Maternal risk factors—use of teratogenic drugs, mother with diabetes mellitus, phenylketonuria, and rubella infection.
- Fetal risk factors—Trisomy (21,18,13), Turner syndrome, and 22q11 deletion syndrome.
- Familial predisposition of genetic syndromes like Noonan, Marfan, and tuberous sclerosis.

Pulse Oximetry Screening

Pulse oximetry screening has been proved as a simple, quick, painless, cost-effective, and accurate screening tool to detect critical congenital heart defects in neonatal period. POS screen facilitates early detection of critical congenital heart disease (CCHD) by identifying those with low oxygen saturations. POS by American College of Cardiology and European Pulse Oximetry Screening Workgroup has set following recommendations for POS:

All-well infants and neonatal intensive care unit (NICU) infants must be screened for CCHD by pulse oximetry in the first week of life as outlined in **Flowchart 1**.

- Motion-tolerant pulse oximeters should be used to screen for CCHD with neonatal sensing probes.
- Screening age between 24 hours and 48 hours of life, or as late as possible if discharge prior to 24 hours of life is planned. European POS Workgroup has set screening time as earliest at or after 6 hours of life or before discharge from the birthing center.
- There must be two screening sites—(1) the right hand (preductal) and (2) one foot (post-ductal).

Flowchart 1: Pulse oximetry screening for critical congenital heart disease as per American Heart Association (AHA) recommendation.

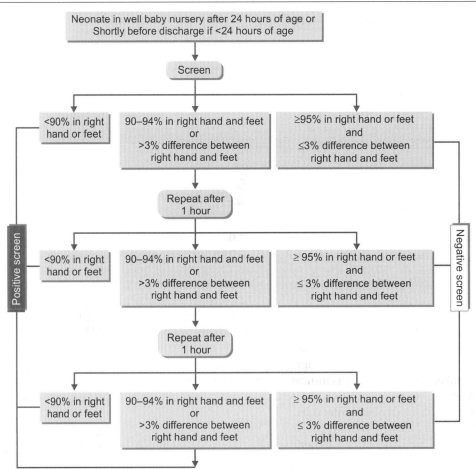

Babies who tested positive by POS must undergo detailed echocardiographic examination to identify any congenital heart defects as soon as possible. The major defects identified with POS include hypoplastic left heart syndrome, pulmonary atresia (with intact septum), TOF, TAPVR, transposition of the great vessels, tricuspid atresia, and truncus arteriosus which amounts to be about 17–31% of all CHD. These seven conditions require intervention soon after birth which is benefited by early diagnosis.

Diagnostic Tests

Echocardiography is the definitive investigation that gives quick information about the cardiac structure and its function. As majority of healthcare facility do not have the required equipment and trained personal, initial evaluation with chest X-ray, electrocardiogram (ECG) and blood gas analysis may help in narrowing down or ruling out certain group of cardiac lesions.

Pulse Oximetry

Pulse oximetry is indispensable in evaluation of a neonate presenting with cyanosis.

Blood Gas Analysis and Hyperoxia Test

When a neonate presents with cyanosis or resting saturations are less than 90%, hyperoxia test is used to differentiate mainly cardiac cause from respiratory cause of cyanosis. Principle of hyperoxia test lies in the fact that extra amount of oxygenation in the pulmonary circulation will not alter saturation in presence of right-to-left shunt in cyanotic heart disease whereas in case of a respiratory cause, it can be increased by increasing the inspired oxygen. Baseline preductal PaO_2 is recorded followed by oxygen administration by hood for 10 minutes. A repeat arterial blood gas (ABG) analysis is done after exposure to 100% FiO_2. PaO_2 is unlikely to rise above 200 mm Hg in presence of cardiac disease and reflects cyanosis to be respiratory in origin. In cardiac pathology, PaO_2 fails to rise beyond 150 mm Hg and termed as failed test. False failed test may be seen in PPHN and TAPVR.

Chest X-ray

This bedside test can comment upon the cardiac size and pulmonary vascularity, which can help in differentiating various cyanotic heart diseases. However, normal size does not exclude cardiac anomaly.

- *Cardiac size:* Cardiac size and cardiac contour are secondary to differential enlargement of chamber and great vessels can give an insight to specific cardiac anomaly. Massive cardiomegaly (Box shaped Heart) with oligemic lung field is seen in Ebstein's anomaly. Chest X-ray in transposition of great arteries shows classical egg on string appearance with narrow mediastinum due to anteroposterior relationship of aorta and pulmonary artery. Boot-shaped heart with upturned right ventricular apex, no cardiomegaly, and pulmonary oligemia indicate presence of TOF physiology. The typical figure of eight appearance (snowman sign) suggestive of supracardiac variety of TAPVR in older infants is usually not observed in neonatal period.
- *Vascularity:* Normal vasculature usually does not narrow down the differential. It represents state of unaltered pulmonary blood or pressures from either milder or earlier forms of

congenital heart defects or anomalies not affecting pulmonary circulation, e.g. simple valvular abnormalities of coarctation of the aorta. Increased pulmonary vasculature may result from increased blood flow or increased pulmonary venous pressure. Increased blood flow is seen in left-to-right shunts with increased right ventricular output, which is seen as enlarged and tortuous vessels extending up to at periphery. Left cardiac dysfunction or obstruction results in pulmonary venous congestion as interstitial edema. Oligemic lung field usually results from the underfilled pulmonary circulation secondary to right ventricular outflow obstruction with an associated right-to-left shunt. All other cyanotic heart diseases (pulmonary atresia, tricuspid atresia, and TOF) have decreased pulmonary vascularity and normal or only slightly increased heart size.

Electrocardiogram

Findings in an ECG can give information regarding the cardiac rhythm, QRS axis, and ventricular hypertrophy. Tricuspid atresia is likely to have a superior QRS axis while pulmonary atresia and TOF often have right axis deviation. Critical PS or pulmonary atresia with intact ventricular septum usually have axis in 0–90 quadrant whereas axis in TOF have axis 90–180.

Echocardiogram

The two-dimensional echocardiogram along with color Doppler remains the primary modality for anatomic details. The echocardiogram is operator dependent and may require prolonged study even by experience cardiologist. Advantages include noninvasive test, bedside availability, and ability to use for serial monitoring. Disadvantages include operator dependent test, poor window of examination in hyperinflated lung condition, and possibility of sick neonate becoming unstable during study.

Cardiac Catheterization

This invasive method helps in exploring cardiac anatomy and for assessing cardiac hemodynamic status where echocardiography fails to identify anatomy like in case of aorticopulmonary collaterals and coronary arteries. This can also be utilized for therapeutic intervention if required.

Evaluation of Additional Organ Systems

Genetics

Syndromic association is found in approximately 25% of CHD, so detailed search for any genetic syndrome should be done. This helps in prognostication. Karyotype should be done to look for chromosomal disorder when a syndrome is suspected.

Central Nervous System

Brain imaging should be done to look for cranial malformations in syndromic infants, hypoxic ischemic injury secondary to decompensated hemodynamics, to rule out intraventricular hemorrhage prior to systemic heparinization during extracorporeal membrane oxygenation (ECMO) or therapeutic intervention.

Renal

Renal ultrasound should be done as higher incidence of renal anomalies (hydronephrosis, ureteral duplication, and unilateral renal agenesis) has been seen in infants with CHD, such as in VACTERL association.

Approach to a child with suspected CHD: **Table 2** summarizes the basic outline for evaluation of child with suspected heart disease.

MANAGEMENT

Initial Stabilization

For babies presenting as circulatory failure or congestive cardiac failure, oxygenation, fluid management, and correction of metabolic acidosis should be done to stabilize the baby.

Prostaglandin E1

Prostaglandin infusion should be started to reopen the closed ductus arteriosus if there is sudden onset of severe cyanosis or shock. This is started at an initial dose of 0.01 µg/kg/min and titrated every 20 minutes up to 0.1–0.3 µg/kg/min if there is no improvement in saturations. Initial doses do not put infant on risk of apnea, but require pre-emptive ventilation and/or treatment with aminophylline prior to transport on prostaglandin or on reaching maximum infusion dose. Noncardiac pathology or obstructed TAPVR will not respond to prostaglandin therapy.

Interventional Catheterization

Cardiac catheterization-based emergency procedures like balloon atrial septostomy can be done by pediatric cardiologists to allow interatrial mixing to help improve the patients' condition prior to definitive surgery.

Surgery

Definitive or palliative surgery followed by definitive surgery can be offered in selective cases as outlined in **Table 3**, details of which are out of scope of this chapter.

Table 3: Interventions for congenital heart disease.	
Procedures	*Conditions*
Interventional catheterization Balloon dilatation	Pulmonic stenosis, aortic stenosis, and coarctation of the aorta
Balloon atrial septostomy	Transposition of the great arteries
Coil embolization	Pulmonary and coronary arteriovenous fistulae
Device closure	ASD, VSD, PDA
Arterial switch procedure	Transposition of the great arteries

Contd...

Contd…

Procedures	Conditions
Blalock-Taussig shunts	Pulmonary atresia Pulmonary stenosis Tricuspid atresia Tricuspid stenosis
Norwood procedure	Hypoplastic left heart syndrome

(ASD: atrial septal defect; PDA: patent ductus arteriosus; VSD: ventricular septal defect)

KEY POINTS

➢ Antenatal echocardiography and postnatal POS are the screening tools in detecting critical CHD, which helps in planning postnatal management.

➢ High index of suspicion and systematic approach are vital for early diagnosis of CHD.

➢ Nonspecific clinical presentation poses challenge to clinician to differentiate from other common neonatal conditions like sepsis, respiratory pathology, and metabolic disorders.

➢ Detailed history and methodical physical examination will help in narrowing down the differentials.

➢ Echocardiogram remains the gold standard noninvasive investigation but does not mandate to delay management in acute life-threatening situation.

➢ Prostaglandin infusion is the lifesaving intervention while waiting for a definitive diagnosis.

➢ Karyotype and/or specific genetic tests should be carefully considered.

SELF ASSESSMENT

1. **Which of the following situation will warrant immediate reference for an echocardiogram during routine POS?**
   a. Preductal saturation 95%
   b. Preductal saturation <90%

2. **What is the usual starting dose of prostaglandin E1 infusion?**
   a. 0.05–0.1 µg/kg/min
   b. 0.1–0.5 µg/kg/min
   c. 1–2 µg/kg/min
   d. 1–5 µg/kg/min

3. **Which of the following cardiac defects shows superior axis deviation?**
   a. Tetralogy of Fallot
   b. Transposition of great arteries
   c. Tricuspid atresia
   d. TAPVC

FURTHER READING

1. Chitra N, Vijayalakshmi IB. Fetal echocardiography for early detection of congenital heart diseases. J Echocardiogr. 2017;15(1):13-7.
2. Fahed AC, Roberts AE, Mital S, et al. Heart failure in congenital heart disease: A confluence of acquired and congenital. Heart Fail Clin. 2014;10(1):219-27.
3. Ferguson EC, Krishnamurthy R, Oldham SA. Classic imaging signs of congenital cardiovascular abnormalities. Radiographics. 2007;27(5):1323-34.
4. Kemper AR, Mahle WT, Martin GR, et al. Strategies for implementing screening for critical congenital heart disease. Pediatrics. 2011;128(5):e1259-67.
5. Liu H, Zhou J, Feng QL, et al. Fetal echocardiography for congenital heart disease diagnosis: A meta-analysis, power analysis and missing data analysis. Eur J Prev Cardiol. 2015;22(12): 1531-47.
6. Lynch TA, Abel DE. Teratogens and congenital heart disease. J Diagn Med Sonogr. 2015;31(5):301-5.
7. Pacileo G, Di Salvo G, Limongelli G, et al. Echocardiography in congenital heart disease: Usefulness, limits and new techniques. J Cardiovasc Med (Hagerstown). 2007;8(1):17-22.
8. Thangaratinam S, Brown K, Zamora J, et al. Pulse oximetry screening for critical congenital heart defects in asymptomatic newborn babies: A systematic review and meta-analysis. Lancet. 2012;379(9835):2459-64.
9. van der Linde D, Konings EE, Slager MA, et al. Birth prevalence of congenital heart disease worldwide: A systematic review and meta-analysis. J Am Coll Cardiol. 2011;58(21):2241-7.
10. Wren C, Richmond S, Donaldson L. Presentation of congenital heart disease in infancy: Implications for routine examination. Arch Dis Child Fetal Neonatal Ed. 1999;80(1):F49-53.

13

Chapter

Patent Ductus Arteriosus in Preterm Infants

Naveen Parkash Gupta, Sonalika Mehta

INTRODUCTION

- During fetal life, most of the pulmonary arterial blood is shunted right-to-left through the ductus arteriosus into the aorta.
- Functional closure of the ductus normally occurs soon after birth, but if the ductus remains patent when pulmonary vascular resistance falls, aortic blood then is shunted left-to-right into the pulmonary artery.
- In term infants, it normally constricts after birth and becomes functionally closed by 72 hours of age.
- Patent ductus arteriosus (PDA) is a major morbidity in preterm infants: <28 weeks and <1,000 g. It can have significant effects on myocardial function as well as systemic and pulmonary blood flows.
- Currently there is continued controversy regarding how to treat, when to treat, and whom to treat. In this review, we shall attempt to discuss these controversies and current trends in PDA management.

NATURAL COURSE OF DUCTUS

Gestation (weeks)	Closed on day 4 (%)	Closed on day 7 (%)	Closed at discharge (%)
Full term	100	100	100
≥29	90	98	100
27–28	20	36	NA
25–26	20	32	NA
24	8	13	NA

Weight (g)	Closed on day 4	Closed on day 7	Closed at discharge
1,000–1,500	35	67	94
<1,000	21	34	NA

From above table, we can infer that PDA is a problem especially in infants <29 weeks.

FACTORS CONTROLLING DUCTAL ARTERIOSUS CLOSURE

Factors which constrict ductal arteriosus	Factors which prevent ductal arteriosus closure
Increase in arterial oxygenation (PaO$_2$)	Hypoxia
Decrease in pulmonary pressures	Increased pulmonary pressure
Decrease in circulating PGE2	Increased sensitivity to vasodilating effects of PGE2
Decrease in PGE2 receptors	Fluid

(PGE2: prostaglandin E2)

WHAT IS HAPPENING WHEN DUCTUS IS HEMODYNAMICALLY SIGNIFICANT IN A PRETERM BABY? (FIG. 1)

- With significant left-to-right shunt through the ductus arteriosus, part of stroke volume of left ventricle (LV) is preferentially diverted through the ductus toward pulmonary artery (low resistance circulation) leading to pulmonary overperfusion and systemic hypoperfusion or systemic steal (less blood to gut, kidneys, and other organs).
- It leads to increased pulmonary venous return and more blood enters left atrium (LA) leading to increased left atrial diameter (same parameter that is ratio of LA to aorta is calculated in echocardiography to classify severity of left-to-right shunt).
- Eventually LV does more work since it is receiving large volume of blood leading to first increase in left ventricular output followed by left ventricular dilatation.

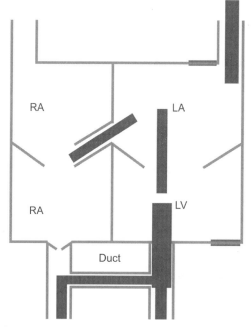

Fig. 1: Circulatory changes in hemodynamically significant patent ductus arteriosus.
(LA: left atrium; LV: left ventricle; RA: right atrium; RV: right ventricle)

PROBLEMS ASSOCIATED WITH PERSISTENT HEMODYNAMICALLY SIGNIFICANT PATENT DUCTUS ARTERIOSUS

- Cardiac failure
- Prolonged ventilator dependence
- Hypotension (usually beyond 48 hours of life)
- Pulmonary hemorrhage
- Periventricular leukomalacia, necrotizing enterocolitis, and abnormalities of cerebral perfusion.

How to Diagnose?

Hemodynamically significant patent ductus arteriosus (hsPDA) can be diagnosed clinically or echocardiographically. Echocardiographic signs precede the clinical signs by approximately 48 hours. Echocardiography remains gold standard to diagnose hsPDA.

Clinical Findings

- Bounding peripheral pulses (diagnosed clinically by easily palpable dorsalis pedis)
- Wide pulse pressure (>25 mm Hg)
- Decreased systolic and diastolic pressures
- Hyperactive precordium (visible precordial pulsations in more than 2 rib spaces)
- Loud systolic murmur (seen in 20–40%) usually ejection systolic; rarely pansystolic or continuous
- Persistent tachycardia
- In a ventilated infant—fluctuating FiO_2, increasing pressure requirements, unexplained CO_2 retention or metabolic acidosis, recurrent apnea suggests a symptomatic ductus.

Radiological Findings

- Cardiomegaly with apex of the heart pointing down suggesting LV dilatation.
- Cardiomegaly and pulmonary plethora in 30% of hsPDA.
- Elevation of left main stem bronchus from dilated LA (pancaking LA).
- Carinal angle >90° had 85% sensitivity and specificity for diagnosis of PDA.

TWO-DIMENSIONAL ECHOCARDIOGRAPHY WITH COLOR DOPPLER FLOW MAPPING (FIGS. 2A AND B)

Two-dimensional echocardiography with color flow Doppler is the gold standard for diagnosis.
- In all infants in whom treatment of PDA is considered, echocardiography before treatment is essential to establish the diagnosis as well as to rule out other structural heart disease.
- Post-treatment echocardiography is required to document the response to treatment and assess the ductus.
- It should not be used in isolation to decide on treatment, which should always be in conjunction with clinical symptoms.
- Short axis view:
  - Direct visualization of the ductus.
  - Classically described as "three-legged stool" appearance.

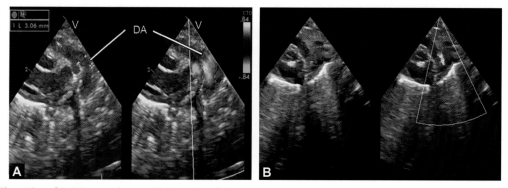

Figs. 2A and B: (A) Large ductus; (B) Constricted ductus.
(DA: ductus arteriosus)

- ◆ In color Doppler—continuous flare in the main pulmonary artery (MPA).
- ◆ Pulsed Doppler—turbulence in MPA due to left-to-right shunt jet flowing into MPA.
- Four chamber view:
  - ◆ Bowing of interatrial septum to right with enlarged LA and LV.
- Long axis view:
  - ◆ LA/Ao ratio >1.5:1.
  - ◆ Raised left ventricular stroke volume.

DEFINITION OF hsPDA ON ECHOCARDIOGRAPHY

- Left atrium to aortic root dimension ratio of more than 1.5:1.
- Ductal diameter of >1.5 mm.
- Reversal of forward blood flow in the descending aorta during diastole.
- End-diastolic flow velocity in the left pulmonary artery ≥0.20 m/s.

Proposed Staging System (Adapted from McNamara PJ, Sehgal A)

Clinical		Echocardiographic	
C1	Asymptomatic	E1	No evidence of ductal flow on Doppler
C2	Mild	E2	Small non-significant
	Oxygenation difficulty (OI <6)		Diameter <1.5 mm
	Need for nCPAP or mechanical ventilation		Restrictive continuous transductal flow (DA Vmax > 2 m/s)
	Feeding intolerance (>20% gastric aspirates)		LA:Ao < 1.5:1
	Radiologic evidence of increased pulmonary vascularity		Normal end organ (superior mesenteric artery, middle cerebral artery) diastolic flow
C3	Moderate	E3	Moderate hsPDA
	OI 7–14		Diameter 1.5–3 mm
	MAP 9–14		Nonrestrictive pulsatile transductal flow (DA Vmax < 2 m/s)
	Marked abdominal distension		LA:Ao 1.5–2:1

Contd...

Contd...

Clinical		Echocardiographic	
	Oliguria		Absent end diastolic flows in end organ vessels (superior mesenteric artery, middle cerebral artery)
	Systemic hypotension		
	Single cardiotropic agent		
	Mild metabolic acidosis (pH 7.1–7.25)		
C4	*Severe*	E4	*Severe hsPDA*
	OI >15		Diameter >3 mm
	MAP >12/High frequency ventilation		Nonrestrictive pulsatile transductal flow (DA Vmax <2 m/s)
	Profound or recurrent pulmonary hemorrhage		LA:Ao >2:1
	Necrotizing enterocolitis (NEC) like abdominal distension/tenderness		Reversal of end diastolic flows in end organ vessels (superior mesenteric artery, middle cerebral artery)
	>1 cardiotropic agent		
	Severe acidosis (pH < 7.1)		

MANAGEMENT OF hsPDA

There are basically four components of treating a hemodynamically significant ductus arteriosus **(Flowchart 1)**:
1. Medical management
2. Surgical management
3. Management strategies (timing)
4. Whether to treat or not.

Pharmacological Management

The pharmacological basis for medical therapy is the use of nonselective cyclooxygenase (COX) inhibitors, which inhibits prostaglandin synthesis and causes ductal constriction. Recent evidence in the use of nonselective COX inhibitor (peroxidase sites)—paracetamol, can be given orally or intravenously.

Drug	Dose	Comments	Side effects
Indomethacin (IV)	0.2 mg/kg IV followed by 0.1 mg/kg IV at 24, 48 hours	If duct remains open after third dose, continue with fourth and fifth doses of 0.1 mg/kg to be given 24 and 48 hours after third dose.	• Renal: Oliguria, rising creatinine • GI: Bleeding, perforation, NEC, electrolyte imbalance
Ibuprofen IV or enteral (standard dose)	10 mg/kg followed by 5 mg/kg/dose 24 hourly (total 20 mg/kg)	If the duct remains open after third dose, continue with fourth and fifth dose of 5 mg/kg to be given 24 and 48 hours after third dose	Oliguria, rising creatinine Higher serum bilirubin Bleeding less common

Contd...

Contd...

Drug	Dose	Comments	Side effects
Ibuprofen IV or enteral (high dose)	20 mg/kg followed by 10 mg/kg q 24 hourly (total 40 mg/kg)	If the duct remains open after third dose, continue with fourth and fifth dose of 5 mg/kg to be given 24 and 48 hours after third dose	Same as with standard dose of ibuprofen
Paracetamol (IV or oral)	15 mg/kg/dose q 6 hourly for total of 48–72 hours		Elevated liver enzymes

Flowchart 1: Algorithm for treatment of ductus.

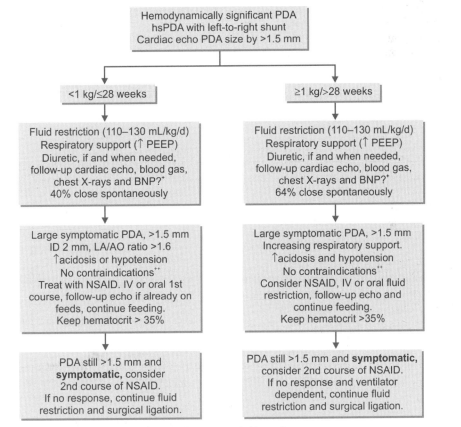

*BNP values vary considerably and not a reliable biomarker.
** Contraindications: NEC, thrombocytopenia (< 60,000 platelets), serum creatinine >1.6 mg/dL and rising >0.3 mg/dL in 24 h, and oliguria <1 mL/kg/h.

(PEEP: positive end expiratory pressure; BNP: brain natriuretic peptide; LA/AO: left atrial to aortic root; PDA: patent ductus arteriosus; NSAID: nonsteroidal anti-inflammatory drug; NEC: necrotizing enterocolitis)

Surgical Ligation

- It is reserved for infants with symptomatic hsPDA with failure of medical therapy or when medical therapy is contraindicated. Over the years, surgical closure of ductus has come down dramatically.
- Studies have also shown that in preterm infants <28 weeks, need for surgical ligation of PDA is an independent risk factor for increased rates of chronic lung disease (CLD), rate of retinopathy of prematurity (ROP), and adverse neurodevelopmental outcome.
- *Complications:* Severe hypotension (25%), unilateral vocal cord paralysis, and scoliosis.

Treatment Strategies

Treatment strategy	Explanation	Evidence
Prophylactic	Indomethacin IV on D1 in babies at risk of hsPDA without doing echocardiography	• Most extensively studied • Reduction in incidence of symptomatic PDA, surgical ligation, major periventricular-intraventricular hemorrhage (PVH), periventricular leucomalacia and pulmonary hemorrhage • No difference in late outcomes (late morbidity, mortality or neurosensory impairment) • *Concerns:* Unnecessary exposure in 30–40% of babies • *Conclusion:* Not advocated
Early targeted (based on echocardiographic findings)	Doing Echo in first 24 hours in babies <28 weeks gestation and treating ductus based on size (>1.5 mm) *Rationale:* Avoids unnecessary exposure which was associated with prophylaxis	• Meta-analysis of three small studies—reduction in symptomatic PDA, reduced duration of supplemental oxygen • Detect study demonstrated a significant reduction in pulmonary hemorrhage • *Conclusion:* Many of ductus might have closed if left untreated. Further studies are desirable which should take adequate end points (or primary outcome)
Early symptomatic (2–5 days) and late symptomatic (10–14 days) treatment	Treating ductus when there are clinical and echocardiographic signs of hemodynamically significant ductus	Although majority of neonatologists are treating ductus in this group, it has not been so well studied Needs further trials with proper end points
Supportive treatment	• Antenatal corticosteroids • Meticulous fluid management (Total fluids around 130 mL/kg/day in premmies from 4 days to 7 days) • Respiratory care [high positive end-expiratory pressure (PEEP)]	• Not evaluated well • However, recent trials have suggested that with modest fluid restriction, ductus may be well tolerated for 1–2 weeks without adverse outcome • Needs further studies

To Treat or Not to Treat

- Longstanding ductus is associated with various morbidities but evidence for long-term benefits of pharmacological closure of PDA is inconclusive and debatable.

- There is emerging school of thought advocating conservative approach.
- Medical therapy reserved for hemodynamically significant PDA with clinical symptoms attributed to large ductal shunt.
- Decision to treat depends on:
    - Rate of spontaneous closure (majority of babies >28 weeks do not need treatment in view of high rates of spontaneous closure).
    - Adverse effects of ductal patency.
    - Risk benefit of treatment.

KEY POINTS

- Patent ductus arteriosus is a major morbidity in preterm infants: <28 weeks and <1,000 g.
- It can have significant effects on myocardial function as well as systemic and pulmonary blood flows.
- Echocardiographic signs precede the clinical signs by approximately 48 hours. So, to diagnose ductus in early days, echocardiography is gold standard.
- Medical therapy is indicated in hemodynamically significant PDA with clinical symptoms attributed to large ductal shunt.
- Surgical ligation is reserved for infants with symptomatic hsPDA with failure of medical therapy or when medical therapy is contraindicated.
- There is emerging school of thought advocating conservative approach to PDA.

SELF ASSESSMENT

1. **Which of the following is not a clinical sign of hsPDA?**
   a. Bounding peripheral pulses (diagnosed clinically by easily palpable dorsalis pedis)
   b. Narrow pulse pressure
   c. Decreased systolic and diastolic pressures
   d. Hyperactive precordium (visible precordial pulsations in more than 2 rib spaces)

2. **Which of the following is not a parameter true to hsPDA?**
   a. Left atrium to aortic root dimension ratio of more than 1.5:1
   b. Ductal diameter of >1.5 mm
   c. Reversal of forward blood flow in the descending aorta during diastole
   d. End-diastolic flow velocity in the left pulmonary artery <0.20 m/s

FURTHER READING

1. de Waal K, Kluckow M. Functional echocardiography; from physiology to treatment. Early Hum Dev. 2010;86(3):149-54.
2. Evans N. Preterm patent ductus arteriosus: A continuing conundrum for the neonatologist? Semin Fetal Neonatal Med. 2015;20(4):272-7.

Neonatal Shock

Ashish Jain, Brajesh Jha

INTRODUCTION

Neonatal shock is a common entity encountered in neonatal intensive care, having a fatal outcome, if not managed immediately. The scope of this chapter is to cover briefly: (1) The unique pathophysiology associated with shock in newborns; (2) Conventional and newer modalities for hemodynamic monitoring in shock; and (3) A logical protocol to manage neonatal shock based on recent evidence.

DEFINITION

- Shock is a pathophysiologic state of inability of the circulatory system to meet the metabolic needs of the tissues for oxygen and nutrients and for removal of toxic metabolites. Shock is not synonymous with hypotension/fall in blood pressure (BP).
- Shock may be "compensated" or "uncompensated".
  - *Compensated shock*: This occurs early and is characterized by surge of the neuro-endocrine compensatory mechanisms which increase tissue oxygen extraction, leading to maintenance of BP in the normal range. The compensated phase may have signs such as tachycardia, prolonged capillary refill time (CRT), and decreased urine output.
  - *Uncompensated shock*: This occurs later and is characterized by a decrease in vital and nonvital organ perfusion evidenced by fall in BP and development of lactic acidosis.

INCIDENCE

While the true incidence is not known, a retrospective cohort study of 3,800 neonates admitted to the NICU over a 6-year period reported septic shock in 1.3% of admitted neonates with an associated mortality peaking at 71% for extremely low birth weight (ELBW) neonates <1,000 g.

TYPES AND PATHOPHYSIOLOGY

- Management of shock largely includes supportive care and specific management targeted toward the causation. Understanding the pathogenesis of shock and classifying **(Table 1)** helps in rationalizing the management of shock.

Table 1: Types and pathophysiology.

Type of shock	Important etiologies (In each category)	Mechanism for poor tissue perfusion
Hypovolemic	• Maternal abruption • Fetomaternal or fetoplacental hemorrhage • Tight nuchal cord • Necrotizing enterocolitis • Pulmonary hemorrhage • Subgaleal bleeding • Intracranial hemorrhage • Diarrhea	Inadequate blood volume
Cardiogenic	• Congenital heart disease • Heart failure • Arrhythmia • Cardiomyopathy • Postcardiac surgery • Postpatent ductus arteriosus (PDA) ligation	Defects of the pump
Distributive	• Sepsis • Endothelial injury	Abnormalities within the vascular beds
Obstructive	• Cardiac tamponade • Pneumothorax • High pulmonary vascular resistance restricting blood flow such as in pulmonary hypertension	Flow restriction

- Blood loss from the body, evident by dehydration and weight loss, leads to inadequate blood volume and hypovolemic shock. Blood volume from the intravascular compartment lost to the extravascular space (third space) within the body because of endothelial damage can lead to distributive shock. In distributive shock, there may be no evident weight loss or dehydration. Cardiogenic shock is the result of pump failure due to heart disease. When the heart is contracting well, but there is high afterload (either at the pulmonary or the aortic end), it can lead to decreased cardiac output and cause *obstructive shock*. Even though, each may be associated with specific etiologies, not uncommonly different type of shock may be caused by single etiology, e.g. neonatal sepsis.

DIAGNOSIS

- Shock cannot be recognized by a single parameter (e.g. BP). An individual finding has a very low sensitivity and specificity to recognize shock in neonates.
- Some of the clinical clues to shock are **(Table 2)**—lethargy/apnea/cyanosis, cold peripheries, pallor—without blood loss, CRT >3 sec [in very low birth weight (VLBW) infants, CRT may be normally prolonged up to 4 seconds and unreliable], tachycardia/bradycardia or increasing heart rate (HR) on serial monitoring.
- Invasive BP monitoring can offer continuous real time assessment of the cardiac output. However, lack of consensus definition of hypotension in neonates is a major hindrance to the use of BP as an adequate measure for such an assessment. Mean BP (MBP) value more than the gestational age in weeks is often considered adequate in the first few days of life. Below the MBP of 30 mm Hg, cerebral blood flow may be inadequate and this is considered to be critical.

Table 2: List of the parameters/signs used for assessment of neonatal shock.

Conventional parameters/signs (mostly clinical)	• Prolonged CRT • Cold peripheries • Decreased urine output • Heart rate (tachycardia or bradycardia) • Hypotension • Presence of lactic acidosis • Central venous pressure • Mixed venous saturation • Arteriovenous oxygen difference
Newer parameters now being used in clinical practice	• Functional echocardiography • Near infrared spectroscopy (rSO$_2$)
Naïve parameters that may have a role	• Perfusion index • Visible-light spectroscopy • Electrical-cardiometry • Functional cardiac MRI

(CRT: capillary refill time; MRI: magnetic resonance imaging)

■ Other invasive measurements like central venous pressure (CVP) monitoring, arterial blood gas (ABG) analysis, and arterial-venous oxygen difference are used in some sick babies to monitor the severity of shock.

FUNCTIONAL ECHOCARDIOGRAPHY

■ "Functional echocardiography (f-ECHO)" is now being increasingly used in intensive care setting. Studies have shown that clinical management may change in 30–60% cases in response to echocardiography. It can assist a treating neonatologist in evaluating the fluid status, cardiac function, cerebral blood flow, and presence of persistent pulmonary hypertension of newborn (PPHN)/patent ductus arteriosus (PDA). However, there are no head-on comparative studies looking at real outcomes with or without use of f-ECHO in management of neonatal shock.

■ Having an objective assessment of these parameters **(Table 3)** adds confidence, uniformity, and rationale to the management of shock. However, there remains concerns regarding significant intraobserver and interobserver variability in assessing many of these parameters and lack of normative data across different gestations.

MANAGEMENT

There cannot be a universally adapted protocol for the management of shock in all neonates. An optimal management requires an in-depth understanding of the underlying pathophysiology specific for the neonate being treated.

A scheme of stepwise approach is described below for easy understanding:

Step 1 (Early identification of shock): There should be serial measurement of the vitals in all the sick neonates for earliest identification of shock (e.g. serial HR monitoring and change in the HR).

Table 3: Some important cardiac function and echo parameters used in management of shock in neonates.

Hypovolemia	• Kissing small LV cavity • RV size • Normal or small RA
Fluid responsiveness	• >15% variation in left ventricular outflow tract velocity time integral (VTI) during inspiration and expiration • IVC collapsibility index >55% • IVC distensibility index exceeding 18%
LV function	• Decreased fractional shortening • Altered Doppler pattern of LV filling
RV function and pulmonary hypertension	• Increased pulmonary artery pressure • Bending of the interventricular septum to the left • Right to left shunt at foramen ovale and PDA
Systemic perfusion	• Decreased RV and LV output • Decreased SVC flows
Significant PDA	• Size of the duct (>1.5 mm at the point of maximum constriction is considered significant)/ (LA:Ao ratio over 1.4)

(IVC: inferior vena cava; LA:Ao: left atrium to aortic root; LV: left ventricle; RA: right atrium; RV: right ventricle; SVC: superior vena cava; PDA: patent ductus arteriosus)

Step 2 (Determine the cause of shock):
- A detailed history including that of antenatal period is important in identifying the setting of shock and rationalizing management. Some important settings are; preterm ELBW with shock in first 48 hours of life with increased systemic vascular resistance and poor cardiac output, birth asphyxia for asphyxiated cardiomyopathy, extreme prematurity for PDA, meconium aspiration syndrome for PPHN, and maternal chorioamnionitis in neonate presenting with features of early onset sepsis and shock.
- A detailed thorough physical examination should be undertaken. A duct-dependent lesion should be suspected in any newborn presenting with shock and hepatomegaly, cyanosis, a cardiac murmur or differential lower and upper extremities pressures or saturations. Inborn errors of metabolism resulting in hyperammonemia and hypoglycemia may also mimic septic shock.

Step 3 (Initiate supportive measures): This is the most important step in the management of shock and the outcome largely depends on how fast and optimal the supportive care is administered. This consists of:
- *Provide warmth*: Radiant warmer care in servo mode with regular monitoring of temperature.
- *Feeds*: The feeds of the baby should be withheld in acute stage of shock and a feeding tube should be inserted and kept open in case there is distension.
- *Maintain adequate gas exchange:* Provide supplemental oxygen. In case of poor respiratory efforts, the baby should be ventilated with minimal pressures to maintain saturation between 91% and 95%.
- *Establish reliable IV line:* An IV line should be established and the blood samples for blood counts/hematocrit/sepsis screen, blood sugar, blood culture, serum electrolytes, ABG,

blood grouping, and cross matching should be drawn. Placement of central line is always preferred. Intraosseous route particularly in preterm infants is not the preferred route for drug administration.

- *Order for chest X-ray*: Look for pneumonia/air leaks, cardiomegaly (C:T ratio >0.6)—heart disease, small heart—volume depletion, ground glass appearance—hyaline membrane disease (HMD) or obstructed total anomalous pulmonary venous connection (TAPVC).
- *Consider echocardiogram and Doppler study*: This will assist in determining high or low output state, contractility, superior vena cava (SVC) flow and other hemodynamics, apart from ruling out a duct-dependent congenital heart lesion.
- *Volume expansion*: Normal saline (NS) 10 mL/kg should be immediately infused over 30 minutes in preterm neonates (10 minutes if there is definitive evidence of fluid or blood loss). The response to the bolus, viz. reducing tachycardia, improving BP, CRT, and SpO$_2$ should be assessed. The close monitoring of the liver size is important. The boluses should not be repeated unless there is a strong evidence to suspect hypovolemia. A septic baby may need more of boluses.
- *Antibiotics*: Should be administered as early as possible when sepsis is suspected.

Step 4 (Measures dedicated to management of shock): All the efforts should be made to identify the severity and the pathogenesis of the shock. The objective should be to reverse the shock as soon as possible and prevent the fatality. The initial hours are the most important and aggressive monitoring and management should be undertaken.

- A central venous line (CVL) should be established to measure the CVP, especially if there is no improvement in shock after the bolus.
- Arterial line may be established for the measurement of the invasive BP, as the noninvasive blood pressure (NIBP) is not reliable in the sick neonate.
- The urine output should be monitored in all these babies. All the babies in shock should be preferably catheterized.
- The packed cell volume (PCV) in these babies should be maintained above 35%, to build up an adequate oxygen carrying capacity.

Step 5 (Initiation of appropriate inotropes): Second line of therapy after fluid bolus should be initiated promptly. One should understand the basic mechanism and receptor action of inotropes **(Table 4)** to get the desired results. Mechanism of action of these agents is complex and influenced by developmental maturation of receptors thus explaining different actions in neonates as compared to older children.

A brief review of common inotropes is given in **Box 1**.

The selection of the initial inotrope would depend on the most likely etiopathogenesis of the shock. When dopamine is used as the first-line drug in the setting of PPHN, its effect on the pulmonary vascular resistance should be considered. A combination of low dose of dopamine (<8 µg/kg/min) with the dobutamine in the dose of 10 µg/kg/min is initially recommended. If the baby does not respond to these interventions, then epinephrine (0.05–0.3 µg/kg/min) can be infused to restore the BP. A guideline to the choice of inotropes is given in **Table 5**.

Table 4: Receptor stimulated effect of vasopressor inotropes and lusitropes.

	Type of receptors (adrenergic, dopaminergic, vasopressin)					
	Receptors on vessels		Receptors on heart		Dopaminergic receptors	Vascular
	α1/α2	β1/β2	α1	β1/β2	DA1/DA2	V1a
Dopamine	++++	++	++	+++	++++	0
Dobutamine	+/0	++	++	++++	0	0
Epinephrine	++++	+++	++	++++	0	0
Norepinephrine	++++	0/+	++	++++	0	0
Vasopressin	0	0	0	0	0	++++

Milrinone is phosphodiesterase III inhibitor

Box 1: Most common used ionotropes.

Dopamine (Flowchart 1):
- Dopamine is most commonly used sympathomimetic agent in clinical practice. It is naturally synthesized and a precursor of epinephrine and norepinephrine. Effects are dose-dependent and vary in preterm babies as compared to older children and adults.
- *Dose:* In VLBW infant, start at dose of 2–5 µg/kg/min and titrate according to blood pressure. Do not use more than 20 µg/kg/min because it may increase afterload by intense vasoconstriction leading to decrease in cardiac output.
- *Side effects:* Tachycardia, hypertension, increased urinary sodium, phosphorus, and free water losses.

Dobutamine (Flowchart 2):
- Synthetic sympathomimetic amine. It does not rely on release of endogenous catecholamines for its positive inotropic actions in contrast to dopamine. It causes peripheral vasodilation via peripheral beta receptors, increase in myocardial contractility by stimulation of cardiac beta receptors, and the net effect is increase in cardiac output and systemic blood flow.
- *Dose:* Start at 10 µg/kg/min and titrate according to systemic blood flow. Maximum dose is 20 µg/kg/min.
- *Side effects:* Tachycardia, sometimes fall in blood pressure due to decreased diastolic pressure.

Epinephrine (Flowchart 3):
- Epinephrine is an endogenous catecholamine released from adrenal medulla in response to stress. It can be used in hypotension refractory to volume expansion and dopamine.
- *Dose:* 0.05 µg/kg/min–1 µg/kg/min have been tried in neonates.
- *Side effects:* Tachycardia, systemic hypertension, decreased systemic perfusion, and rise in lactate at higher doses owing to intense vasoconstriction.

Milrinone:
- Milrinone is phosphodiesterase 3 inhibitor and therefore increases intracellular cyclic adenosine monophosphate (cAMP) concentrations. It is an inodilator. It exerts its effect predominantly by lowering systemic vascular resistance (lusitrope) and increasing myocardial contractility (ionotrope). It may be useful in preterm babies who have diastolic dysfunction of heart owing to increased systemic vascular resistance on day 1 of life and low cardiac output syndrome (LCOS) in infants postsurgery.
- *Dose:* 50–75 µg/kg/hr over 30–60 minutes and then a continuous IV infusion of 30–45 µg/kg/hr.

Vasopressin:
- It exerts direct vasoconstrictive effect by acting on V1 receptors found on vascular smooth muscle thereby increasing blood pressure. It can be used as rescue therapy for hypotension refractory to dopamine, epinephrine, and hydrocortisone in the setting of warm septic shock.
- *Dose:* 0.02 units/kg/hr; increase as required to not more than 0.1 units/kg/hr.

Table 5: The different scenarios and the choice of inotropes.

Type of infant	Association	Action
ELBW (<24 hours)	Low SVC flow Large ductus High PVR Poor myocardial contractility	NS 10–20 mL/kg Dobutamine (10–20) to maintain SVC flow >40 mL/kg/min, RVO > 120 mL/kg/min Second line—add dopamine Third line—add adrenaline 0.05 µc/kg/min
Preterm infant	Low BP Low systemic VR Poor myocardial contractility	Dopamine (5–15) titrate to the BP Adrenaline add as second line Consider hydrocortisone in refractory shock
Asphyxia	Low SBF High PVR Poor myocardial contractility	Normal saline Dobutamine (as in case 1) Second line—dopamine or adrenaline
Sepsis (warm)	Low BP Low PVR + Fluid leak High SVF/RVO	Normal saline may need large volumes Dopamine (titrate to BP) Second line adrenaline (noradrenaline better)
Sepsis (cold)	Low BP Low SVC/RVO High PVR	Normal saline bolus Dobutamine Second line (low flow) adrenaline Second line (hypotension) dopamine or adrenaline
Infant with RDS	Pulmonary hypertension Low to normal BP High PVR	Dobutamine Second line adrenaline Consider milrinone

Source: David Osborn, Nick Evans and Martin Kusckow. Diagnosis and treatment of low systemic blood flow in preterm infants. Neoreviews. 2004;5;e109:5-3. doi: 10.1542/neo.5-3-e109.
(BP: blood pressure; ELBW: extremely low birth weight; NS: normal saline; RDS: respiratory distress syndrome; RVO: right ventricular output; PVR: pulmonary vascular resistance; SBF: systemic blood flow; SVC: superior vena cava; VR: vascular resistance)

Flowchart 1: Dopamine: Dose-dependent effect in neonates.

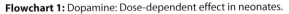

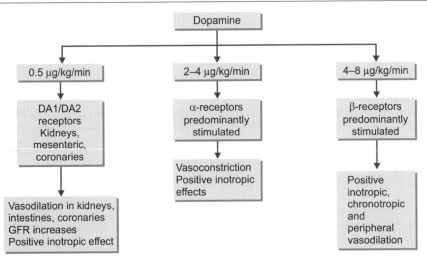

(GFR: glomerular filtration rate)
Source: Modified from Seri I. Management of hypotension and low systemic blood flow in the very low birth weight neonate during the first postnatal week. J Perinatol. 2006;26:S8-13.

Flowchart 2: Effect of dobutamine in neonates.

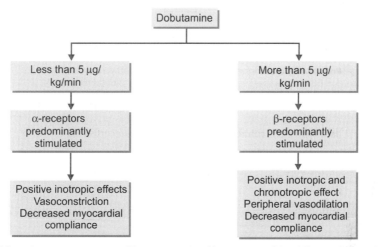

Source: Modified from Seri I. Management of hypotension and low systemic blood flow in the very low birth weight neonate during the first postnatal week. J Perinatol. 2006;26:S8-13.

Flowchart 3: Effect of epinephrine in neonates.

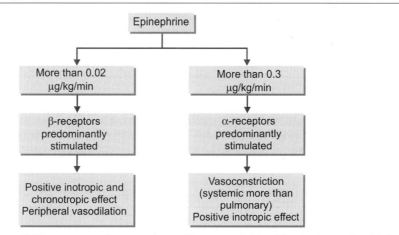

Source: Modified from Seri I. Management of hypotension and low systemic blood flow in the very low birth weight neonate during the first postnatal week. J Perinatol. 2006;26:S8-13.

GUIDELINES FOR MANAGEMENT OF NEONATAL SHOCK

The protocols for management of shock are described in **Flowcharts 4 and 5**.

Flowchart 4: Algorithm for treatment of shock in term infants.

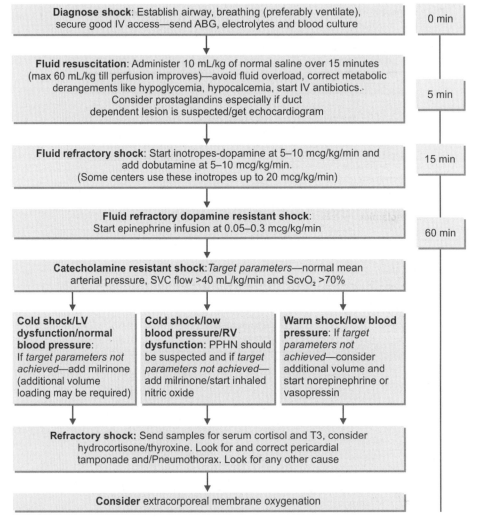

(IV: intravenous; ABG: arterial blood gas; SVC: superior vena cava; LV: left ventricle; RV: right ventricle; PPHN: persistent pulmonary hypertension of newborn)
Source: Modified from Wynn JL, Wong HR. Pathophysiology and treatment of septic shock in neonates. Clin Perinatol. 2010;37(2):439-79.

Flowchart 5: Algorithm for treatment of shock in preterm infants.

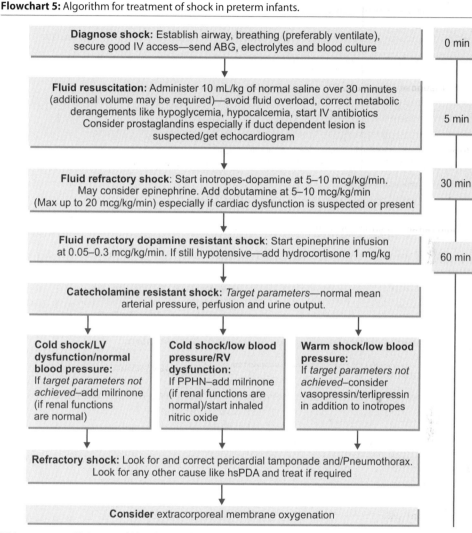

(IV: intravenous; ABG: arterial blood gas; LV: left ventricle; RV: right ventricle; hsPDA: hemodynamically significant PDA; PPHN: persistent pulmonary hypertension of newborn)
Source: Modified and printed in Wynn JL, Wong HR. Pathophysiology and treatment of septic shock in neonates. Clin Perinatol. 2010;37(2):439-79.

KEY POINTS

➢ Understanding etiology and pathophysiology of neonatal shock is most important step in managing babies with shock.
➢ Hypovolemia is very rare as cause of shock on first day of life unless there is history of blood loss.
➢ Dobutamine is preferred as first-line inotrope in first 48 hours of life in preterm VLBW babies presenting with shock.
➢ Dopamine and epinephrine remains inotrope of choice for septic shock.

SELF ASSESSMENT

1. **Which of the following parameter/s best define shock?**
   a. Increase in heart rate
   b. Low blood pressure for age
   c. Deranged capillary refill time
   d. Decrease in oxygen supply to tissues

2. **A preterm 28 weeks weighing 1 kg on D1 of life is having hypotension with deranged capillary refill time. You decide for intravascular volume expansion. Select the most appropriate choice:**
   a. Normal saline
   b. 5% albumin
   c. Ringer lactate
   d. Fresh frozen plasma

3. **What is the drug of choice in vasopressor resistant hypotension**
   a. Milrinone
   b. Vasopressin
   c. Norepinephrine
   d. Hydrocortisone

4. **First-line inotrope to be used in preterm very low birth weight baby with shock:**
   a. Milrinone
   b. Dobutamine
   c. Dopamine
   d. Epinephrine

FURTHER READING

1. Davis AL, Carcillo JA, Aneja RK, et al. American College of Critical Care Medicine Clinical Practice Parameters for Hemodynamic Support of Pediatric and Neonatal Septic Shock. Crit Care Med. 2017;45(6):1061-93.
2. Singh Y, Katheria AC, Vora F. Advances in diagnosis and management of hemodynamic instability in neonatal shock. Front Pediatr. 2018;6:2.
3. Subhedar NV, Shaw NJ. Dopamine versus dobutamine for hypotensive preterm infants. Cochrane Database Syst Rev. 2003;(3):CD001242.
4. Wynn JL, Wong HR. Pathophysiology and treatment of septic shock in neonates. Clin Perinatol. 2010;37(2):439-79.

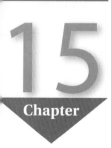

Necrotizing Enterocolitis

Anup Thakur

INTRODUCTION

Necrotizing enterocolitis (NEC) is a devastating gastrointestinal inflammatory process occurring predominantly although not exclusively in preterm infants, characterized by intestinal necrosis of variable extension that can lead to perforation **(Fig. 1)**, generalized peritonitis, and death.

INCIDENCE

- 1–3 per 1,000 live birth.
- About 5–10% in very low birth weight (VLBW) infants.
- Approximately 10% of all NEC occurs in term infants.

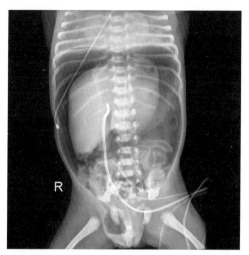

Fig. 1: Patient with perforation due to necrotizing enterocolitis.

IMPORTANT RISK FACTORS

Preterm infants	Late preterm and term infants
• Prematurity—inverse relation with gestation and birth weight • Birth weight—higher incidence in VLBW and extremely low birth weight (ELBW) infants • Formula feeding—increased risk as compared to human milk feeding • Absent/reverse end diastolic flow in umbilical artery—increases the risk by 2–3 folds • Red cell transfusion—increases risk by 3–4 folds • Patent ductus arteriosus (PDA), indomethacin, and steroid use • H_2 blocker use/sepsis	• Congenital heart disease • Polycythemia/Hyperviscosity • Severe perinatal asphyxia • Intrauterine growth restriction • Sepsis • Exchange transfusion

PATHOGENESIS

Current evidence suggests that NEC is a multifactorial disease with complex pathophysiological model. In brief, mucosal injury in the intestine and dysbiosis results in translocation of luminal organism across the epithelial barrier that leads to toll-like receptor (TLR) activation, triggering an exaggerated local and systemic inflammatory response mediated by cytokines and hosts of other inflammatory mediator. The detailed discussion is beyond the scope of this book.

CLINICAL FEATURES

The manifestations of NEC can be protean as summed up below:

Generalized	Respiratory	Cardiovascular	Gastrointestinal
• Temperature instability • Lethargy • Irritability • Generalized edema/capillary leak syndrome	• Desaturation/apnea • Oxygen/ventilatory requirement	• Bradycardia/tachycardia • Low blood pressure • Poor perfusion • Prolonged capillary refill time (CRT) • Weak pulses • Decreased urine output	• Abdominal distension • Emesis • Increased gastric residua • Billous/hemorrhagic aspirates • Diminished/absent bowel sounds • Increased abdominal girth • Abdominal erythema/discoloration of abdominal wall/abdominal tenderness • Right lower quadrant abdominal masses • Bloody stool

INVESTIGATIONS

• Laboratory parameters
  – Complete blood count—thrombocytopenia/anemia/leukopenia
  – Arterial blood gas (ABG)—metabolic acidosis
  – Electrolytes—hyponatremia
  – Biomarkers—see table further for biomarkers
• Blood culture and sensitivity for isolation of microorganism. Bloodstream infection may be present in 40–50% cases
• Abdominal X-ray and ultrasonography (USG)—refer to table further on imaging.

Contd...

Contd...

Radiological and ultrasound features of NEC	

Radiology:
- Ileus-distended loops of bowel filled with gas
- Thickening of bowel wall
- Pneumatosis intestinalis—pathognomonic of NEC, reflecting presence of gas within bowel wall
- Persistent fixed bowel loop for 24–36 hours—impending perforation
- Portal venous gas—occurs when gas becomes absorbed in the mesenteric circulation. Associated with severe disease
- Pneumoperitoneum—American football sign, with the appearance of a longitudinal strip of sutures from a football caused by the falciform ligament
- Ascites and a gas-less abdomen

Duke's abdominal assessment scale:
Score findings:
0. Normal gas pattern
1. Mild diffuse distension
2. Moderate distension or normal with bubbly lucencies likely corresponding to stool
3. Focal moderate distension
4. Separation or focal thickening of bowel loops
5. Featureless or multiple separated bowel loops
6. Possible pneumatosis with other abnormal findings
7. Fixed or persistent dilatation of bowel loops
8. Highly probable or definite pneumatosis
9. Portal venous gas
10. Pneumoperitoneum

Ultrasound:
Early stage:
- Thickening of bowel wall >2.6 mm
- Abnormal bowel wall echoic pattern
- Increased wall perfusion
- Initial signs of pneumatosis intestinalis (PI)—microbubbles inside bowel wall appearing as hyperechoic spots usually without posterior reverberation (X-ray will not show PI at this stage)

Intermediate stage:
- Extensive air bubbles in bowel wall as multiple hyperechoic spots some with circumferential pattern affecting one or more loops
- Portal pneumatosis—hyperechoic spots irregularly distributed in liver parenchyma often moving during examination
- Extraintestinal gas—small hyperechoic spots between liver and abdominal wall or between bowel loops—initial sign of perforation (may not be evident on X-ray)

Advanced NEC:
- Bowel wall ischemia and thinning—bowel wall thickness less than 1 mm and decreased vascularity to its disappearance
- Free fluids in between loops especially with internal echoes and septa

Biomarkers	
Nonspecific biomarkers	*Characteristics*
C-reactive protein	• Increases 12–24 hours after inflammation, low specificity
Serum amyloid A (SAA)	• It may increase 1,000 folds in 8–12 hours following inflammation • Mild correlation of levels with severity of NEC
Apo SAA	• Plasma level of SAA combined with apoprotein C II (Apo C2) • Early diagnosis of NEC and sepsis
IL-6, IL-8	• Early biomarkers for sepsis and NEC
Nonspecific biomarkers	*Characteristics*
Urinary intestinal fatty acid binding protein (I-FABP) and liver FABP	• Marker of cell wall integrity • Significantly raised in NEC • Significantly raised in patients with NEC who required surgery or died versus who did not
Trefoil factor 3	• Plasma levels increased in NEC

Contd...

Contd…

Nonspecific biomarkers	Characteristics
LIT score	• Combination of **L**iver FABP, **I**ntestinal fatty acid binding protein (I-FABP) and **T**refoil factor 3 • Improved sensitivity and specificity to diagnose surgical NEC
Claudin-3	• Tight junction protein indicating cell wall integrity • Elevated in NEC
Plasma inter-alpha inhibitor protein	• Regulates systemic inflammation • Lowered in NEC
Fecal calprotectin	• Calcium and zinc binding protein excreted in stool • Marker of intestinal inflammation • Raised in NEC and further raised in those with severe disease
Fecal Calgranulin C	• Pro-inflammatory molecule • Found useful in small studies but wide variation in results
Others—urinary fibrinogen peptides and fecal volatile organic compounds	• Require expensive tests and time consuming • No place currently in clinical practice

DIFFERENTIAL DIAGNOSIS

- Sepsis
- Ileus due to other causes like prematurity per se, electrolyte imbalance or infection
- Gastrointestinal (GI) anomalies like focal intestinal perforation, intestinal atresia, volvulus, and Hirschsprung disease
- Spontaneous intestinal perforation.

MANAGEMENT

Management depends on stage of NEC (Bell's staging, **Table 1**) and associated complications. The basic management is described below:

- Discontinue enteral feeds (duration depends on stage of NEC and clinician's assessment) and place a nasogastric tube for gut decompression.
- Continue parenteral nutrition.
- Central lines should be secured especially in sick infants.
- *Intravenous antibiotics*: Broad-spectrum antibiotic with anaerobic coverage such as Piperacillin tazobactam or Meropenem can be started. Depending on culture reports, antibiotics may be modified.
- *Mechanical ventilation:* Low threshold for intubation and mechanical ventilation for infants showing respiratory embarrassment.
- *Inotropes:* Infants with NEC often have massive third space losses and may require fluid boluses or increased maintenance fluid to maintain intravascular volume. Hemodynamically unstable infants may require inotropes to maintain blood pressure and perfusion.
- Obtain serial laboratories such as sodium, potassium, glucose, and periodic complete blood count (CBC). Frequent abdominal imaging may be required to assess disease progression and detect perforation. Manage fluid, electrolyte balance, and glucose homeostasis.

Table 1: Bell's staging for necrotizing enterocolitis.

Stage	Systemic signs	Intestinal signs	Radiologic signs	Treatment
IA—suspected NEC	Temperature instability, apnea, bradycardia, lethargy	Elevated pregavage residuals, mild abdominal distension, emesis, guaiac-positive stool	Normal or intestinal dilation, mild ileus	NPO, antibacterials for 3 days
IB—suspected NEC	Same as IA	Same as above plus bright red blood in stool	Same as IA	Same as above
IIA—definite NEC (mildly ill)	Same as IA	IA and IB signs plus absent bowel sounds. Patient also may have abdominal tenderness	Intestinal dilation, ileus, pneumatosis intestinalis	NPO, antibacterials for 7–10 days
IIB—definite NEC (moderately ill)	Same as IA plus mild metabolic acidosis and mild thrombocytopenia	IA, IB, and IIA signs. Patient also may have abdominal cellulitis or right lower quadrant mass	Same as IIA plus portal vein gas. Patient also may have ascites	NPO, antibacterials for 10–14 days
IIIA—advanced NEC (severely ill— bowel intact)	Same as IIB plus hypotension, bradycardia, respiratory acidosis, metabolic acidosis, disseminated intravascular coagulation, and neutropenia	IA, IB, IIA, IIB signs plus peritonitis, marked abdominal tenderness and distension	Same as IIB plus definite ascites	NPO, antibacterials for 10–14 days, fluid resuscitation, inotropic support, ventilator therapy, paracentesis
IIIB—advanced NEC (severely ill—bowel perforation)	Sam as IIIA	Same as IIIA	Same as IIB plus pneumoperitoneum	Same as IIA plus surgery

(NEC: necrotizing enterocolitis; NPO: nil by mouth)

- Packed cells, platelets or fresh frozen plasma (FFP) transfusion may be required in infants who are bleeding or have disseminated intravascular coagulation (DIC).
- *Surgery:* Involve pediatric surgeon in decision making. Pneumoperitoneum is an absolute indication for laparotomy. Clinical signs indicating intestinal necrosis, such as tender ecchymotic abdomen, persistent dilated loop on serial X-rays or rapidly deteriorating clinical status, refractory thrombocytopenia, metabolic acidosis, hyponatremia, and shock may require prompt operative exploration. Surgery usually consists of removal of necrotic bowel and proximal diversion with an enterostomy. Reports on primary peritoneal drain (PPD) versus laparotomy are conflicting. PPD alone is associated with higher mortality compared to laparotomy (OR 5–6) and neurodevelopmental impairment.

COMPLICATIONS AND SEQUELAE

Acute	Subacute or late
• Fulminant sepsis • Refractory shock • Multiorgan dysfunction • Disseminated intravascular coagulation • Mortality—20–50%	• Recurrent NEC—5% • Intestinal strictures/adhesions 10–35% • Short bowel syndrome—10% • Dysmotility, malabsorption, and cholestasis • Growth retardation • Neurological sequelae—psychomotor retardation, cerebral palsy, microcephaly, visual, hearing, and cognitive impairment. In ELBW infants, surgical NEC and medical NEC are associated with almost 40% and 25% chances of severe neurodevelopmental disability, respectively

PREVENTION OF NECROTIZING ENTEROCOLITIS

Intervention	Current status and evidence
Antenatal steroids	Decreases risk of NEC
Human milk	Strong evidence—mother's own milk as well as donor human milk beneficial
Minimal enteral feeds	• Lesser time to reach full enteral feeds • Shorter hospital stay • No effect on NEC
Delayed initiation of feeds or slow advancement	Does not prevent NEC
Standardized feeding regime	Significant reduction in NEC
Probiotics supplementation	• Meta-analysis shows decreased risk of severe NEC and death • Recent large RCT-PIPS trial showed no benefit in reduction of NEC
Prebiotics	Promising results in preclinical trials—large clinical trials awaited
Oral lactoferrin	Insufficient data in prevention of NEC
Oral immunoglobulins	Insufficient data in prevention of NEC
Enteral antibiotics	Reduction in NEC and NEC-related deaths but concerns over antimicrobial resistance
L-arginine and glutamine	Insufficient data in prevention of NEC
Recombinant cytokines and epidermal growth factor	Biological plausibility and advantageous in preclinical studies

KEY POINTS

➤ Necrotizing enterocolitis is a gastrointestinal emergency in neonates and has high morbidity and mortality.
➤ The management is mainly supportive with appropriate surgical intervention when indicated.
➤ Adequate follow-up is required to detect and manage its complications, sequelae, and optimize neurodevelopmental outcomes.

1. **Which of the following is not a risk factor for NEC in preterm infant?**
   a. Absent/reverse end diastolic flow in umbilical artery
   b. Red cell transfusion
   c. Antenatal steroids
   d. H_2 blocker use/sepsis

2. **Which of the following does not prevent NEC?**
   a. Standardized feeding protocol
   b. Human milk feeding
   c. Probiotics
   d. Minimal enteral feeds

FURTHER READING

1. Esposito F, Mamone R, Di Serafino M, et al. Diagnostic imaging features of necrotizing enterocolitis: a narrative review. Quant Imaging Med Surg. 2017;7(3):336-44.
2. Markiet K, Szymanska-Dubowik A, Janczewska I, et al. Agreement and reproducibility of radiological signs in NEC using The Duke Abdominal Assessment Scale (DAAS). Pediatr Surg Int. 2017;33(3):335-40.

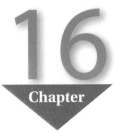

16 Neonatal Unconjugated Hyperbilirubinemia

Chapter

Sanjiv B Amin

INTRODUCTION

- Unconjugated hyperbilirubinemia (UHB or jaundice) is a common neonatal condition requiring monitoring, evaluation, and treatment (if required) during the first few weeks after birth to prevent severe jaundice.
- Kernicterus (bilirubin encephalopathy), a severe life-long neurologically debilitating condition characterized by hearing disorders, cerebral palsy, upward gaze palsy, language delay, etc. is a preventable condition.
- Therefore, it is essential to monitor premature and term infants for UHB and implement appropriate therapy in a timely manner.

INCIDENCE

- One in two infants develops UHB or jaundice.
- Prevalence of severe jaundice or UHB varies depending on the characteristics of the population and compliance with timely follow-up and evaluation.
- The prevalence of severe jaundice is low in most developed countries; however, the prevalence is relatively high in countries with high prevalence of hemolytic jaundice and inadequate follow-up.

PATHOPHYSIOLOGY OF UNCONJUGATED HYPERBILIRUBINEMIA

- Bilirubin is produced from the catabolism of heme, which is present in hemoglobin, myoglobin, and other hemoproteins such as cytochromes and catalase.
- Although hemoglobin is the primary source, other sources may account up to 20% of the bilirubin load, specifically in preterms.

Unconjugated hyperbilirubinemia is common in neonates because of the reasons as described in **Box 1**.

Boxes 2 to 5 discuss briefly the differentiation of unconjugated or conjugated hyperbilirubinemia, course of UHB in term and premature neonates, etiology of UHB and underlying mechanism, and clinical evaluation.

Box 1: Reasons for increased risk of unconjugated hyperbilirubinemia in neonates.

- Increased bilirubin production:
  - Increased red blood cell (RBC) volume
  - Decreased RBC survival (80 days versus 120 days in adults)
  - Ineffective erythropoiesis—cessation of hematopoiesis
- Decreased hepatic uptake
  - Decreased transporters, ligandin
- Decreased bilirubin conjugation
  - Decreased uridine diphosphoglucuronate glucuronosyl transferase activity for first few days
- Increased enterohepatic circulation
  - In very premature infants, this may account up to 25% of bilirubin load

Box 2: Differentiation of unconjugated or conjugated hyperbilirubinemia.

- Hyperbilirubinemia is classified based on the relative proportions of bilirubin forms in the blood:
  - Unconjugated bilirubin not bound to albumin (also called free unconjugated bilirubin)
  - Unconjugated bilirubin bound to albumin
  - Free conjugated bilirubin
  - Conjugated bilirubin bound to albumin
- The biochemical assays commonly used to measure and differentiate between forms of bilirubin use are—a direct reaction to detect free conjugated bilirubin (but not conjugated bilirubin bound to albumin), while the indirect reaction reflects unconjugated bilirubin (bound or free)
- Unconjugated hyperbilirubinemia is defined as an indirect serum bilirubin concentration of greater than or equal to 2 mg/dL.

Box 3: Course of unconjugated hyperbilirubinemia (UHB) in term and premature neonates.

- Normal course of UHB
  - Term neonates:
    » UHB peaks on days 2–5 of life
    » Peak total serum bilirubin (TSB) of 10–12 mg/dL among Asians; 6 mg/dL among non-Asians
    » UHB then decreases over the next few weeks to levels <2 mg/dL
  - Preterm neonates:
    » UHB peaks on days 2–5
    » Peak TSB unknown because usually treatment initiated at lower level of TSB than term neonates
    » Duration often prolonged and may need recurrent intervention for rebound jaundice
- Abnormal course of UHB:
  - UHB occurring within the first 24 hours of life
  - UHB is exaggerated (TSB > 12 mg/dL)
  - UHB beyond 14 days in late preterm and term infants

LABORATORY EVALUATION

- All premature infants should have total serum bilirubin (TSB) measured during the first week until the resolution of UHB.
- All infants ≥35 weeks gestational age (GA) with clinical jaundice should have transcutaneous bilirubin (TcB) and/or TSB and fractionated bilirubin concentrations measured.

Box 4: Etiology of unconjugated hyperbilirubinemia (UHB) and underlying mechanism.

Increased bilirubin production:
- Hemolytic diseases:
    - Red cell membrane defects
        » Hereditary spherocytosis
        » Hereditary elliptocytosis
        » Hereditary stomatocytosis
    - Red cell enzyme defects:
        » Glucose 6-phosphate dehydrogenase deficiency
           (Exposure to fava beans, sulfa drugs, or naphthalene in mothballs)
        » Pyruvate kinase deficiency
    - Hemoglobinopathies:
        » α thalassemia
        » β thalassemia
- Hemolysis due to external factors such as blood group incompatibility:
    - ~30% with ABO incompatibility have a positive direct Coombs test
    - ~20% with ABO incompatibility develop moderate to severe UHB
- Increased red cell mass—polycythemia
- Extravascular collection of blood:
    - Cephalohematoma, extensive bruising
    - Internal hemorrhages such as intracranial bleed, pulmonary hemorrhage, etc.

Decreased hepatic bilirubin clearance:
- Genetic diseases
    - Crigler-Najjar syndrome type 1 and 2
    - Gilbert syndrome
- Metabolic diseases
    - Hypothyroidism
    - Hypopituitarism

Increased enterohepatic circulation:
- Breast feeding and breast milk jaundice
- Breast feeding jaundice is seen during first week in primiparous mothers, with c-section deliveries, and in late preterms
- Structural obstruction in the gastrointestinal tract such as atresia, pyloric stenosis, Hirschsprung disease

- For ≥35 weeks GA infants, TSB should be plotted on an American Academy of Pediatrics (AAP) hourly nomogram to predict probability of developing severe UHB and the need for intervention (AAP, 2004).
- Determine the underlying cause for UHB and rule out hemolysis as shown in **Flowchart 1**.
- If hemolysis is unexplained by blood group incompatibility, investigate for G6PD deficiency, etc.
- Rate of rise in TSB of >0.5 mg/dL/hr (>0.25 mg/dL/hr in premature infants), umbilical cord TSB >5 mg/dL, or increase in TSB despite phototherapy indicates hemolysis.
- Serum albumin is measured to evaluate bilirubin-binding capacity if infant requires phototherapy.
- Risk factors that increase the risk of neurotoxicity such as acidosis, hypoxia, hypothermia, and sepsis should be evaluated if applicable.

Management of Unconjugated Hyperbilirubinemia

Management of UHB depends on level of serum bilirubin and presence or absence of risk factors for neurotoxicity. It should be based on standard guidelines as indicated in **Box 6**.

Box 5: Clinical evaluation.

History: Factors associated with an increased risk of UHB and neurotoxicity—
- *Gestational age:* Premature infants are at higher risk of jaundice and related complications
- Blood group of the mother, if known, to rule out hemolytic jaundice
- Any symptoms suggestive of intrauterine infections such as maternal fever, rash, or foul-smelling discharge
- Perinatal complications such as a difficult delivery and/or birth trauma—cephalohematoma, caput, extensive bruising, intracranial hemorrhage are associated with increased risk of jaundice
- Use of oxytocin during labor
- Any family history of jaundice, gallstones, genetic diseases in the family; certain hemolytic jaundice such as G6PD and hereditary spherocytosis are hereditary disorders
- Any history of neonatal jaundice in the siblings and whether that required intervention
- *Race and ethnicity:* G6PD deficiency is more common among Asians than Caucasians
- *Gender of the child:* Male gender carries increased risk
- Breast milk carries a higher chance of jaundice than formula feed

Physical examination: To formulate a differential diagnosis and management—
- Extent of clinical jaundice on skin (generalized jaundice is suggestive of TSB >12 mg/dL)
- Pallor secondary to hemolysis; cephalohematoma; bruising
- Hepatosplenomegaly for hemolytic anemia
- Signs of sepsis—temperature instability, lethargy, poor feeding. Sepsis increases the risk of bilirubin-induced toxicity
- Any signs of dehydration—lethargy, significant weight loss (more than 10% of birth weight), dry mucous membranes, decreased urine output, poor capillary refill, sunken eyes and fontanelle, and poor skin turgor
- Any signs of bilirubin encephalopathy—altered tone, opisthotonos (extreme extension of the body with spasm), lethargy, apnea, fever, poor feeding, high-pitched or shrill cry, and/or seizure

Screening transcutaneous bilirubinometry: Used as a screening tool to estimate TSB in late preterm and term neonates not exposed to phototherapy. Obtain TSB if transcutaneous bilirubin (TcB) ≥75th percentile on the AAP nomogram or TcB ≥13 mg/dL

(TSB: total serum bilirubin; UHB: unconjugated hyperbilirubinemia)

Flowchart 1: Laboratory evaluation.

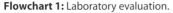

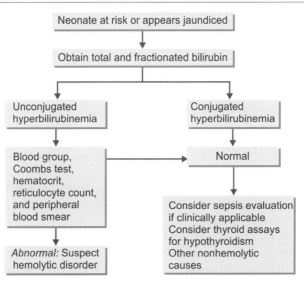

Box 6: Management of unconjugated hyperbilirubinemia (UHB).

Follow American Academy of Pediatrics (AAP) and/or Institutional guidelines for the Management of UHB

Phototherapy
Mechanism of action:
- *Geometric isomerization:* Native bilirubin (4Z 15Z bilirubin) is converted to 4Z 15E and 4E 15Z isomers for rapid excretion. This is a reversible process and the geometric isomers can be reconverted back into native bilirubin
- *Structural isomerization:* Exposure to phototherapy irreversibly changes bilirubin structurally to a compound called lumirubin which is excreted rapidly in the bile without conjugation

Factors influencing effectiveness:
- *Intensity of the phototherapy:* Intensive phototherapy provides irradiance of 30 µ watt/square cm. LED lights provide higher intensity
- *Distance of the phototherapy lights:* The lesser the distance of the infant from the photo lights, the more effective is phototherapy. The distance can be as close as 10–15 cm. When using non-LED phototherapy, monitor temperature of the infant. To facilitate intensive phototherapy, place white linen or aluminum foil in the side walls of the bassinet to reflect the light back on the infant
- *The amount of the surface area exposed:* Use of a Biliblanket underneath the infant may be required to increase the surface area exposed

Exchange transfusion: Exchange transfusion is associated with many complications such as acid-base imbalance, electrolyte imbalance, clotting factor deficiencies, volume overload, death, etc. and therefore, it should be performed with utmost care and by experienced personnel only

Indications:
- When total serum bilirubin (TSB) crosses the threshold for exchange transfusion as per AAP guidelines
- If the infant demonstrates any signs of acute bilirubin encephalopathy, even if the TSB is falling

Intravenous immunoglobins (IV IgG)
Block the site of attachment of the antibodies and thus prevent the antigen-antibody reaction and resultant hemolysis from Rh or ABO incompatibility

Indications for ABO or Rh incompatibility:
- TSB levels continue to rise at a rapid rate despite intensive phototherapy
- TSB within 2–3 mg/dL of the TSB level when exchange transfusion is indicated

Phenobarbitone: Increases the conjugation of bilirubin by stimulating the hepatic enzymes and may be useful in Crigler-Najjar type II

NEUROLOGICAL COMPLICATIONS OF UNCONJUGATED HYPERBILIRUBINEMIA

1. *Acute bilirubin encephalopathy (ABE):* The clinical manifestations of ABE are characterized into three stages:
   i. Phase 1 characterized by poor suck, hypotonia, and high-pitched cry.
   ii. Phase 2 manifested by irritability, fever, and increase in the tone of extensor muscles leading to opisthotonus, retrocollis, and rigidity.
   iii. Phase 3 or advanced stage—infants show exaggeration of extensor hypertonia leading to profound opisthotonus, central apnea, seizures, coma, and even death.
2. *Bilirubin-induced auditory toxicity:*
   i. Auditory toxicity may be the earliest manifestation of bilirubin-induced neurotoxicity.
   ii. All infants with severe jaundice should have comprehensive auditory evaluation using auditory brainstem-evoked response and otoacoustic-emission test during the

neonatal period and behavioral audiometry at 6–9 months of age to rule out sensorineural hearing loss and/or neural hearing loss (also known as auditory neuropathy).
3. *Kernicterus:* Chronic manifestation of injury to basal ganglia, brainstem nuclei, cerebellum, auditory pathway, etc. and is characterized by hearing disorders, choreoathetoid cerebral palsy, language delay, and upward gaze palsy.

KEY POINTS

➤ Unconjugated hyperbilirubinemia is a common neonatal condition requiring monitoring, evaluation, and treatment (if required) during the first few weeks after birth to prevent severe jaundice.
➤ Phototherapy is the standard treatment in cases of UHB.
➤ Exchange transfusion is required in few cases: When TSB crosses the threshold for exchange transfusion as per AAP guidelines or if the infant demonstrates any signs of acute bilirubin encephalopathy, even if the TSB is falling.
➤ Neurological complications of UHB include acute bilirubin encephalopathy, bilirubin-induced auditory toxicity, and kernicterus.

SELF ASSESSMENT

1. **Reasons for increased risk of UHB in neonates include all except:**
    a. Increased bilirubin production
    b. Decreased hepatic uptake
    c. Decreased bilirubin conjugation
    d. Decreased enterohepatic circulation

2. **All are true about transcutaneous bilirubinometry except:**
    a. Based on principle of spectrophotometry
    b. Used as a screening tool to estimate TSB in late preterm and term neonates not exposed to phototherapy
    c. Obtain TSB if transcutaneous bilirubin (TcB) ≥75th percentile on the AAP nomogram or TcB ≥13 mg/dL
    d. Good correlation with TSB in preterm infants

FURTHER READING

1. American Academy of Pediatrics Subcommittee on Hyperbilirubinemia. Management of hyperbilirubinemia in the newborn infant 35 or more weeks of gestation. Pediatrics. 2004;114(1): 297-316.
2. Amin SB. Bilirubin binding capacity in the preterm neonate. Clin Perinatol. 2016;43(2):241-57.
3. Volpe JJ (Ed). Bilirubin and Brain Injury. Neurology of the Newborn, 5th edition. Philadelphia, PA: Saunders; 2008. pp. 635-7.

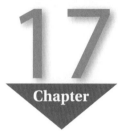

17

Chapter

Neonatal Cholestasis

Nishant Wadhwa, Jaswinder Kaur

INTRODUCTION

Cholestasis is defined:
- Physiologically as a measurable decrease in bile flow.
- Pathologically as the histologic presence of bile pigment in hepatocytes and bile ducts.
- Clinically as the accumulation in blood and extrahepatic tissues of substances normally excreted in bile (bilirubin, bile acids, and cholesterol).

Cholestatic jaundice is always pathologic and indicates hepatobiliary dysfunction. Persistent jaundice in any infant beyond 2 weeks of age needs evaluation for cholestasis with estimation of total and direct serum bilirubin. A direct bilirubin level >1.0 mg/dL or >17 mmol/L needs to be considered for further evaluation. An opinion from a pediatric gastroenterologist or hepatologist may be sought in such cases.

INCIDENCE

- In infancy, it affects approximately 1 in every 2,500 term infants.
- Biliary atresia accounts for approximately 25% of all cases of neonatal cholestasis (NC) and genetic disorders for another 25% of cases.
- Parenteral nutrition (PN) related cholestasis can be seen in approximately 20% of neonates receiving PN for more than 2 weeks.

ETIOLOGY

Disorders associated with cholestasis in the neonate are diverse. Early recognition of the treatable disorders such as sepsis and specific metabolic disorders allows initiation of appropriate treatment to prevent progression of liver damage. **Table 1** outlines the wide variety of known etiologies of neonatal cholestasis.

CLINICAL FEATURES

Cholestasis should be suspected in an infant with jaundice who is passing dark yellow urine and/pale stools. In an infant with cholestasis, certain clinical features can help in evaluation and diagnosis:

Table 1: Classification of the etiologies of neonatal cholestasis.

• Bile duct obstruction • Extrahepatic biliary atresia • Choledochal cyst • Alagille syndrome • Nonsyndromic bile duct paucity • Inspissated bile • Neonatal sclerosing cholangitis • Spontaneous perforation of bile duct	• Metabolic disorders • Galactosemia • Congenital disorders of glycosylation • Tyrosinemia • A1-antitrypsin deficiency • Bile acid synthetic defects • Storage disorders: Niemann-Pick type C, Gaucher, Wolman disease • Mitochondrial hepatopathies • Peroxisomal disorders • Cystic fibrosis • Neonatal hemochromatosis • Endocrinopathies: Hypopituitarism, hypothyroidism
• Neonatal hepatitis • *Viral:* TORCH, coxsackie, enteroviruses • *Bacterial:* Sepsis, urinary tract infection • Idiopathic	• Cholestatic syndromes • Progressive familial intrahepatic cholestasis (PFIC) type 1 and 2 • Benign recurrent intrahepatic cholestasis (BRIC)
• Toxic • Parenteral nutrition • Drugs	• Cardiovascular • Shock/hypoperfusion • Congestive heart failure • Perinatal asphyxia

- Persistent pale stools in a well thriving baby suggest extrahepatic obstruction such as caused by extrahepatic biliary atresia (EHBA).
- Infants with irritability, lethargy, poor feeding or vomiting should be evaluated for sepsis or metabolic disorders.
- History of cholestasis during pregnancy in the mother may point toward progressive familial intrahepatic cholestasis (PFIC) 2 in the infant.
- Dysmorphism is seen in Alagille syndrome, trisomies.
- Micropenis is seen in hypopituitarism.
- In infants who are small for gestational age (SGA) at birth and have failure to thrive, congenital infections should be suspected.
- Renal disease is seen in tyrosinemia type 1, congenital hepatic fibrosis, Alagille syndrome, and arthrogryposis renal cholestasis (ARC) syndrome.
- Splenomegaly may be suggestive of either early cirrhosis with portal hypertension, congenital infection or storage disorders.
- History of consanguinity suggests autosomal recessive, genetic disorders like PFIC, cystic fibrosis, etc.
- Family history of similar disease may be found in alpha-1-antitrypsin deficiency, cystic fibrosis, and Alagille syndrome.
- Early onset severe liver dysfunction is seen in metabolic disorders as listed in **Box 1**.

LABORATORY EVALUATION

Box 2 and **Flowcharts 1 and 2** outline a staged approach that excludes treatable life-threatening conditions early and then considers investigations relevant for more common conditions and finally those targeted at specific conditions.

Box 1: Early onset severe liver dysfunction.

- Neonatal iron storage disease (gestational alloimmune liver disease)
- Herpes simplex virus
- Tyrosinemia type 1
- Galactosemia
- Niemann-Pick C
- Hemophagocytic lymphohistiocytosis
- Mitochondrial respiratory chain dysfunction
- Bile acid synthetic disorders

Box 2: Diagnostic evaluation of neonatal cholestasis.

- Initiate investigations to detect readily treatable disorders:
  - Liver function test, prothrombin time/INR
  - Complete blood count
  - Bacterial cultures of blood/urine as indicated
  - Thyroid-stimulating hormone (TSH)
- Investigations for conditions requiring prompt specific therapy as indicated:
  - Ultrasound abdomen
  - Ophthalmologic examination—posterior embryotoxon, retinopathy, cataract
  - HIDA scan
  - Urine reducing substances (by both Benedicts and Glucostix), GALT assay
  - Serum iron ferritin
  - *Viral PCR:* CMV, HSV, HHV-6, enterovirus
  - Urine succinylacetone
  - Liver biopsy
  - Per-operative cholangiogram
- Investigations for less common causes as indicated:
  - Serum bile acids
  - Serum ammonia
  - Urine and plasma amino acids
  - Serum cholesterol
  - Cardiac evaluation- 2D echocardiography: Peripheral pulmonary stenosis in Alagille syndrome
- Other specific tests if indicated:
  - Karyotype
  - Very long chain fatty acids
  - Plasma acylcarnitines
  - Bone marrow examination
  - *Genetic testing:* Cystic fibrosis, Alagille syndrome, PFIC disorders

(CMV: cytomegalovirus; GALT: galactose-1 phosphate uridyltransferase; HHV-6: human herpesvirus 6; HIDA: hepatobiliary iminodiacetic acid; HSV: herpes simplex virus; PCR: polymerase chain reaction; PFIC: progressive familial intrahepatic cholestasis; INR: international normalized ratio)

- Elevated aminotransferases indicate primarily hepatocellular damage.
- Elevations of alkaline phosphatase (ALP) and gamma-glutamyltransferase (GGT) indicate biliary tract injury or obstruction.
- Gamma-glutamyltransferase is elevated in most cholestatic disorders. A low or normal GGT merits further work-up for rarer entities as listed in **Box 3**.

Flowchart 1: Algorithm for evaluation of neonatal cholestasis.

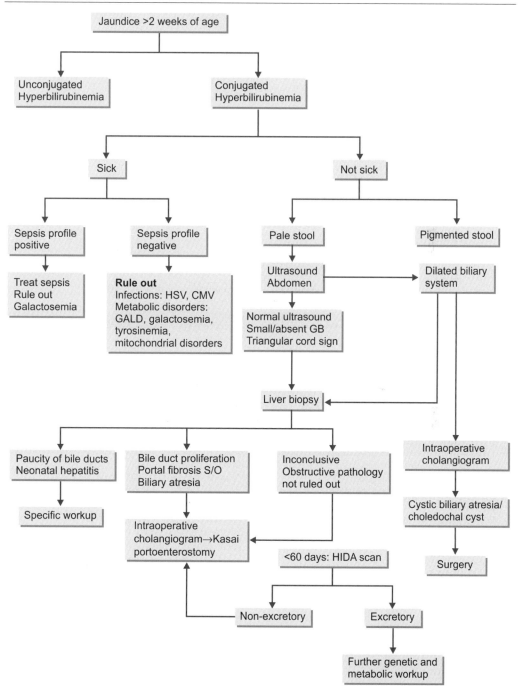

(HSV: herpes simplex virus; CMV: cytomegalovirus; GALD: gestational alloimmune liver disease; GB: gall bladder; HIDA scan: hepatobiliary iminodiacetic acid scan)

Flowchart 2: Algorithm for evaluation of neonatal cholestasis.

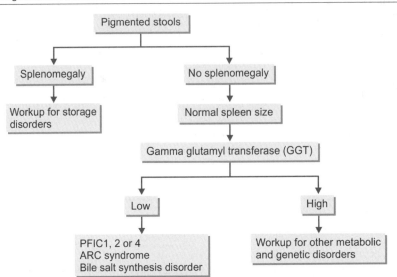

(PFIC: progressive familial intrahepatic cholestasis; ARC: arthrogryposis–renal–cholestasis)

Box 3: Causes of low gamma-glutamyltransferase (GGT) cholestasis.

- Low/normal GGT cholestasis
  - Progressive familial intrahepatic cholestasis type 1 and 2
  - Bile acid synthetic defects
  - Endocrine causes
  - Arthrogryposis-renal tubular dysfunction-cholestasis syndrome
  - Lymphedema cholestasis syndrome (Aagenaes syndrome)

Table 2: Medical management of neonatal cholestasis.

Malabsorption/Malnutrition: • Optimize calorie intake • Medium chain triglycerides (MCT): 30–50% of total fat as MCT • Enteral tube feeding/parenteral nutrition	*Vitamin supplementation:* • Vitamin A: 5,000–25,000 U/day • Vitamin D: 400–1,200 IU/day • Vitamin E: 15–25 IU/kg/day • Vitamin K: 2.5–5 mg/day • Water-soluble vitamin: 1–2 times of recommended daily allowance (RDA) • Ca/P/Mg/Zn/Fe supplementation
Pruritus: • Ursodeoxycholic acid • Cholestyramine • Rifampicin • Naloxone • Partial external biliary diversion	*Ascites:* • Sodium restriction • *Diuretic therapy*: Spironolactone, furosemide • Antibacterial prophylaxis • Albumin transfusion • Therapeutic paracentesis
• Portal hypertension and variceal • Hemorrhage • Endoscopic variceal ligation/sclerotherapy • Surgical shunt procedure • Liver transplantation	• End stage liver disease/refractory symptoms • Liver transplantation

Table 3: Specific management of cholestatic disorders.

Extrahepatic biliary atresia	*Kasai portoenterostomy*
Hypothyroidism	Thyroxine replacement
Hypopituitarism	Hormone replacement therapy
Galactosemia	Galactose-free diet
Tyrosinemia	NTBC [2-(2-nitro-4-trifluoromethylbenzoyl)-1,3 cyclohexanedione], low tyrosine diet
Congenital cytomegalovirus (CMV)	Ganciclovir
Herpes simplex infection	Acyclovir
Neonatal hemochromatosis	IVIg, plasmapheresis, antioxidant cocktail

MANAGEMENT OF NEONATAL CHOLESTASIS

Two main components:
1. General principles applicable to all patients **(Table 2)**: Cholestasis results in decreased concentration of bile acids in the small intestines resulting in reduced micelle formation and hence absorption of long-chain fat and accompanying fat-soluble vitamins. This results in early malnutrition and poor growth. Early and aggressive nutritional management is vital in improving overall outcome.
2. Specific management related to individual entities **(Table 3)**.

KEY POINTS

➢ Any infant noted to be jaundiced after 2 weeks of age should be evaluated for cholestasis with measurement of total and direct serum bilirubin.
➢ An elevated serum direct bilirubin level (direct bilirubin levels >1.0 mg/dL or >17 mmol/L) warrants timely consideration for evaluation and referral to a pediatric gastroenterologist or hepatologist.
➢ Early recognition of the treatable disorders such as sepsis, specific metabolic disorders allows initiation of appropriate treatment to prevent progression of liver damage.
➢ Early and aggressive nutritional management is vital in improving overall outcome.
➢ Finding the cause is important to treat the specific disorder.

SELF ASSESSMENT

1. **Which of the following is false?**
   a. Clinically cholestasis is the accumulation in blood and extrahepatic tissues of substances normally excreted in bile (bilirubin, bile acids, and cholesterol).
   b. Cholestatic jaundice is always pathologic and indicates hepatobiliary dysfunction.
   c. Any infant noted to be jaundiced after 2 weeks of age should be evaluated for cholestasis with measurement of total and direct serum bilirubin.
   d. The cutoff to define cholestasis is direct bilirubin level >2.0 mg/dL or >20% of the total serum bilirubin (TSB) if TSB is <5 mg/dL.

Impaired platelet function:

Qualitative defect	Quantitative defect
• Bernard-Soulier syndrome • Glanzmann thrombasthenia • Collagen receptor deficiency	• TAR syndrome • Wiskott–Aldrich syndrome • Autosomal dominant thrombocytopenia, May-Hegglin anomaly, macrothrombocytopenia

Coagulation Protein Disorders

Congenital coagulation factor deficiencies	Acquired deficiencies
X-linked recessive: Hemophilia A and B *Autosomal recessive:* Factors V, VII, X, XI, XII, XIII, afibrinogenemia	Vitamin K deficiency

Combined Platelet and Coagulation Factor Disorders

- Disseminated intravascular coagulation (DIC)
- Hepatic dysfunction (primary or secondary) to shock, infection.

Disorders of Vascular Integrity

For example, hemangiomas or vascular malformations (Kasabach–Merritt syndrome) which may rupture and directly bleed or sequester platelets and secondarily cause bleeding.

CLINICAL AND DIAGNOSTIC EVALUATION OF A BLEEDING NEONATE

Questions to be Asked?

- Is the baby sick or well?
- Was vitamin K given at the time of birth?
- Type of bleeding—generalized or localized? Generalized is almost secondary to coagulopathy or platelet disorders.
- Is there a family history of bleeding? (More relevant in a well baby with bleeding.)
- Maternal history of thrombocytopenia, infection, connective tissue disorder, and use of drug.
- Age of onset of bleeding [Immune thrombocytopenia (ITP) presents in first 24 hours and vitamin K deficiency usually presents between 2nd and 4th day of life (DOL)].
- Small petechial bleed with mucosal involvement (suggests thrombocytopenia) or large bleed (suggests coagulopathy).
- Other coexisting signs like jaundice, hepatosplenomegaly, and sepsis.

Examination

Assess the baby whether "sick" or "well". Bleeding in a well neonate suggests vitamin K deficiency, coagulopathy, and birth trauma. Bleeding in a sick baby suggests perinatal asphyxia, sepsis, and DIC. Look for symptoms of hypovolemia and infection. Look for vascular malformations and hemangioma **(Flowchart 1)**.

Investigation

Initial screen:

- Complete blood count (CBC), differential count, smear
- Platelet count
- Prothrombin time (PT)
- Fibrinogen
- Activated partial thromboplastin time (aPTT).

Flowchart 1: Algorithm for diagnostic considerations and workup of a neonate with bleeding.

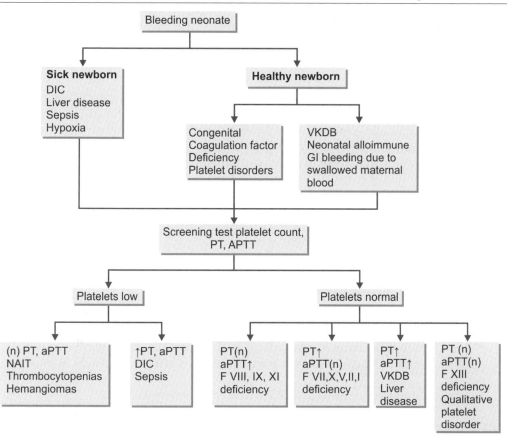

(aPTT: activated partial thromboplastin time; DIC: disseminated intravascular coagulation; F: Factor; GI: gastrointestinal; NAIT: neonatal alloimmune thrombocytopenia; PT: prothrombin time; VKDB: vitamin K deficiency bleeding; VWD: von-Willebrand disease)

Depending on the above-mentioned test, following conclusions can be made:

Clinical condition	Platelet	PT	aPTT	Diagnosis
Sick neonate	Decreased	Increased	Increased	Disseminated intravascular coagulation
	Decreased	Normal	Normal	Sepsis, necrotizing enterocolitis
	Normal	Increased	Increased	Liver disease
	Normal	Normal	Normal	Compromised vascular integrity (associated with hypoxia, prematurity, acidosis, hyperosmolarity)
Well neonate	Decreased	Normal	Normal	Immune thrombocytopenic purpura, occult infection, thrombosis
	Normal	Increased	Increased	Hemorrhagic diseases of newborn (Vitamin K deficiency), common pathway defect
	Normal	Normal	Increased	Hereditary clotting factor deficiency
	Normal	Normal	Normal	Swallow blood, trauma, qualitative platelet defect, Factor XIII deficiency

Platelet count can be false low in certain normal conditions like, platelet adherent to heel after needle prick, error in dilution, adherence to tube and dilution with EDTA.

Prothrombin time and activated partial thromboplastin time can be falsely high in decrease plasma/citrate ratio, contamination with heparin from indwelling lines, improper storage and transport and sample contamination with tissue thromboplastin from difficult vein puncture.

Antiplatelet Antibodies

Antibodies against maternal and fetal platelets (autoimmune thrombocytopenia):
- Immune thrombocytopenic purpose (ITP)
- Drug-induced
- Systemic lupus erythematosus (SLE)
- Gestational or incidental thrombocytopenia.

Antibodies against Fetal Platelets

- *Neonatal alloimmune thrombocytopenia (NAIT):* Maternal platelet is normal while baby's platelets are low. Screen for human platelet antigen 1 (HPA-1) antibody in neonate is positive.
- Isoimmune thrombocytopenia associated with erythroblastosis fetalis.

TREATMENT

Principal of Therapy

- Goal should be the well-being of infant rather than correcting the laboratory abnormalities.

- Therapy should be focused on treating the underlying disease such as septicemia, infection, shock, etc.
- Inj. vitamin K 1 mg IV if not given earlier.
- Use blood components rather than whole blood when required.

Supportive Treatment

- Ensure normal temperature, correct acidosis, hypovolemia, hypoxia, and electrolyte imbalance.

Severe Life-threatening Bleeding

- Maintain adequate circulating blood volume. Send blood for clotting study.
- If clotting defect is not known, consider giving all of the following:
  - Vitamin K 1 mg IV
  - Fresh frozen plasma (FFP) 10 mL/kg over 5–10 minutes
  - Platelet 1 unit and cryoprecipitate 1 unit
  - Obtain hematology consultant if bleeding is not controlled.

Indication for Platelet Transfusion

Less than 50,000/mm³:
- Any preterm <33 weeks in 1st week of life.
- Clinically unstable infant in 1st week of life.
- Any infant undergoing invasive procedure.

Less than 20,000/mm³: All stable infants after 1 week of life without active bleeding.

Less than 100,000/mm³: In presence of neonatal alloimmune thrombocytopenia with intra-cranial hemorrhage.

Products for treatment of coagulopathies

Products	Factor content	Usual dose	Indications
Fresh frozen plasma	All factors	10–20 mL/kg	DIC, liver disease, protein C deficiency
Exchange transfusion	All factors + platelets	Double volume	Severe DIC, liver disease
Factor VIII concentrate	Factor VIII	25–30 U/kg	Hemophilia A
Factor IX concentrate	Factor IX	50–100 U/kg	Factor IX deficiency
Vitamin K		1–2 mg	Vitamin K deficiency
Platelet concentrate	Platelets	As discussed above	As discussed above
Intravenous immunoglobulin (IVIG)	IgG	1–2 g/kg	Severe sepsis, thrombocytopenia due to transplacental antibodies

KEY POINTS

➤ A bleeding neonate may present with very wide spectrum of clinical conditions starting from an entirely normal situation to a serious life-threatening situation.

➤ A good clinical history, relevant examination, and some simple investigations can help in narrowing the diagnosis in most situations.

➤ Common disorders to be considered are: Vitamin K deficiency, sepsis, DIC, and immune thrombocytopenia. Rarely inherited coagulation disorders can also present in neonatal period.

➤ For significant bleeding, resuscitation with fluid therapy followed by blood component therapy helps in most situations.

➤ Current emphasis is to use blood component therapy mainly in bleeding neonates only and not to use just to correct laboratory values.

SELF ASSESSMENT

1. **Which of the following is not responsible for combined platelet and coagulation disorder?**
   a. Disseminated intravascular coagulation
   b. Hepatic failure following sepsis
   c. Vitamin K deficiency
   d. Kasabach-Merritt syndrome

2. **Which of the following bleeding neonates need further evaluation?**
   a. A well neonate vomiting blood which is apt test positive for maternal blood.
   b. A female neonate with vaginal bleed in first week of life.
   c. A neonate having hematoma after intramuscular hepatitis B vaccination.
   d. A neonate with bilateral subconjunctival bleed after cesarean delivery.

FURTHER READING

1. Avila L, Barnard D. Bleeding in the neonate. In: Blanchette VS, Brandão LR, Breakey VR, Revel-Vilk S (Eds). SickKids Handbook of Pediatric Thrombosis and Hemostasis. Basel: Karger; 2013. pp. 23-41.
2. Gleason C, Ballard R. Avery's Disease of Newborn, 8th edition. US: Saunders; 2004. pp. 1-1664.
3. Hansen AR, Eichenwald EC, Stark AR, Martin CR. Cloherty and Starks Manual of Neonatal Care, 8th edition. Philadelphia: Lippincott Williams & Wilkins; 2017.
4. Jaffray J, Young G1, Ko RH. The bleeding newborn: a review of presentation, diagnosis, and management. Semin Fetal Neonatal Med. 2016;21(1):44-9.
5. Ogundeyi MM, Ogunlesi TA. Approach to the management of a bleeding neonate. Niger J Med. 2009;18(3):238-43.

Anemia in Neonate

Raktima Chakrabarti, Sanjay Wazir

By definition, anemia is a downward shift by >2 standard deviation of mean hemoglobin or hematocrit for gestational and postnatal age.

EPIDEMIOLOGY

- Neonatal anemia is common in neonatal intensive care units (NICUs) especially in preterm babies (<34 weeks and <1,500 g babies).
- The incidence of anemia in preterm infants is 25–30%, which is much higher than term babies (15–20%).

Causes of neonatal anemia:
- *Blood loss:*
  - *Obstetric cause*—placenta previa, placental abruption, trauma to placenta or umbilical cord during delivery, and rupture of anomalous placental vessel
  - Fetomaternal transfusion
  - Twin-to-twin transfusion in monozygotic twin—donor has anemia and recipient has polycythemia
  - Fetoplacental transfusion
  - Hemorrhage—intraventricular, intra-abdominal, adrenal hemorrhage
  - Early cord clamping
  - Iatrogenic blood loss due to sampling—the most common cause
- *Increased red blood cell (RBC) destruction:*
  - *Intrinsic*—hereditary RBC disorders, e.g. G6PD deficiency, pyruvate kinase deficiency
  - *Extrinsic*—immune hemolysis, blood group incompatibility, acquired hemolysis due to infection, vitamin E deficiency, and malaria infestation
- *Decreased RBC production:*
  - Anemia of prematurity
  - Nutritional causes like iron, vitamin B_{12}, and folic acid deficiency
  - Bone marrow suppression due to infection or drug or genetic disorders like Diamond Blackfan syndrome, congenital dyserythropoietic anemia (CDA), etc.

PATHOGENESIS

- Red blood cell production starts in the yolk sac (2 weeks of life), liver (5 weeks), and in bone marrow (by 13–15 weeks of life). Bone marrow becomes the major organ for production by 30 weeks of intrauterine life.

Table 1: Hemoglobin changes after birth.			
Week	*Term*	*Preterm (1.2–2.5 kg)*	*Preterm (<1.2 kg)*
0	17	16.4	16.0
1	18.8	16.9	14.8
3	15.9	13.5	13.4
6	12.7	10.7	9.7
10	11.4	9.8	8.5
50	12.0	11.5	11.0
Lowest hemoglobin	10.3 (9.50–11.0)	9.0 (8.0–10.0)	7.1 (6.5–9.0)
Time of nadir	6–12 weeks	5–10 weeks	4–8 weeks

- After delivery, the tissue oxygenation increases and this decreases the stimulus to erythropoiesis over time.
- This leads to decrease in hemoglobin with nadir occurring at 6–12 weeks of extrauterine life. This nadir tends to be more severe and earlier in preterm infants. This is known as physiological anemia of infancy. This is shown in **Table 1**.
- Due to relative hypoxemia secondary to fall in hemoglobin, the erythropoiesis resumes again.
- Red blood cells in neonates have shorter life span (60–70 days), being the shortest in most premature neonates.
- Neonatal anemia occurs if this change is aggravated due to blood loss, destruction of RBC or impaired production.

CLINICAL EFFECTS/FEATURES OF ANEMIA

- Pallor
- Poor feeding and lethargy
- Decreased weight gain in neonatal period
- Apnea (association is weak and doubtful)
- Jaundice (hemolytic anemia)
- Hypotension (acute hemorrhagic anemia with more than 20% blood loss)
- Tachycardia and tachypnea (more common in acute hemorrhagic and hemolytic anemia)
- Hepatosplenomegaly (hemolytic anemia).

DIAGNOSIS

- *History:*
  - Maternal history—placenta previa, abruption placentae, peak systolic velocity of fetal middle cerebral artery on Doppler ultrasound more than 1.5 multiples of median (MoM) for gestation suggest antenatal fetal anemia. In addition, sinusoidal fetal heart pattern on cardiotocography may suggest severe fetal anemia.
  - Birth history—traumatic or instrumental delivery.
  - Family history—genetic disorder affecting RBC, significant neonatal jaundice in the sibling.

- *Timing:*
    - ◆ Within 24 hours:
        - • Hydrops
        - • Decreased production—CDA, Diamond Blackfan syndrome, Parvovirus
        - • Immune hemolysis
        - • Traumatic hemorrhage
- *Laboratory examinations:* Complete blood count, reticulocyte count, peripheral blood film (PBF), bilirubin, blood grouping, hemoglobin electrophoresis, and Kleihauer–Betke test to identify fetomaternal hemorrhage.
    - ◆ Reticulocyte count:
        - • Normal or low—nutritional, hypoplastic
        - • High—hemolysis, chronic blood loss
    - ◆ Mean corpuscular volume:
        - • Decreased—alpha thalassemia, CDA
        - • Normal—infection, bone marrow (BM) failure syndrome
        - • Increased—B_{12}, folate deficiency.
- Ultrasonography to detect internal bleeding.

MANAGEMENT

Strategies for Management of Anemia in Newborn

- Simple replacement transfusion
- Partial exchange transfusion
- Exchange transfusion
- Nutritional supplementation
- Erythropoietin injections
- Treatment of underlying condition.

Indications for Simple Replacement

- Acute hemorrhage
- Ongoing deficit replacement
- Maintenance of effective oxygen carrying capacity.

Target hemoglobin would vary according to the age of infant after birth. Standard guidelines for packed red blood cell (PRBC) transfusion are depicted in **Table 2**.

Volume of Blood for Transfusion

Although there is no consensus regarding the optimum volume of the blood to be transfused, 20 mL/kg PRBC transfusion should be given unless the pretransfusion hemoglobin is 9 g/dL or more or signs of fluid overload are already present in which case the volume should be restricted to 10 mL/kg. Time taken for transfusion should be 2–4 hours. In case of congestive cardiac failure (CCF), the rate of transfusion should be 2 mL/kg/hr. Each 10 mL/kg of PRBC transfusion increases hemoglobin by 3 g/dL.

Time of Collection

There is no difference in the neonatal outcomes whether the blood is fresh or more than 1 week old. Hence, there is no need to press the blood bank for fresh blood if a routine replacement

Table 2: Standard transfusion guidelines.

		BCSH* guideline (Hb: g/L)	Australian guideline (Hb:g/L)	Canadian guideline (Hb:g/L/HCT)
First 24 hours		Ventilated: <120 On oxygen/NIPPV: <120 Off oxygen: <100		
≤week 1 (1–7 days)	Respiratory support	Ventilated: <120 On oxygen/NIPPV: <100	110–130	115(35)#
	No respiratory support	<100	100–120	100(30)
Week 2 (2–14 days)	Respiratory support	Ventilated: <100 On oxygen/NIPPV: <95	100–125	100(30)#
	No respiratory support	<75	85–110	85(25)
≥week 3	Respiratory support	Ventilated: <100 On oxygen/NIPPV: <85	85–110	85(25)#
	No respiratory support	<75	70–110	75(23)

(HCT: hematocrit; NIPPV: nasal intermittent positive pressure ventilation)
*BCSH: British Committee for Standards in Hematology.
#Respiratory support is defined as inspired oxygen requirement in excess of 25% or need for mechanical increase in airway pressure.

transfusion is being planned. In fact, in studies the use of fresh blood leads to more donor exposures. PRBC could be used for up to 42 days after donation.

Special Considerations

■ *Prevention of cytomegalovirus (CMV) infection:* This can be achieved by using CMV seronegative donors or using inline filters during transfusion, which removes 99.9% white blood cell (WBC) reducing although not completely eradicating the risk of CMV infection. Filters are recommended in neonates to reduce the risk of CMV transmission, especially in infants less than 30 weeks gestation or weight less than 1,500 g and those with congenital or acquired immune deficiency.

■ *Irradiation:* Irradiation of blood with 25–50 Gy is not sufficient to kill the viruses but can remove the donor lymphocytes to reduce the risk of graft-versus-host disease (GVHD). Blood should be irradiated for preterm infants and in those with congenital immune deficiency. Donations from first or second-degree relatives should be avoided. Blood should be irradiated within 14 days of donation and used within 48 hours of irradiation.

■ *Hematocrit of the donor blood:* It should be around 55–60%.

■ *G6PD of the donor blood:* For exchange transfusion, screening of donor blood for G6PD results in reduced need for number of exchanges in areas where G6PD has a high prevalence but for routine transfusion, there is no guideline. However, if transfusion is being planned in a sick child it is better to screen the blood for G6PD as most immature livers are not able to handle the bilirubin load due to hemolysis in G6PD blood.

■ *Reconstitution of RBC and fresh frozen plasma (FFP):* It should be done in the blood bank preferably and should be used within 24 hours of reconstitution. Ideally, the FFP from the same donor should be used but if not available, then AB plasma which has no antibodies can be used.

NONTRANSFUSION APPROACH FOR PREVENTION OF ANEMIA

- Delayed umbilical cord clamping at the time of delivery and if not feasible then cord milking and exploring the possibility of using the cord blood for baseline investigation in NICU.
- *Enteral iron:* During neonatal period or early infancy this intervention is of no value for prevention of anemia, but it is important to start iron at the rate of 2–4 mg/kg from 2 weeks to 4 weeks of age in preterm babies (by the time they are on full feed) to reduce the risk of iron deficiency. Other nutritional components like B_{12} and folate should also be supplemented.
- *Erythropoietin and other erythropoietic stimulant agent:* Because of the low plasma erythropoietin concentrations in infants, recombinant human erythropoietin (r-HuEPO) and other erythropoietic-stimulating agents have been suggested for the treatment of neonatal anemia. It reduces the number of donor exposures in a preterm infant, however, routine use is not supported by current evidence.
- *Reducing iatrogenic blood loss:* Two strategies can be adopted—point of care bench-top laboratory analyzer for laboratory tests in which small volume of blood will be sufficient and secondly, limiting and rationalizing laboratory investigations.
- Use of restrictive approach for blood transfusion can be adopted.

ALGORITHM OF ANEMIA IN NEWBORN

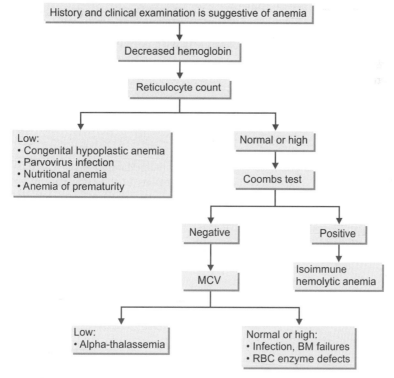

(MCV: mean corpuscular volume; BM: bone marrow; RBC: red blood cell)

KEY POINTS

➢ Anemia is a common occurrence in term neonates and even more common in preterm neonates.
➢ Common causes are—phlebotomy losses, isoimmune hemolytic anemia, and hemorrhagic anemia.
➢ Good clinical history, simple laboratory investigations like Hb, reticulocyte count and RBC indices help in narrowing the differential diagnosis.
➢ It is important to have departmental transfusion policy, which should be updated from time to time based on recent evidence.
➢ Special precautions like leukocyte filters and gamma irradiation are needed to reduce the transfusion-associated infections and GVHD in preterm and very low birth weight (VLBW) neonates.
➢ Delayed cord clamping, restrictive sampling, and transfusion policies are the need of the hour.

SELF ASSESSMENT

1. **Which is the correct definition of anemia in neonates?**
   a. Hemoglobin <14 g% in neonates.
   b. Hemoglobin <14 g% in full term neonates and <13 g% in preterm neonates.
   c. Hemoglobin level associated with signs or symptoms like failure to thrive, features of congestive heart failure or apnea.
   d. Hemoglobin level <2 SD for that gestation and age of the neonate.

2. **Rate of blood transfusion in cases of anemia with congestive heart failure:**
   a. 5 mL/kg/hr
   b. 2 mL/kg/hr
   c. 10 mL/kg/hr
   d. 15 mL/kg/hr

FURTHER READING

1. Neonatal Anemia. Intensive Care Nursery House Staff Manual. UCSF Children's Hospital at UCSF Medical Center. Oakland, California: The Regents of the University of California; 2004. pp. 108-10.
2. Ohlsson A, Aher SM. Early erythropoiesis-stimulating agents in preterm or low birth weight infants. Cochrane Database Syst Rev. 2017;11:CD004863.
3. von Lindern JS, Lopriore E. Management and prevention of neonatal anemia: current evidence and guidelines. Expert Rev Hematol. 2014;7(2):195-202.

Polycythemia in Neonates

Raktima Chakrabarti, Sanjay Wazir

INTRODUCTION

- The term polycythemia signifies increased cell number (poly—increased and cythemia—cell number). In neonates, it reflects increased red blood cell (RBC) mass which is characterized by increased venous hemoglobin or hematocrit (Hct) for gestational and postnatal age.
- It is defined as a Hct greater than two standard deviations (SD) above the normal value for gestational and postnatal age. Normal term babies have Hct around 51± 7%.
- In case of a term infant, polycythemia is considered if the Hct from a peripheral venous sample is greater than 65% or the hemoglobin is greater than 22 g/dL. This has been chosen as a cutoff because the blood viscosity increases exponentially after this.
- *Incidence of polycythemia:* About 1-5% (higher at higher altitudes). Incidence is higher in small for gestational age (SGA) and large for gestational age (LGA) babies and rare amongst those born appropriate for gestational age (AGA) less than 34 weeks of gestation.

RISK FACTORS

Risk factors of polycythemia are mentioned in **Table 1**.

PATHOPHYSIOLOGY

The symptoms in polycythemia are due to the increased viscosity. Almost 50% of the babies with polycythemia have hyperviscosity whereas only 25% of the babies with hyperviscosity

Table 1: Risk factors for polycythemia.			
Increased fetal erythropoiesis			
Placental insufficiency	*Endocrine*	*Genetic*	*Increased transfusion*
• Gestational hypertension • Mother having cyanotic heart disease • Maternal smoking • Postdated pregnancy • Renovascular disease • Intrauterine growth restriction • Perinatal asphyxia	Congenital thyrotoxicosis, infant of diabetic mother	• Trisomies 13/18/21 • Beckwith-Wiedemann syndrome	• Placental transfusion in delayed cord clamping • Twin-to-twin transfusion

Table 2: Signs and symptoms of polycythemia.	
General	Lethargy, irritability, priapism, hypoglycemia, hyperbilirubinemia
Cardiorespiratory	Cyanosis, tachycardia, increased pulmonary vascular resistance
Respiratory	Respiratory distress
Gastrointestinal	Vomiting, poor feeding, necrotizing enterocolitis
Neurological	Hypotonia, abnormal cry, jitteriness, lethargy, seizure, tremor, cerebrovascular accident
Hematological	Thrombocytopenia
Renal	Decreased glomerular filtration rate, oliguria, hematuria, proteinuria, renal vein thrombosis

have polycythemia. Other causes of hyperviscosity include increased plasma proteins, decreased deformation of RBC membrane, changes in platelet and increased WBC count. When this viscous blood flows through the microcirculation of the neonate, it tends to cause the hypoperfusion of most organs (kidney and lungs) whereas the decreased oxygen delivery in brain is due to increased arterial oxygen content causing vasospasm. This viscous blood is also likely to cause thrombosis of end organs due to stasis of blood.

DIAGNOSIS

- *History:* Presence of risk factor/s.
- *Physical examination:*
    - Most of the cases are asymptomatic (75–90%).
    - In case of symptomatic neonates, most symptoms are nonspecific and may reflect the underlying condition leading to polycythemia or may reflect the symptoms related to hypoperfusion of the organs.
    - Most common signs are gastrointestinal symptoms (poor feeding or vomiting), hypoglycemia, and cyanosis/apnea.
- *Other signs:* Other signs and symptoms are shown in **Table 2**.

LABORATORY EXAMINATIONS

Hematocrit measurement is essential for confirmation of diagnosis. Its measurement depends on factors such as:
- *Site of blood sampling:* Hct values are highest in capillary samples followed by peripheral veins and lowest in umbilical vein samples.
- *Age at the time of sampling:* Hct increase from birth to maximum at 2 hours of age and then starts receding to reach the cord blood level by 18 hours.
- *Method of Hct measurement:* Centrifuged machine values are higher than automated analyzers.

Laboratory Screening

- Screening is done only for symptomatic cases with risk factors as mentioned in **Table 1**. Asymptomatic term babies even if they have growth restriction are not screened as there is no data to show the benefit of treating the asymptomatic ones.
- Screening is recommended at 2 hours of age. If the value is <65% at 2 hours, then no further screening is required but if it is >65% then further screening at 12 and 24 hours is required.

- Warmed capillary samples may be used for screening, but all high values should be confirmed by a venous sample. Venous samples usually have lower values of Hct by 5–15%.
- *Other investigations:* In sick neonates with polycythemia, additional laboratory tests such as serum glucose, calcium, bilirubin, arterial blood gas, and sepsis screen as clinically indicated should be done. Coagulation profile, platelet counts, and USG/renal Dopplers or neuroimaging may be required in suspected thrombosis/thromboembolism.

DIFFERENTIAL DIAGNOSIS

Symptomatic polycythemia can mimic any organ dysfunction. Diseases which can present with similar signs/symptom are:
- Pneumonia
- Congenital heart disease
- Persistent pulmonary hypertension
- Intracranial hemorrhage
- Venous thrombosis
- Intracranial anomalies
- Metabolic abnormalities
- Moderate/severe dehydration.

MANAGEMENT

Management depends on value of Hct and presence/absence of symptoms **(Flowchart 1)**. Other conditions that could cause similar symptoms such as sepsis, pneumonia, and hypoglycemia should be excluded.
- *For symptomatic infants:* Partial exchange transfusion (PET) should be done in case the Hct is more than 65%.
- *For asymptomatic infants:*
  - *Hematocrit 65–70%:* Monitor closely for cardiorespiratory status. Maintain adequate hydration and glucose intake. Monitor oral intake, weight, and urine output. Repeat Hct and glucose in next 6–12 hours for at least 24 hours or until the Hct starts to decline.
  - *Hematocrit 70–75%:* Maintain hydration with intravenous (IV) fluids if required. Improving hydration would result in reducing the viscosity of blood by causing hemodilution. Monitor cardiorespiratory status closely. Hct and serum glucose should be monitored every 6 hourly.
  - *Hematocrit >75%:* These infants should be managed by PET.
- *Partial exchange transfusion:* Isovolumetric partial exchange transfusion reduces viscosity by hemodilution without causing hypovolemia. The target hematocrit is usually set at 55%.
- The amount of blood (mL) required to be exchanged is:

Volume to be exchanged = [Blood volume × (observed hematocrit – desired hematocrit)] ÷ observed hematocrit (Blood volume is estimated to be 80–90 mL/kg in term babies and 90–100 mL/kg in preterm).

- In general, the exchange volume is 15–20 mL/kg body weight.
  Fluids used for replacement are usually crystalloid like normal saline. One could use peripheral route or the central route for exchange. Peripheral route involves pushing blood

Flowchart 1: Management of polycythemia.

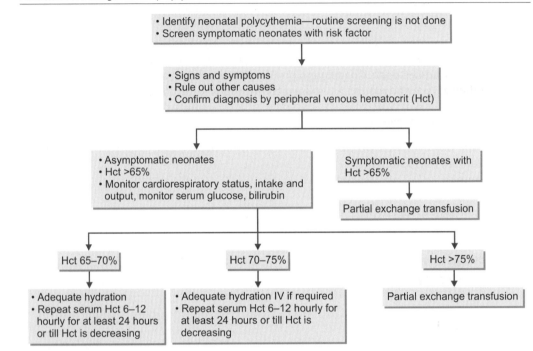

• Identify neonatal polycythemia—routine screening is not done
• Screen symptomatic neonates with risk factor

• Signs and symptoms
• Rule out other causes
• Confirm diagnosis by peripheral venous hematocrit (Hct)

• Asymptomatic neonates
• Hct >65%
• Monitor cardiorespiratory status, intake and output, monitor serum glucose, bilirubin

Symptomatic neonates with Hct >65%

Partial exchange transfusion

Hct 65–70%

Hct 70–75%

Hct >75%

• Adequate hydration
• Repeat serum Hct 6–12 hourly for at least 24 hours or till Hct is decreasing

• Adequate hydration IV if required
• Repeat serum Hct 6–12 hourly for at least 24 hours or till Hct is decreasing

Partial exchange transfusion

(IV: intravenous)

through a peripheral vein and drawing blood through a peripheral arterial line. Central route involves pushing through a peripheral vein and drawing the blood through the umbilical vein or artery or else use of umbilical vein for both pushing and withdrawing of blood. Central route is more invasive and possibly fraught with slightly increased risk of necrotizing enterocolitis (NEC) and hence preferably avoided. Risk of NEC may be increased in infants with polycythemia treated with PET, however, the evidence is not conclusive.

- *Long-term outcome of polycythemia and its treatment:*
    - Effect of polycythemia or hyperviscosity on the long-term outcome in neonates is uncertain because of conflicting reports. It is generally believed that the outcome is largely related to the underlying cause for polycythemia rather than the hyperviscosity itself.
    - Improved long-term outcomes have not been demonstrated with PET, but most clinicians perform PET due to fear of hyperviscosity and its presumed clinical effects.

KEY POINTS

➢ Polycythemia is defined as Hct of more than 65% or Hb of >22 g%.
➢ Incidence is higher in SGA, LGA infants, infants of diabetic mother or mothers with gestational hypertension.
➢ Screening is recommended only for symptomatic infants with risk factors.
➢ Signs and symptoms are nonspecific.
➢ Management depends on symptoms and level of Hct.
➢ Partial exchange transfusion has not shown to improve outcomes.

SELF ASSESSMENT

1. **Which statements are true regarding hematocrit estimation done by different methods/at different sites?**
   a. Peripheral venous Hct > Capillary Hct > Umbilical cord venous Hct.
   b. Capillary Hct > Peripheral venous Hct > Umbilical cord venous Hct.
   c. Umbilical cord venous Hct > Capillary Hct > Peripheral venous Hct.
   d. Centrifuged Hct > Automated analyzer Hct.
   e. Automated analyzer Hct > Centrifuged Hct.

2. **Calculate the amount of blood for partial exchange transfusion in a symptomatic polycythemic neonate with birth weight of 3 kg, observed Hct 77 and desired Hct 55.**

FURTHER READING

1. Luchtman-Jones L, Wilson DB. Hematologic problems in the fetus and neonate. In: Martin RJ, Fanaroff AA, Walsh MC (Eds). Fanaroff and Martin's Neonatal-Perinatal Medicine, 9th edition. St. Louis: Mosby; 2010. p. 1303.
2. Morag I, Strauss T, Lubin D, et al. Restrictive management of neonatal polycythemia. Am J Perinatol. 2011;28(9):677-82.

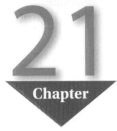

Hypoxic-ischemic Encephalopathy

Chapter 21

Sindhu Sivanandan, M Jeeva Sankar

INTRODUCTION

Hypoxic-ischemic encephalopathy (HIE) is an important cause of mortality and neurologic morbidity in neonates. Hypoxia (decreased oxygen delivery) and ischemia (decreased blood flow) to the fetus in-utero or at birth results in injury to brain and dysfunction of other organs. HIE secondary to perinatal asphyxia is the most important cause of neonatal encephalopathy (52%).

INCIDENCE OF BIRTH ASPHYXIA

- Two to three per 1,000 live term births in developed countries
- Twenty-six per 1,000 live births in low middle income countries.

ETIOLOGY

Asphyxiating event can occur during intrapartum period (56%), antepartum (13%), both ante-intrapartum periods (10%), and postnatally (2%). The factors that increase the risk of asphyxia are listed in **Table 1**.

PATHOGENESIS

When fetal blood flow is compromised, there is redistribution of blood flow to vital organs such as brain, heart, and adrenal glands at the expense of decreased blood flow to less vital organs

Table 1: Risk factors for asphyxia in fetus and neonate.		
Maternal	*Placental*	*Neonatal*
• Maternal diseases such as diabetes, hypertension, PIH, renal diseases • Hypotension • Antepartum hemorrhage • Rupture uterus • Chorioamnionitis	• Abruption • Cord prolapse • True knot • Velamentous insertion of cord • Feto-maternal hemorrhage	• Seizures, meningitis, or neurological disorders • Cardiopulmonary arrest, shock, and blood loss • Airway anomalies

(PIH: pregnancy-induced hypertension)

such as kidney, intestine, skin, and muscle (an adaptive response called "diving reflex"). When systemic blood flow is further compromised, even vital organs are affected, especially the brain. In some situations, blood flow is acutely cut off (cord occlusion, prolapse, abruption, and uterine rupture) allowing less or no time for adaptive response to occur resulting in acute total asphyxia.

Biochemical and pathological changes in neuronal cells in an asphyxiated neonate include:
- Reduced oxygen supply
- Anaerobic glycolysis
- Decrease in high-energy phosphates
- Accumulation of lactate
- Failure of Na-K ATPase pump
- Cell swelling and necrosis
- Calcium entry into cells and activation of various enzymes
- Excitotoxic injury due to glutamate excess
- Formation of free radicals, nitric oxide synthesis, and lipid peroxidation.

Asphyxial brain injury occurs in four phases:
1. *Primary energy failure*: First 60 minutes following ischemic injury; energy-rich adenosine triphosphate (ATP) is depleted; apoptosis or necrosis of cells occurs.
2. *Latent phase*: 1–6 hours of injury; resuscitation partially restores cerebral perfusion and oxygenation with partial restoration of energy sources.
3. *Secondary energy failure*: 6–48 hours; reperfusion brings in inflammatory mediators and free radicals promoting inflammation, and oxidative and excitotoxic damage.
4. *Tertiary energy failure*: Late cell death and gliosis take place.

NEUROPATHOLOGY

The neuropathological features of HIE depend on the gestational age of the infant, severity and duration of injury, and whether or not timely intervention is offered. Asphyxial injury can also occur in preterm neonates but in contrast to term neonates, the white matter is the main site of injury **(Table 2)**.

DIAGNOSIS

Birth asphyxia or HIE as the etiology of neonatal encephalopathy can be strongly suspected based on maternal antepartum or intrapartum history, condition of neonate at birth, need for resuscitation, and postnatal clinical examination.

Table 2: Site of neuronal injury in term and preterm neonates with asphyxia.

	Term neonate	Preterm neonate
Site of injury	• *Acute severe asphyxia:* Basal ganglia and thalamus • *Partial prolonged asphyxia:* Parasagittal cerebral injury (watershed areas) • *Very severe and prolonged:* Diffuse cerebral cortex and deep nuclear	• Periventricular white matter • White matter injury subsequently affects cerebral cortical development
Type of injury	• *Main:* Selective neuronal necrosis (neuron is the predominant cell involved) • Focal and multifocal ischemic necrosis	• Preoligodendrocytes are predominantly affected • Myelination is affected

- *History of antenatal and intrapartum events with high likelihood for asphyxia*: Antepartum hemorrhage or abruption, uterine rupture, cord prolapse, fetal heart rate decelerations, poor biophysical profile, chorioamnionitis, difficult or prolonged labor, and meconium-stained liquor
- *Perinatal depression and need for resuscitation*:
  - Born apneic, gasping or bradycardic; need for positive-pressure ventilation or chest compressions at birth
  - Low Apgar scores (10-minute Apgar score ≤ 5)
  - Acidosis in cord gas (pH < 7, BE > –12)
- *Neonatal encephalopathy*: The severity of encephalopathy in the first week of life is the most important clinical predictor of prognosis after birth asphyxia. The modified Sarnat staging system can be used. This staging has six components—level of consciousness, activity, posture, tone, primitive reflexes and autonomic dysfunction. Any of the abnormal clinical sign in three of the six components are required to classify a neonate into mild, moderate or severe encephalopathy **(Table 3)**. Around half of those with moderate encephalopathy and nearly all those with severe encephalopathy develop poor outcome (death or neuro-developmental impairment).
- *Seizures*: Occur in up to half of all asphyxiated neonates and indicates that HIE severity is moderate or severe. Onset is early within 24 hours after the asphyxiating injury. Seizures may be subtle, tonic, or clonic types and can often be subclinical. Electroencephalography (EEG) aids in diagnosis of seizures.
- *Features of multiorgan dysfunction*: See **Table 4**.
- *Neuroimaging*
  - *Cranial ultrasound and computer tomography (CT)*: Has low sensitivity and specificity; can identify features of cerebral edema and help to rule out intracranial hemorrhage.
  - *Magnetic resonance imaging (MRI)*: Best modality to determine the severity and extent of asphyxia injury. Lesions progress over time and timing of imaging and modality

Table 3: Modified Sarnat staging for grading the severity of encephalopathy.

Assessment components		Severity of encephalopathy		
		Mild	Moderate	Severe
Level of consciousness		Hyperalert	Lethargic	Stupor or coma
Spontaneous activity		Normal. May be increased	Decreased activity	Absent
Posture		Normal	Distal flexion, complete extension	Decerebrate
Tone (Check in trunk and limbs)		Normal or increased	Hypotonia	Flaccid
Primitive reflexes	Suck reflex	Normal or incomplete suck	Weak suck	Absent
	Moro reflex	Strong, low threshold	Incomplete Moro	Absent
Autonomic system		Pupils equal and reacting to light; normal heart rate and respirations	Pupils constricted bradycardia irregular breathing	Pupils non-reactive variable heart rate apnea

Table 4: Multiorgan dysfunction in hypoxic-ischemic encephalopathy—clinical and laboratory findings.

Organ system	Clinical features	Lab evaluation or imaging findings
Acute kidney injury—most common	Oligoanuria, fluid retention	Elevated blood urea, creatinine, hyponatremia, hyperkalemia, and acidosis. Fractional excretion of Na$^+$ helps differentiate prerenal from acute kidney injury. Urine beta-2 microglobulin level is a marker of proximal tubular dysfunction
Myocardial dysfunction	Myocardial ischemia, cardiac failure, pulmonary edema, hypotension	*ECG*: ST depression and T-wave inversion in left precordial leads *Echocardiography*: Decreased ejection fraction, poor contractility, tricuspid regurgitation, and pulmonary hypertension *Elevated creatine kinase*: MB (myocardial bound) fraction. Elevated cardiac troponin I and T levels
Pulmonary dysfunction	Hypoxia, persistent pulmonary hypertension of newborn (PPHN), pulmonary hemorrhage, and pulmonary edema	
Hematologic	Bleeding diathesis, DIC	Complete blood count, coagulation profile
Liver dysfunction	Jaundice (rare), hypoglycemia, bleeding diathesis	Elevated liver enzymes, prolonged prothrombin time
Gastrointestinal injury	Gut ischemia, necrotizing enterocolitis	X-ray abdomen

(DIC: Disseminated intravascular coagulation; ECG: electrocardiogram)

used should be considered while interpreting. It is also used to rule out other causes of encephalopathy [inborn errors of metabolism, structural central nervous system (CNS) malformations, antenatal insult, etc.]

- *Diffusion weighted MRI (DWI)*: Areas of restricted diffusion appear as hyperintense which can be picked up by DWI in a very early stage (1–2 days).
- *Conventional T1- and T2-weighted sequences*: Changes best apparent between 3 days and 7 days. Injury may continue to progress over the first 2 weeks.
- *Areas involved*:
  - *Basal ganglia predominant pattern*—basal ganglia, thalamus, and perirolandic cortex
  - *Watershed pattern*—parasagittal gray and white matter
  - *Total pattern*—both the above areas
- *Magnetic resonance spectroscopy*: Detects abnormalities in brain metabolism from specific areas; lactate (from anaerobic metabolism) levels are elevated and N-acetylaspartate (NAA) levels decrease; abnormalities noted between 1 days and 3 days.
- *Amplitude-integrated EEG*
  - For continuous bedside brain function monitoring
  - Two leads record raw EEG signal that is amplified, filtered to minimize artifacts, and time compressed

◆ *Uses*:
  • *Prognostication*: Abnormal EEG background pattern during the first 3–6 hours of asphyxia and delayed recovery of background beyond 48 hours are highly predictive of an adverse outcome. Background patterns associated with poor outcome include low voltage activity, isoelectric background, and persistent burst suppression pattern. Medications such as sedatives and anticonvulsants can alter the amplitude-integrated EEG (aEEG) tracing but not therapeutic hypothermia.
  • *Seizure detection*: It is not as good as conventional EEG, but can still be used to identify subclinical seizures and initiate treatment.

MANAGEMENT

Supportive Therapy

- *Temperature*: Maintain in normal range (36.5°C–37.5°C). During therapeutic hypothermia, monitor rectal temperatures. Avoid hyperthermia.
- *Airway and breathing*: Intubate and mechanically ventilate, if apnea or gasping or shallow respiration is noted. Maintain $PaCO_2$ in the normal range. Hypercapnia ($PaCO_2 > 55$ mm Hg) or hypocarbia ($PaCO_2 < 25$ mm Hg) should be avoided. Oxygen saturation should be maintained between 90% and 95% using pulse oximetry.
- *Circulation*: Monitor heart rate, capillary refill time, and blood pressures (BP). Insertion of an umbilical venous and arterial catheter may aid in venous access, and arterial BP monitoring and blood gas analysis. Inotropes may be needed to maintain BP.
- *Maintain euglycemia*: Blood sugar should be maintained in normal range. Both hypoglycemia and hyperglycemia can exacerbate brain injury.
- *Fluid and electrolytes*: Judicious fluid management is needed to avoid both fluid overload and underload. Acute kidney injury as well as syndrome of inappropriate antidiuretic hormone (ADH) secretion can cause fluid retention and dilutional hyponatremia. Monitor sodium, body weight, and urine-specific gravity to adjust fluids. Electrolyte abnormalities are common and need monitoring.
- *Seizure control:* Seizures in HIE usually begin early within 12 hours of birth, can be subclinical, increase in frequency over time, and often difficult to control. Seizures increase brain injury and need to be controlled. Rule out and treat hypoglycemia, hypocalcemia, and hyponatremia as causes of seizure **(Table 5)**.

If seizures still persist, IV lorazepam or midazolam (IV or infusion) can be considered.

Table 5: Drugs used for management of seizure in hypoxic-ischemic encephalopathy.		
Drug name	*Loading dose*	*Maintenance*
Phenobarbital—drug of choice	20 mg/kg IV. Additional 5–10 mg/kg up to a maximum of 40 mg/kg	3–5 mg/kg/day orally (PO) or IV 12 hours after loading in two divided doses
Phenytoin—seizures persisting after phenobarbital	15–20 mg/kg IV	4–8 mg/kg/day in 2–3 divided doses
(PO: per oral; IV: intravenous)		

MANAGEMENT OF OTHER ORGAN DYSFUNCTION

- *Gastrointestinal (GI)*: Delay feeds until hypotension is resolved and bowel sounds are heard.
- Monitor platelets and coagulation profile, and watch for active bleeding.
- Monitor liver function, renal function, and urine output.
- Prevent and treat infection.

Neuroprotective Strategies

- *Therapeutic hypothermia (TH)*: It involves selective cooling of the head or whole body to a temperature of 33.5°C–34.5°C maintained for 72 hours followed by slow rewarming over 8–12 hours. In term and late preterm infants with moderate-to-severe encephalopathy due to birth asphyxia, TH decreases the combined poor outcome of mortality or major neurodevelopmental disability at 18 months of age by 25% [relative risk (RR) 0.75; 95% confidence interval (CI) 0.68–0.83].
- *Criteria for initiating TH*: All the three criteria should be satisfied:
    - Gestational age > 35 weeks and age less than 6 hours
    - Evidence of acute perinatal event or intrapartum asphyxia (any one)
        - Cord pH ≤ 7 or base deficit ≥ 16 mmol/L.
        - Acute perinatal event—cord prolapse, cord rupture, uterine rupture, maternal trauma, hemorrhage, or cardiorespiratory arrest or late decelerations
        - 10-minute Apgar score of ≤5
        - Need for positive-pressure ventilation beyond 10 minutes of age
    - Evidence of moderate-to-severe neonatal encephalopathy based on clinical examination and classified based on modified Sarnat staging (moderate or severe encephalopathy) (stages 2 and 3). Amplitude EEG is not mandatory for decision to start TH.
- *Exclusion*: TH is not offered in the presence of major congenital abnormality, severe growth restriction (birth weight ≤ 1,800 g), and severely moribund infants.
- *Protocol*: Cool before 6 hours of age. Obtain parental consent. Units offering TH should have trained personnel and equipment for providing comprehensive intensive care and also offer continued follow-up services. Cooling blankets or phase changing material have been used to maintain the core body temperature of 33.5°C (33.5°C–34.5°C) for 72 hours. Arterial access and central venous access are must. Address pain relief and sedation during cooling. Monitor core body temperature continuously using rectal thermometer to avoid fluctuations. Both hyperthermia and overcooling below 33°C are harmful. Monitor hemodynamic and respiratory parameters. Ensure nutrition, fluid, and electrolyte balance. Based on clinical status, either nil per oral or trophic feeds (10 mL/kg/day) can be considered during cooling. Rewarm at the end of 72 hours at the rate of 0.5°C/hr.
- *Novel therapies*: A number of therapies such as xenon inhalation, erythropoietin, melatonin, topiramate, calcium channel blockers, magnesium, and free radical scavengers have shown promise as an add-on to therapeutic hypothermia in clinical trials.

OUTCOME OF ASPHYXIATED NEONATES

The outcome of asphyxiated neonates depends on the severity of HIE. The overall incidence of poor outcome (death or neurological sequelae) even among infants who are cooled for

HIE is 30–50%. Those with mild encephalopathy have a nearly normal outcome, half of those with moderate encephalopathy have a poor outcome. Those with severe encephalopathy have the worst outcome; 50% die and the other 50% have disability. The outcomes have significantly improved after TH. The benefits of therapeutic hypothermia persists into childhood.

- *Neurodevelopmental impairment (NDI) includes*: Cerebral palsy (CP), hearing loss, visual impairment, cognitive deficits, learning disability, attention deficit, behavioral issues, and autistic spectrum disorders.
- *Prognostic markers*:
  - *Neurological examination*:
    - *Moderate or severe encephalopathy*: Severe grades of encephalopathy and persistence of abnormal neurological examination beyond 1 week predict poor outcome.
    - *Clinical or electrographic seizures*: Increases risk of cerebral palsy, mortality, and NDI.
  - *Neurophysiological*: Amplitude EEG done within 6 hours of age showing a severely abnormal voltage and background pattern predicts a poor NDI outcome at 18 months of age but less so among cooled neonates.
  - *Neuroimaging*: Best modality for determining prognosis is MRI brain. The type and severity of disability correlates well with the site of injury in MRI. In the basal ganglia-thalamus pattern of injury, 50% had spastic quadriplegia while in the watershed predominant pattern, 11% had CP and cognitive deficits are more common. Abnormal signal intensity in the posterior limb of the internal capsule (PLIC) on T1/T2 imaging predicted abnormal ND outcomes with high sensitivity and specificity.

PREVENTION

- Antenatal management of maternal medical problems
- Institutional delivery
- Intrapartum monitoring and timely intervention for fetal distress, meconium-stained liquor, prolonged labor, antepartum hemorrhage, and cord accidents
- Timely resuscitation of neonate in delivery room by skilled care providers.

KEY POINTS

- ➤ Hypoxic-ischemic encephalopathy is an important cause of mortality and neurologic morbidity in neonates.
- ➤ Infants with HIE can present with variable degree of encephalopathy and features of multiorgan dysfunction.
- ➤ MRI, especially diffusion weighted, can pickup early brain lesions.
- ➤ Supportive management is important and therapeutic hypothermia is a proven neuroprotective strategy.
- ➤ Units offering therapeutic hypothermia should have trained personnel and equipment for providing comprehensive intensive care and also offer continued follow-up services.

SELF ASSESSMENT

1. **The most common organ involved in perinatal asphyxia is:**
   a. Heart
   b. Kidney
   c. Lungs
   d. Liver

2. **Which of the following is not a component of therapeutic hypothermia program?**
   a. Selective cooling of the head or whole body to temperature of 33.5°C–34.5°C maintained for 72 hours.
   b. It should be followed by slow rewarming.
   c. It should only be performed in units with facility of amplitude EEG to guide response to therapy.
   d. It should be initiated in term and late preterm infants with moderate-to-severe encephalopathy.

FURTHER READING

1. Bhat BV, Adhisivam B. Therapeutic cooling for perinatal asphyxia-Indian experience. Indian J Pediatr. 2014;81(6):585-91.
2. Glass HC, Wusthoff CJ, Shellhaas RA. Amplitude-integrated electro-encephalography: the child neurologist's perspective. J Child Neurol. 2013;28(10):1342-50.
3. Inder TE, Volpe JJ. Mechanisms of perinatal brain injury. Semin Neonatol. 2000;5(1):3-16.
4. Jacobs SE, Berg M, Hunt R, et al. Cooling for newborns with hypoxic ischaemic encephalopathy. Cochrane Database Syst Rev. 2013(1):CD003311.
5. Kurinczuk JJ, White-Koning M, Badawi N. Epidemiology of neonatal encephalopathy and hypoxic-ischaemic encephalopathy. Early Hum Dev. 2010;86(6):329-38.
6. Miller SP, Ramaswamy V, Michelson D, et al. Patterns of brain injury in term neonatal encephalopathy. J Pediatr. 2005;146(4):453-60.
7. Pierrat V, Haouari N, Liska A, et al. Groupe d'Etudes en Epidémiologie Périnatale. Prevalence, causes, and outcome at 2 years of age of newborn encephalopathy: population based study. Arch Dis Child Fetal Neonatal Ed. 2005;90(3):F257-61.
8. Rainaldi MA, Perlman JM. Pathophysiology of birth asphyxia. Clin Perinatol. 2016;43(3):409-22.
9. Shalak LF, Laptook AR, Velaphi SC, et al. Amplitude-integrated electroencephalography coupled with an early neurologic examination enhances prediction of term infants at risk for persistent encephalopathy. Pediatrics. 2003;111(2):351-7.
10. Shankaran S, Laptook AR, Ehrenkranz RA, et al. National Institute of Child Health and Human Development Neonatal Research Network. Whole-body hypothermia for neonates with hypoxic-ischemic encephalopathy. N Engl J Med. 2005;353(15):1574-84.

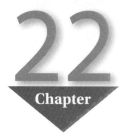

22 Chapter

Neonatal Seizure

Vivek Choudhury, Susanta Kumar Badatya

INTRODUCTION

Neonatal seizure can be described as a paroxysmal and abnormal neurologic manifestation (motor, behavioral, or autonomic function) secondary to an excessive electrical discharge of neurons within the central nervous system.

INCIDENCE

- 1.5–5.5 per 1,000 live births
- 14–57.7 per 1,000 in very low birth weight infants.

CLASSIFICATION

Seizure classification according to seizure semiology:

Subtle seizure	• Most common type (40–50%) • Motor (repetitive buccolingual movements, orbital—ocular movements, unusual bicycling, or pedaling) • Autonomic (tachycardia or bradycardia) activities • Inconsistently associated with an electrocortical activity
Focal clonic	• Second most common type (25–30%) • Repetitive, rhythmic contractions (1–4 Hz) of focal muscle group(s) • Electroencephalogram (EEG) correlation is a characteristic feature
Multifocal clonic	• Simultaneous clonic movements of more than one random muscle groups • Uncommon variety (approximately 3–5%) • Ictal EEG correlation is inconsistent
Myoclonic	• Shock-like quicker muscle contractions, predominantly flexor muscles • Around 15–20% of all neonatal seizures • EEG correlation is usually present
Tonic	• Sustained contraction of a group(s) of muscles • Uncommon variety (approximately 5%) • Ictal EEG correlation is inconsistent

ETIOLOGY

- Most common causes include hypoxic-ischemic encephalopathy (38%), arterial or venous ischemic stroke (18%), and intracranial hemorrhage (12%).
- Other causes include brain malformation (4%), intracranial infection (4%), inborn error of metabolism (3%), and benign familial neonatal seizure (3%).
- Hypoglycemia, hypocalcemia, and hypomagnesemia are transient metabolic disturbances that can cause seizures in the neonatal period.

Correlation of age of onset and etiology:

	Age of onset		
	1–3 days	*4–7 days*	*8–28 days*
Etiology	Hypoxic-ischemic encephalopathy		
	Hypoglycemia		
	Early hypocalcemia		Late
		Inborn errors of metabolism	
		Intracranial infection	
	Structural central nervous system (CNS) malformation		
	Drug withdrawal		

INVESTIGATIONS

Investigations for neonatal seizure:

First-tier investigation
(For all acute symptomatic neonatal seizure)
• Blood sugar (glucometer measurement should guide treatment, but value to be confirmed by laboratory measurement)
• Serum Na, serum calcium, serum magnesium
• Cerebrospinal fluid (CSF) examination—cytology/biochemistry/culture to rule out meningitis
• Cranial ultrasonography (CUS)—rules out gross brain malformation/intracranial hemorrhages
• Electroencephalogram (EEG)—conventional (gold standard)

Second-tier investigation
(Especially for refractory neonatal seizure)
• EEG—for diagnosis, prognosis, and to decide on antiepileptic drug (AED)
• Neuroimaging CT/MRI/MRI with different modes like—diffusion weighted MRI—detects early infarcts
• Workup for inborn error of metabolism—ABG, serum ammonia, serum lactate, blood, and urine ketone
• Tandem mass spectrometry and urine GC-MS
• CSF for specific biochemical level
– CSF lactate
– CSF glucose (paired with plasma)
– CSF amino acids (paired with plasma)
– CSF neurotransmitters
• Plasma and/or urine sulfocysteine—sulfite oxidase deficiency
• Biotinidase assay
• Urine α-aminoadipic semialdehyde (AASA)—pyridoxine dependent and pyridoxine responsive seizures
• Serum copper, ceruloplasmin—Menkes syndrome
• Investigation for TORCH infection (in case of strong clinical suspicion)

(ABG: arterial blood gas; GC-MS: gas chromatography-mass spectrometry; CT: computed tomography; MRI: magnetic resonance imaging)

A systematic approach to a case of neonatal seizure is as follows:

Evaluation of neonatal seizure		
	History	Significance
Antenatal history	• Intrauterine infection • Maternal narcotic addiction • Excessive fetal movement	• Congenital CNS infection • Stroke (cocaine abuse), neonatal abstinence syndrome • Possible in utero seizures
Perinatal history	• History of fetal distress • Instrumental delivery • Need for resuscitation in the labor room • Cord pH • Risk factor for sepsis • Maternal thrombophilic tendency	• Perinatal asphyxia • Neonatal meningitis • Ischemic stroke
Postnatal history including history of the event	• Onset of seizure • Duration and type of seizure • History of head trauma • Prematurity • History of congenital heart disease, ECMO, PPHN	• Etiological correlation • Seizure classification and prognosis • IVH in term babies • IVH in preterm babies, prognosis • Hypoxic insult
Family history	• History of consanguinity in parents • Early fetal/neonatal deaths • History of seizures in either parent or siblings in neonatal period	• Inborn error of metabolism • Benign familial neonatal seizure
	Clinical examination	Significance
General examination	• Obvious malformations or dysmorphic features/distinctive phenotype • Neurocutaneous marker • Injection mark in scalp • DiGeorge syndrome	• Zellweger syndrome • Underlying CNS malformation as in tuberous sclerosis • Local anesthetic toxicity • Congenital hypoparathyroidism
Central nervous system (CNS) examination	• Features of raised ICT • Cranial nerve involvement	• Cerebral edema • Unilateral hemorrhage or venous sinus thrombosis

(ECMO: extracorporeal membrane oxygenation; ICT: intracranial pressure; IVH: intraventricular hemorrhage; PPHN: persistent pulmonary hypertension of the newborn)

DIFFERENTIAL DIAGNOSIS

The following clinical entities may mislead for seizure activity due to their paroxysmal and repetitive nature:
- Jitteriness
- Benign neonatal sleep myoclonus
- Hyperekplexia.

Absence of electrocortical signature, restrainable nature of movements, and clinical characteristics help in differentiating them from seizures.

MANAGEMENT

Seizure is a medical emergency and demands prompt management.
- Restore normal vitals by addressing abnormal temperature, securing airway, and establishing adequate ventilation and circulation.

- Put intravenous cannula and keep baby nil per orally. Draw appropriate blood samples (serum electrolytes, blood sugar by glucometer/lab, sepsis screen).
- Every seizure episode must be screened for hypoglycemia and even treated empirically (200 mg/kg of glucose intravenous push rapidly) in the absence of facility to measure blood sugar.
- Calcium (2 mL/kg of 10% calcium gluconate) should be given over 10 minutes under strict cardiac monitoring in case of seizure persistence after ensuring normoglycemia.
- Antiepileptics drugs are offered when seizures persist after taking care of transient metabolic derangements such as hypoglycemia/hypocalcemia.
- Phenobarbitone is the first-line antiepileptic drug due to its better dosing schedule and wider therapeutic margin. Second-line anticonvulsants include phenytoin/fosphenytoin, levetiracetam, and benzodiazepines.
- Seizure is considered refractory when it persists despite administration of maximum tolerable doses of two conventional antiepileptics.
- Few cases of refractory seizures include vitamin deficiency seizure. A trial of intravenous therapeutic dose of pyridoxine (100 mg) should be considered for every refractory seizure.
- Escalate the drug dosage and continue antiepileptics till both clinical and electrographic seizures cease.
- If more than one drug is required to control the seizure, drugs should be stopped one by one sparing phenobarbitone for the last.
- During the neonatal period, if neonatal neurological examination becomes normal with normal electroencephalogram (EEG) finding, antiepileptic drug (AED) can be discontinued after >72 hours of seizure-free interval.
- If neonatal neurological examination is persistently abnormal, continue phenobarbitone and discontinue phenytoin if possible. Re-evaluation after 1 month with neurological examination and EEG is needed.
- On 1-month follow-up, if neurological examination has become normal, phenobarbitone should be discontinued over 2 weeks. In case of abnormal neurological examination with overt paroxysmal activity in EEG, reassessment is done for discontinuation of therapy after a 3–6-month period.

MANAGEMENT ALGORITHM

Flowchart 1 illustrates an algorithmic approach to seizures in newborn.

PROGNOSIS

- Mortality—15–20% in preterm infants and 5–10% in term neonates
- Long-term outcome
  - Global developmental delay (45%)
  - Mental retardation (20–35%)
  - Cerebral palsy (20–25%)
- Factors influencing outcome are etiology of underlying seizure, seizure burden, gestational age (term vs. preterm), and neurological examination.

Flowchart 1: Algorithm for management of neonatal seizure.

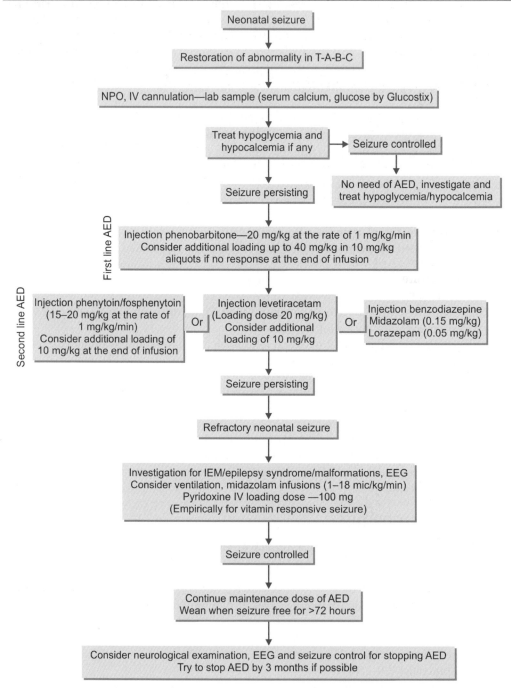

(AED: antiepileptic drug; NPO: nil per orally; IV: intravenous; EEG: electroencephalogram; IEM: inborn errors of metabolism)

KEY POINTS

➤ Neonatal seizure manifests as paroxysmal abnormal neurologic manifestation due to excessive electrical discharge of neurons within the central nervous system.

➤ Neonatal seizures can be classified as subtle, focal clonic, multifocal clonic, and myoclonic and tonic seizures.

➤ The two most common causes of neonatal seizures are hypoxic-ischemic encephalopathy and neonatal stroke.

➤ A detailed history and clinical examination are warranted in all cases of neonatal seizures. Phenobarbitone is the first-line antiepileptic drug due to its better dosing schedule and wider therapeutic margin. Second-line anticonvulsants include phenytoin/fosphenytoin, levetiracetam, and benzodiazepines.

➤ Prognosis depends on etiology of underlying seizure, seizure burden, gestational age, and neurological examination.

SELF ASSESSMENT

1. **The most common type of neonatal seizure is**
   a. Subtle seizure
   b. Clonic seizure
   c. Myoclonic seizure
   d. Tonic seizure

2. **The most common cause of neonatal seizure is**
   a. Hypoxic ischemic encephalopathy
   b. Neonatal stroke
   c. Hypocalcemia
   d. Brain malformation

3. **First-line drug for neonatal seizure is**
   a. Phenytoin
   b. Phenobarbitone
   c. Midazolam
   d. Levetircetam

FURTHER READING

1. Volpe JJ. Neonatal seizures. In: Volpe JJ (Ed). Neurology of the Newborn, 5th edition. Philadelphia: Saunders; 2008. pp. 203-44.
2. WHO. (2011). Guideline on Neonatal Seizure. [online] Available from: http://www.who.int/mental_health/publications/guidelines_neonatal_seizures/en/ [Last accessed on September, 2019].

Intracranial Hemorrhage and Intraventricular Hemorrhage

Chapter 23

Geeta Gathwala

INTRAVENTRICULAR HEMORRHAGE IN THE PRETERM INFANT

INTRODUCTION

- Most common cause of cerebral palsy in preterm infants.
- Incidence has declined with improved care.
- The amount of blood lost may be large enough to result in hypovolemia, hypotension, and death.
- Large hemorrhages are often followed by progressive ventricular enlargement (dilatation) and/or parenchymal hemorrhagic infarction in the adjacent periventricular white matter and these serious complications carry a high risk of subsequent neurodevelopmental impairment.

INCIDENCE

- In the early 1980s, nearly 50% of all infants with birth weight <1,500 g had intraventricular hemorrhage (IVH).
- The incidence of IVH has come down remarkably in infants with birth weights of 1,000–1,500 g.

About 26% of infants with birth weights 500–749 g have IVH with 13% being severe. Factors in the causation of GMH-IVH is shown in **Flowchart 1**.

PATHOLOGY

- During 10–20 weeks of gestation, neuronal precursors are formed from germinal matrix which later forms glial precursor cells. Germinal matrix is dependent on rich blood supply for producing new brain cells, however, structurally these vessels are immature and do not last a lifetime. In preterm infants, endothelial cells of capillaries or small venules are not well supported by pericytes and act as the source of IVH. There are gaps in between

Flowchart 1: Factors in the causation of GMH-IVH.

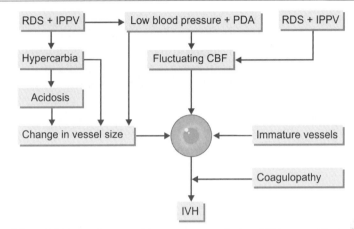

(CBF: cerebral blood flow; IPPV: intermittent positive pressure ventilation; IVH: intraventricular hemorrhage; GMH: germinal matrix hemorrhage; PDA: patent ductus arteriosus; RDS: respiratory distress syndrome)

the endothelial cells and they do not have connective tissue or support of muscle. The basal lamina is immature and there is a deficiency of glial fibrillary acidic protein in the astrocyte-end-feet. By the time the infant has reached term gestation, the germinal matrix has done its job of producing brain cells and almost disappears.

- Diminished autoregulation of blood flow in the cerebral circulation increases the risk of rupturing the germinal matrix vessels. Healthy individuals can (auto) regulate cerebral blood flow so that it remains constant despite variations in blood pressure. However, very preterm infants with respiratory distress syndrome (RDS) are usually unable to autoregulate cerebral blood flow. Struggling to breathe (with or without mechanical ventilation) generates wide swings in intrathoracic pressure, which are transmitted directly to the fragile vessels in the germinal matrix. As a result, the arterial pressure and cerebral blood flow velocity fluctuate.
- Hypercapnia produces cerebral vasodilatation, and acute swings in PCO_2 further destabilize cerebral blood flow.
- Once bleeding has started, it may progress rapidly as the premature skull has the capacity to expand without enough rise in the pressure to tamponade the hemorrhage. Formation of intraventricular clot may consume coagulation factors and platelets, which cannot be rapidly replaced, resulting in secondary coagulopathy. In addition, IVH may lead to obstruction to the terminal vein resulting in periventricular hemorrhagic infarction.
- The venous drainage from the periventricular white matter occurs via the terminal vein through the germinal matrix. A large hematoma at that location will obstruct the terminal vein, thus raising venous pressure in the periventricular white matter. If there is a concurrent episode of hypotension, perfusion in the periventricular white matter will be reduced because of the raised venous pressure leading to a hemorrhagic infarction. Furthermore, because of the raised venous pressure, secondary bleeding can occur into the infarcted area.

CLINICAL FEATURES

- For a clinical diagnosis it is important to identify the predisposing factors, e.g. gestational age, details of labor and delivery, resuscitation details, perinatal asphyxia, positive pressure ventilation, mechanical ventilation, hypercarbia, acidosis, coagulopathy, and hypotension.
- *Catastrophic deterioration:* This can present as a sudden worsening in the baby's clinical condition such as increased respiratory support, hypotension and/or peripheral mottling, pallor and acidosis accompanied by a drop in hematocrit, clinical seizures and a full fontanelle is very suggestive of IVH.
- *Saltatory syndrome:* This is more common and insidious in onset. There may be subtle seizures.
- *Asymptomatic:* Most frequent. About 25–50% of infants with IVH are asymptomatic.

DIAGNOSIS

- Cranial ultrasound is a reliable, portable, and noninvasive technique for the diagnosis of IVH and to study its evolution over time **(Figs. 1 to 4)**.
- *Magnetic resonance imaging (MRI):* For definite diagnosis; has greater role in assessing complications and prognosis.

PAPILE GRADING OF INTRAVENTRICULAR HEMORRHAGE

- *Grade I*: Hemorrhage confined to the subependymal germinal matrix in the caudothalamic groove.
- *Grade II*: Hemorrhage in germinal matrix and a small amount within the ventricular lumen, with the clot occupying less than 50% of the ventricular lumen and not distending the ventricular system.
- *Grade III*: Germinal matrix hemorrhage with a large amount of clot (>50% of ventricular lumen) distending the ventricular system.

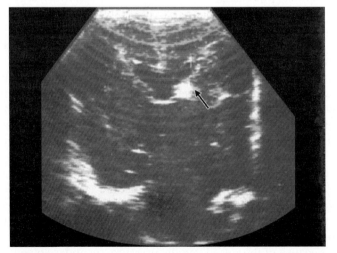

Fig. 1: Coronal ultrasound scan showing a small hemorrhage (arrowed) in the subependymal germinal matrix. Grade 1 intraventricular hemorrhage.

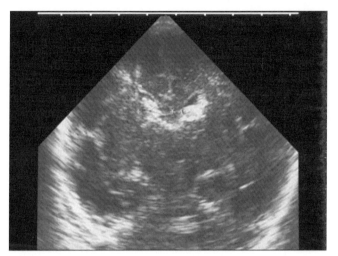

Fig. 2: Coronal ultrasound scan showing small amounts of blood clot in both lateral ventricles without ventricular distension. Grade II intraventricular hemorrhage.

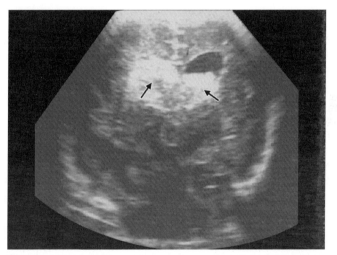

Fig. 3: Coronal ultrasound scan showing large amounts of blood clot (arrowed) in both lateral ventricles with distension. Grade III intraventricular hemorrhage.

- *Grade IV*: Germinal matrix and IVH in apparent continuity with hemorrhage into the periventricular white matter.

COMPLICATIONS

- Posthemorrhagic ventricular dilatation.
- Periventricular hemorrhagic infarction.

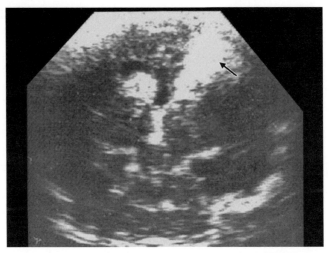

Fig. 4: Coronal cranial ultrasound scan showing a large amount of blood in the third and both lateral ventricles with some distension. In addition, there is a large periventricular echo density (arrowed) in apparent continuity with the lateral ventricle. Grade IV intraventricular hemorrhage.

MANAGEMENT

- *Intervention to decrease the ventriculomegaly:* If there is evidence of raised intracranial pressure (ICP), which is symptomatic (persistent and marked irritability, reduced responsiveness, or clinical seizures), then an intervention is required to lower pressure. If there is no indication of raised ICP, the indications for intervention are not universally agreed upon. However, ventricular width of 4 mm over the 97th percentile (on each side) has been widely used as a criterion for treatment in clinical trials.
- *Evidence-based treatment interventions to decrease ventriculomegaly:* Repeated lumbar puncture/ventricular puncture; diuretic therapy with acetazolamide and furosemide; intraventricular injection of streptokinase; and drainage, irrigation, and fibrinolytic therapy (DRIFT) have been tested in randomized trials. None have shown any short-term benefit, e.g. reduction in shunt surgery, but irrigation and fibrinolytic therapy significantly reduced severe cognitive disability at 2 years and 10 years of age.
- *Treatments used but without evidence from randomized trials:* Tapping a ventricular reservoir, subgaleal shunt insertion, external ventricular drainage, third ventriculostomy, and choroid plexus coagulation have all been used to treat posthemorrhagic ventricular dilatation (PHVD) but without evidence of efficacy in randomized clinical trials.
- *Indications for cerebrospinal fluid (CSF) removal in an infant with a ventricular reservoir:* The purpose for inserting a ventricular reservoir is to enable the removal of sufficient CSF to normalize ICP and to prevent any further enlargement of the ventricles and excessive head enlargement. The standard procedure is to remove 10 mL/kg CSF over 10 (or more) minutes. Rapid removal of CSF can cause midline shift and precipitate secondary bleeding. Taking more than 20 mL/kg CSF at one tap may result in clinical deterioration. The frequency of taps should be adjusted in order to prevent any further ventricular enlargement and to achieve normal head growth over 7 days. When the ventricles are very large, the goal is to reduce ventricular size to 4 mm over the 97th percentile.
- Anticonvulsant therapy (refer to chapter on neonatal seizures).

PREVENTION OF IVH: EVIDENCE-BASED INTERVENTIONS THAT REDUCE THE RISK OF IVH

- Antenatal corticosteroids before preterm delivery have shown a very consistent reduction in IVH, including severe IVH in many randomized trials. For optimal effect, the first dose had to have been given at least 24 hours before delivery.
- Delayed cord clamping is a useful strategy as it leads to placental transfusion and allows for better hemodynamic transition therefore reducing the risk of IVH.
- A meta-analysis on use of antenatal vitamin K did not show a significant benefit.
- Use of pancuronium has shown to reduce the incidence of IVH in preterm infants who are ventilated and have respiratory asynchrony. However, there is uncertainty about long-term pulmonary and neurologic complications with prolonged use of pancuronium in ventilated newborn infants.
- Volume-targeted ventilation may reduce IVH when compared with the more traditional pressure-limited ventilation; however, larger randomized trials are needed.
- Indomethacin promotes maturation of blood vessels in the germinal matrix and blunts swings in blood pressure and cerebral blood flow. Randomized clinical trials have shown a reduction in IVH but a meta-analysis and the largest trial showed no reduction in neurologic disability.
- Phenobarbital modulates blood pressure fluctuations and may have some free radical scavenging function. It has been tested in 11 postnatal trials with inconsistent results. However, the meta-analysis and the largest trial did not find any reduction in IVH.
- Ethamsylate improves platelet function and enhances capillary basement membrane stability but clinical trials showed no reductions in mortality or neurodevelopmental impairment despite the reduction in IVH in infants <35 weeks' gestation.
- Vitamin E has free radical scavenging action. In preterm infants, supplemented with vitamin E, there is decreased risk of intracranial hemorrhage. However, there is increase in risk of infection preventing its routine use especially in high doses and by intravenous route.

PROGNOSIS

Severity of IVH	Incidence of definite neurological sequelae (%)
Grade 1	15
Grade 2	25
Grade 3	50
Grade 3 and periventricular hemorrhagic infarction (PVHI)	75

INTRACRANIAL HEMORRHAGE IN THE TERM INFANT

INCIDENCE

Asymptomatic intracranial hemorrhage (ICH) is quite common and was reported in 8% of term neonates in the first 48 hours. The incidence of symptomatic ICH is much lower and is estimated at around 3 per 10,000 live births.

CLASSIFICATION

Extradural, subdural, and subarachnoid, intraventricular and intraparenchymal bleeding.

RISK FACTORS

- *Difficult delivery:* Difficult ventouse, multiple attempts, multiple applications of instruments, failed instrumentation followed by cesarean section.
- Neonatal bleeding disorders including vitamin K deficiency disorders.
- *Structural anomalies:* Arteriovenous (AV) malformations and aneurysms.
- Extracorporeal membrane oxygenation (ECMO).
- Hemorrhage into an area of venous infarction.

CLINICAL FEATURES

- Seizures
- Apnea
- Neonatal encephalopathy.

INVESTIGATIONS

- Complete blood count may reveal anemia and thrombocytopenia
- Coagulation screen
- *Neuroimaging:*
  - ◆ Cranial ultrasound is a good technique for intraventricular and parenchymal bleeds.
  - ◆ MRI is the imaging modality of choice.

TREATMENT

- Most ICHs can be managed conservatively.
- Seizures should be treated.
- Thrombocytopenia should be corrected with platelet transfusion and deranged coagulation should be treated with vitamin K and fresh frozen plasma.
- Provide respiratory and hemodynamic support as needed.
- In cranial sinus thrombosis, there is a risk of the thrombosis extending, thus producing an increased secondary infarction. This has been the argument for anticoagulation with low-molecular weight heparin but most clinicians have not dared to do this because of fear of rebleeding.
- Serial scanning and head circumference measurements will be needed to detect progressive ventricular dilatation.
- Neurosurgical consultation in cases of symptomatic ICH associated with skull fracture, mid-line shift, signs of raised ICP, and focal neurological signs.

PROGNOSIS

Adverse outcome is associated with intraparenchymal bleeds and accompanying hypoxic ischemic encephalopathy.

KEY POINTS

➤ Intraventricular hemorrhage is the most common cause of cerebral palsy in preterm infants.

➤ Usually seen in infants <32 weeks of gestation.

➤ It may be asymptomatic or have a more gradual saltatory presentation or may present in the form of acute deterioration.

➤ Risk of mortality and neurological sequelae depends on severity of IVH.

SELF ASSESSMENT

1. **All of the following is evidence-based strategy to prevent IVH in preterm infants except:**
   a. Delayed cord clamping
   b. Antenatal steroid therapy
   c. Postnatal steroid therapy
   d. Intravenous indomethacin therapy

2. **Which of the following cutoff has been used in trials as a criterion for treatment for ventriculomegaly based on Levene index?**
   a. Ventricular width 1 mm over the 97th percentile
   b. Ventricular width 2 mm over the 97th percentile
   c. Ventricular width 3 mm over the 97th percentile
   d. Ventricular width 4 mm over the 97th percentile

FURTHER READING

1. Polin R, Yoder M. Workbook in Practical Neonatology, 5th edition. US: Saunders; 2014.
2. Volpe JJ. Neurology of the Newborn, 6th edition. Philadelphia, PA: Saunders; 2017.

24

Chapter

Neonatal Acute Kidney Injury

Kanav Anand, Deblina Dasgupta

INTRODUCTION

Acute kidney injury (AKI) is a sudden deterioration in renal functions resulting in fluid, electrolyte, and acid–base imbalance. It is common in neonates especially very low birth weight (VLBW) neonates and is an important risk factor determining mortality and morbidity.

NEONATAL RENAL PHYSIOLOGY

- Nephrogenesis starts at 5th week of gestation and continues till 34th–36th week of gestation resulting in formation of approximately 2.7 million nephrons.
- At birth, 2.5-4% of cardiac output is supplied to the kidneys compared to 25% of cardiac output supplied in adults. The blood flow to kidneys increases after birth due to increased systemic arterial pressure and decreased renal vascular resistance.
- *Glomerular filtration rate (GFR)* in the first few days of life ranges from 10 mL/min/1.73 m^2 to 20 mL/min/1.73 m^2 and increases gradually to reach adult values by 2 years of age. This dynamicity of GFR has implications in drug dosing and development of AKI in neonates.
- Preterms have lower GFR at birth and slower subsequent rise. The tubular immaturity and consequent defective urinary concentrating ability are other factors to be considered during management of AKI in preterm neonates.

DEFINITION OF NEONATAL ACUTE KIDNEY INJURY

Neonatal AKI has been defined based on the neonatal modified KDIGO (Kidney Disease Improving Global Outcomes) criteria and neonatal RIFLE (Risk, Injury, Failure, Loss of kidney function, and End-stage kidney disease) staging **(Tables 1 and 2)**. Both these staging systems use urine output and serum creatinine for defining and staging neonatal AKI **(Box 1)**.

RISK FACTORS AND ETIOLOGY

- Risk factors for AKI in neonates include VLBW (<1,500 g), low 5 minutes Apgar score, maternal drug administration [nonsteroidal anti-inflammatory drugs (NSAIDs), antibiotics], intubation at birth, respiratory distress syndrome, patent ductus arteriosus (PDA), phototherapy, and neonatal drug administration (NSAID, antibiotic, diuretics).

Table 1: Neonatal modified KDIGO criteria.

Stage	Serum creatinine	Urine output
0	No change in S. Cr or rise <0.3 mg/dL	≥0.5 mL/kg/hr
1	S. Cr rise ≥0.3 mg/dL within 48 hours or rise 1.5–1.9 times reference value within 7 days	<0.5 mL/kg/hr for 6–12 hours
2	S. Cr rise 2.0–2.9 times reference value	<0.5 mL/kg/hr for ≥12 hours
3	S. Cr rise ≥3 times reference value/≥2.5 mg/dL or receipt of dialysis	<0.5 mL/kg/hr for ≥24 hours or anuria for more than 12 hours

(KDIGO: Kidney Disease Improving Global Outcomes)

Table 2: Neonatal RIFLE classification.

	Creatinine	Urine output
Risk	Increased creatinine × 1.5 or GFR decreases >25%	UO < 1.5 mL/kg/hr × 24 hr
Injury	Increased creatinine × 2 or GFR decreases >50%	UO < 1 mL/kg/hr × 24 hr
Failure	Increased creatinine × 3 or GFR decreases >75%	UO < 0.7 mL/kg/hr × 24 hr or anuria × 12 hr
Loss	Persistent failure >4 weeks	
End stage	End-stage renal disease (persistent failure >3 months)	

(GFR: glomerular filtration rate; UO: urine output)

Box 1: The pitfalls of using serum creatinine as the marker for neonatal acute kidney injury (AKI) and newer biomarkers.

- Postnatally, the serum creatinine of neonates is reflective of the maternal serum creatinine and it takes days weeks for the serum creatinine to decline and reach a new equilibrium, the decline being slower in preterms.
- Serum creatinine will rise 48–72 hours after a perturbation in kidney function and this rise occurs only after 50% of the kidney function has been impaired.

Numerous biomarkers have been developed that allow earlier identification of kidney injury. These novel biomarkers include neutrophil gelatinase associated lipocalin, cystatin C, urine interleukin 18, kidney injury molecule 1, urine liver fatty acid binding protein, urine aprotinin, urine netrin 1.

- The etiologies can be broadly categorized into prerenal azotemia, intrinsic AKI, and postrenal factors **(Table 3)**. The most common cause is prerenal azotemia accounting for up to 85% of neonatal AKIs. Acute tubular necrosis is found to be the most common cause of intrinsic AKI.

EVALUATION

- Evaluation of a neonate with AKI should be aimed at finding out whether the etiology is prerenal, renal or postrenal.
- A thorough antenatal history including antenatal ultrasounds, exposure to nephrotoxic medications is mandated along with history of birth and resuscitation details, body weight changes, and postnatal exposure to medications and interventions.
- Important examination findings include hypotension/hypertension, signs of hypovolemia/fluid overload, neurological status, and seizures.

Table 3: Etiologies of acute kidney injury (AKI) in a neonate.

Prerenal AKI	Intrinsic AKI	Postrenal AKI
• Loss of effective blood volume • Absolute loss • Blood loss • Dehydration • Relative loss (capillary leak) • Sepsis • Necrotizing enterocolitis • Respiratory distress syndrome • Hypoalbuminemia • ECMO • Renal hypoperfusion • Congestive heart failure • Drugs • Indomethacin • ACE inhibitors/ARB (angiotensin receptor blocker)	• Acute tubular necrosis • Severe renal ischemia • Nephrotoxins • Infections • Congenital infections • Pyelonephritis • Bacterial endocarditis • Renal vascular causes • Renal artery thrombosis • Renal vein thrombosis • Nephrotoxins • Aminoglycosides • Indomethacin • Amphotericin B • Radiocontrast dyes • Acyclovir • Intrarenal obstruction • Uric acid nephropathy • Myoglobulinuria • Hemoglobinuria • Congenital malformations • Bilateral renal agenesis • Renal dysplasia • Polycystic kidney disease	• Congenital malformations • Tight phimosis • Urethral stricture • Posterior urethral valve • PUJ obstruction (B/L) • VUJ obstruction (B/L) • Extrinsic compression • Sacrococcygeal teratoma • Hematocolpos • Intrinsic obstruction • Renal calculi • Fungus balls • Neurogenic bladder

(ACE: angiotensin-converting enzyme; ECMO: extracorporeal membrane oxygenation; PUJ: pelviureteric junction; VUJ: vesicoureteric junction)

Table 4: Prerenal vs. intrinsic acute kidney injury in neonates.

	Prerenal acute kidney injury	Intrinsic acute kidney injury
Urine flow rate (mL/kg/hr)	Variable	Variable
Urine osmolality	>400 mOsm/L	≤400
Urine to plasma osmolal ratio	>1.3	≤1
Urine to plasma creatinine ratio	29.2 ± 1.6	9.7 ± 3.6
Urine Na (mEq/L)	10–50	30–90
FeNa (%)	<0.3 (1.3 ± 0.6)	>3.0 (4.3 ± 2.2)
Renal failure index (urine Na × plasma creatinine/ urine creatinine)	<3.0 (1.3 ± 0.8)	>3.0 (11.6 ± 9.5)
Response to fluid challenge	Improved tachycardia, increased urine output	No effect on tachycardia or urine output

- Urine output needs to be strictly quantified and assessed in all newborns at risk for AKI. Blood urea, creatinine, serum electrolytes, blood gas, hemoglobin, and platelet count along with routine urine analysis, urine culture are important investigations.

To differentiate between prerenal and intrinsic renal injury certain clinical parameters, laboratory markers, and interventions can help as shown in **Table 4**. However, these parameters are less sensitive in premature newborns owing to the immaturity in their tubular function and defective urinary concentrating capacity.

- Ultrasound examination of the kidneys and urinary tract is needed to look for features of obstructive uropathy and renal anomalies. In cases with hypertension and/or hematuria, renal doppler is mandated to look for renal vein thrombosis/renal artery stenosis.
- Micturating cystourethrography can help to delineate the urinary tract anatomy and detect vesicoureteral reflux (VUR), bladder outlet obstruction especially if antenatal USGs were suggestive of hydronephrosis.
- Radioisotope imaging with MAG-3 and DTPA is used for assessing renal function and urinary tract obstruction (PUJ/VUJ obstruction) whereas DMSA scans can help in renal cortical function evaluation.

MANAGEMENT

There is no specific medical therapy for AKI and management depends on the underlying etiology. For prerenal azotemias, appropriate fluid management is essential. Relieving obstruction followed by surgical correction is needed for AKIs due to obstructive uropathy.

Fluid Management

- Prerenal azotemias are treated with adequate hydration and/or fluid boluses. In case of hemorrhagic shock, packed cell transfusion is mandated. For other cases of hypovolemic shock, KDIGO AKI guidelines recommend rapid fluid boluses with crystalloid solutions over colloid solutions. In case of fluid refractory hypotension, catecholamines and other inotropes with or without low dose hydrocortisone help in restoring systemic perfusion.
- Anemia needs to be corrected with packed cell transfusion to improve tissue oxygenation and correction of hypoalbuminemia with albumin infusion also helps in restoring tissue perfusion.
- Loop diuretics have been shown to increase urine output in neonates with intrinsic renal injury in certain studies but at the cost of an increase in serum creatinine. They have not been shown to improve outcomes in critically ill neonates. If diuretics are to be used, continuous infusions are better than large intermittent dosages.
- Studies of low dose dopamine use in AKI in neonates are lacking and hence its use is not recommended.
- In case of neonates with intrinsic renal injury and fluid overload, fluid restriction is necessary along with trial of loop diuretics failing which renal replacement therapies are indicated. In case of nonoliguric AKI or in neonates in the recovery phase of AKI with polyuria, fluid administration has to be liberal based on the gestational age and hydration status to prevent another episode of prerenal AKI.

Management of Dyselectrolytemias

- Hyponatremia is a frequent accompaniment and is due to free water overload. Free water restriction is recommended in absence of clinical signs and symptoms of hyponatremia. If symptomatic or if serum sodium is less than 120 mEq/L, 3% sodium chloride administration should be considered.
- Hyperkalemia can be life-threatening.
  - If electrocardiogram (ECG) changes are present, intravenous (IV) calcium gluconate (10%) 0.5–1 mL/kg is to be administered over 30 minutes for cardioprotection.
  - Oral or rectal potassium binders like sodium polystyrene sulfonate can be given at the dose of 1 g/kg/dose every 6 hours.

- ◆ Potassium excretion can be increased with loop diuretics.
- ◆ Measures to shift potassium to intracellular compartment can be adopted like salbutamol nebulization, IV sodium bicarbonate (3.75% solution given IV at the dose of 1–2 mEq/kg) and insulin dextrose infusions (2 mL/kg 25% dextrose with insulin 0.1 U/kg as intermittent dose over 15–30 minutes or continuous infusion).
- ◆ Definitive management for hyperkalemia is dialysis especially if it is resistant to conservative treatment.
- Hyperphosphatemia can be treated with oral calcium carbonate. Breast milk is low in phosphorus and hence is recommended in neonates with AKI. Severe hyperphosphatemia mandates dialysis.
- Calcium supplementation should be done only if hypocalcemia is symptomatic. 1–2 mL/kg 10% calcium gluconate IV over 20–30 minutes followed by oral or IV supplementation with 100–200 mg/kg/day should be given along with oral or IV calcitriol administration to increase intestinal calcium reabsorption.

Management of Hypertension

- Hypertension is a common association in intrinsic AKI and occurs due to salt and water retention and renin angiotensin system over activity. Salt and water retention can be treated with diuretics and dialysis.
- Long-acting calcium channel blockers like amlodipine can be used starting at doses of 0.1–0.6 mg/kg/day. Beta blockers like propranolol or labetalol can also be used. Use of angiotensin-converting enzyme inhibitors (ACEIs) or angiotensin receptor blockers (ARBs) should be avoided.

Nutrition

- Nutrition requirements are same as in neonates without AKI. Enteral or parenteral nutrition will have to be made nutrient dense to achieve fluid restriction.
- If fluid overload still persists, risks and benefits of dialysis vs. reduced intake of proteins and calories will have to be weighed and discussed with parents. In neonates on renal replacement therapy (RRT), especially peritoneal dialysis, additional 1 g/kg/day of protein needs to be provided.

Management of Acid-base Disorders

Metabolic acidosis is to be treated with bicarbonate replacement (oral or IV).

Renal Dose Modification of Drugs

All drug dosages need to be modified according to the creatinine clearance and if needed the serum trough levels of drugs should be monitored (e.g. vancomycin and amikacin). If the neonate is on dialysis, then the dialysis modality, dialysis interval, and the pharmacokinetic properties of the drug need to be considered before making dosing adjustments.

Special Considerations in Neonates with Severe Perinatal Asphyxia

- Increased levels of adenosine following hydrolysis of adenosine triphosphate (ATP) in perinatal asphyxia can decrease GFR by causing renal vasoconstriction. Theophylline administered within 1 hour of birth has been found to have renoprotective effects in these

> **Box 2:** Indications of renal replacement therapy.
>
> - Refractory fluid overload
> - Refractory hyperkalemia
> - Refractory metabolic acidosis
> - Uremic manifestations in form of uremic encephalopathy, uremic pericarditis
> - Refractory hyperphosphatemia
> - Inability to achieve nutritional goals in an attempt to achieve fluid restriction in oliguric neonates

neonates. KDIGO AKI guidelines recommend a single dose of prophylactic theophylline in severely asphyxiated neonates at risk for AKI.

- Therapeutic hypothermia has also been found to have renoprotective effect in certain retrospective studies but prospective trials remain to be undertaken.

Renal Replacement Therapy

Indications of RRT in neonates with AKI are shown in **Box 2**.

The various modalities include:

- *Peritoneal dialysis:* Preferred modality due to easier insertion techniques and avoidance of anticoagulation. The composition of the dialyzer fluid, cycle duration, and dwell volume can be altered to achieve desired degree of dialysis and ultrafiltration. Contraindications include abdominal surgeries, necrotizing enterocolitis, pleuroperitoneal leakage, and ventriculoperitoneal shunting.
- *Continuous renal replacement therapy:* Preferred in neonates with hemodynamic instability as it achieves controlled removal of fluids and solutes. Only disadvantage is the need for establishing vascular access that is difficult in neonates. Two modes are commonly used—continuous veno-venous hemofiltration (CVVH) where an ultrafiltrate of the neonate's plasma is removed and a portion is replaced back and continuous veno-venous hemodialysis (CVVHD), where a countercurrent dialysate is used that helps in solute removal along with ultrafiltration.
- *Intermittent hemodialysis:* Not preferred in neonates because of the need for anticoagulation, rapid osmolar shifts, and propensity to cause hemodynamic disturbances.

PROGNOSIS

- Acute kidney injury in neonates increases mortality (14–73%), length of hospital stay, and predisposes to development of chronic kidney disease (CKD) subsequently, as has been found in various studies.
- The outcomes are also dependent on the underlying etiology with those neonates having AKI due to renal hypoperfusion that is rapidly corrected having better prognosis whereas those having intrinsic renal injury having the worst outcomes. The prognosis of AKI due to obstructive uropathy is variable depending upon the associated renal dysplasias.
- Factors associated with increased mortality include VLBW, bronchopulmonary dysplasia, lack of antenatal steroids, very high serum creatinine, very high serum blood urea nitrogen (BUN), hyponatremia, hyperkalemia, anuria, mechanical ventilation, dialysis, and fluid refractory hypotension.
- KDIGO AKI guidelines recommend that screening for appearance of or worsening of CKD should be done at 3 months of age in all neonates with past history of AKI. Urine spot

protein: creatinine ratio greater than 0.6 at 1 year of age, serum creatinine greater than 0.6 mg/dL at 1 year of age, and body mass index greater than 85th centile are associated with progressive kidney disease.

- Other long-term sequelae of AKI in neonatal age group include impaired growth of kidneys, hypertension, renal tubular acidosis, and impaired concentrating capacity of the renal tubules.

KEY POINTS

➤ Acute kidney injury is a sudden deterioration in renal functions resulting in fluid, electrolyte, and acid-base imbalance.

➤ Neonatal AKI has been defined based on the neonatal modified KDIGO criteria and neonatal RIFLE staging.

➤ The most common cause of neonatal AKI is prerenal azotemia accounting for up to 85% of cases. Acute tubular necrosis is found to be the most common cause of intrinsic AKI.

➤ Evaluation includes a good clinical history, examinations, kidney function test, USG KUB with renal Dopplers, and additional imaging tests as warranted.

➤ Management is mainly supportive and includes management of fluid and electrolyte balance, acid and base balance, hypertension, nutrition, and RRT in refractory cases.

➤ The outcomes are dependent on the underlying etiology.

SELF ASSESSMENT

1. **Which of the following is false in defining AKI in neonates?**
   a. Postnatally, in the first few days, the serum creatinine of neonates is reflective of the maternal serum creatinine.
   b. As per Neonatal Modified KDIGO Criteria, the rise in serum creatinine of 1.5 times indicates stage 2 AKI.
   c. As per Neonatal Modified KDIGO Criteria, the rise in serum creatinine more than 3 times indicates stage 3 AKI.
   d. Serum creatinine will rise 48–72 hours after a perturbation in kidney function and this rise occurs only after 50% of the kidney function has been impaired.

2. **Which of the following is not an indication of renal replacement therapy in neonatal AKI?**
   a. Refractory fluid overload
   b. Refractory hyperkalemia
   c. Failure to achieve nutritional goal due to oliguria
   d. Serum creatinine >5 mg/dL

FURTHER READING

1. Jetton JG, Boohaker LJ, Sethi SK, et al.; Neonatal Kidney Collaborative (NKC). Incidence and outcomes of neonatal acute kidney injury (AWAKEN): a multicentre, multinational, observational cohort study. Lancet Child Adolesc Health. 2017;1(3):184-94.
2. Kidney Disease. Improving Global Outcomes (KDIGO); Acute Kidney Injury Work Group. KDIGO clinical practice guideline for acute kidney injury. Kidney Int Suppl. 2012;2(1):1-138.
3. Vieux R, Hascoet JM, Merdariu D, et al. Glomerular filtration rate reference values in very preterm infants. Pediatrics. 2010;125(5):e1186-92.

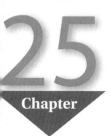

25
Chapter

Interpretation of Arterial Blood Gas

Pradeep Kumar Sharma

IMPORTANCE

- Assess acid–base status in neonates.
- Assess ventilation and oxygenation in sick neonates.

TERMINOLOGY

- There are some values which are directly measured in blood gas and some values which are calculated (not directly measured).
- Measured values (pH, pCO_2, pO_2).
- Calculated values (HCO_3^-, base excess, oxygen saturation, and lactate).

MEASURED VALUES

- *pH:* It reflects the concentration of extracellular hydrogen ion. $pH = -\log [H^+]$. Maintaining pH in normal range is important for maintaining normal function of cell membranes and proteins. pH 6.9–7.6 is compatible with life. Normal range of pH is 7.35–7.45.
  pH <7.35—acidosis
  pH >7.45—alkalosis
- *H^+:* The proton which is highly reactive cation needs to be in a narrow physiologic range for normal cellular function for which various buffering mechanisms have been developed. Normal value is 40 nmol/L.
- *pCO_2:* Partial pressure of CO_2 in blood (dissolved CO_2 in blood).
- *pO_2:* Partial pressure of O_2 in blood (dissolved oxygen in blood).

CALCULATED VALUES

- *Actual HCO_3^- (A):* This is the bicarbonate concentration in the blood. Normal value is 22–26 mmol/L. In newborns it may be lower also.
- *Standard HCO_3^- (st):* $CO_2 + H_2O = HCO_3^- + H^+$. This equation shows that bicarbonate concentration is affected by the carbon dioxide. Therefore, standard bicarbonate is used

which is independent of CO_2. CO_2 is standardized as 40 mm Hg. The bicarbonate value that is calculated from actual H^+ and CO_2 of 40 mm Hg at 37°C is the standard bicarbonate.

- *Buffer base (BB):* Body has developed various mechanisms to keep the pH toward normal. This is called the buffering system. If all the buffers, e.g. HCO_3^-, Hb^+, proteins, sulfates, and phosphates are added up, they constitute the BB. Normal value is 48 ± 5 mmol/L.
- *Base excess (BE):* If alkali is added to the blood, the buffer base is increased. The rise in BB is called BE. If acid is added, the buffers will be used to neutralize the acid and the decrease in BB is called as base deficit, the negative of which is called BE.

Example: If acid is added and BB falls from 48 mmol/L to 40 mmol/L, the base deficit is 8 mmol/ or the BE is –8 mmol/L.

The advantage of base excess over HCO_3^- is that it depicts pure metabolic change and is not affected by CO_2. When CO_2 accumulates as a result of impaired respiration, the following reactions occur:

$$CO_2 + H_2O = H_2CO_3 = HCO_3^- + H^+$$

$$Hb^- + H^+ = HHb$$

The decrease in amount of Hb^- buffer is equal to the amount of HCO_3^- released in the reaction. Therefore, total amount of buffer anion content will not change. Therefore, changes in the $PaCO_2$ will not change BE.

- *SaO_2:* This is the percentage of hemoglobin saturated with oxygen calculated from the hemoglobin–oxygen dissociation curve. SaO_2 is lesser than SpO_2 in neonates if the machine uses adult hemoglobin oxygen dissociation curve for this calculation as oxygen is more tightly bound to fetal hemoglobin.

Acid–base disorders: There are six primary acid–base disorders (shaded areas in the figure).

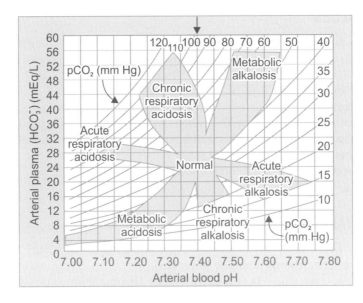

Approach to blood gas analysis:

Step 1	What is pH	• pH <7.35—acidosis • pH >7.45—alkalosis
Step 2	Determine whether it is primarily metabolic or respiratory	• HCO_3 <24—metabolic acidosis • HCO_3 >24—metabolic alkalosis • Normal range of $PaCO_2$—35–45 mm Hg • $PaCO_2$ <35—respiratory alkalosis • $PaCO_2$ >45—respiratory acidosis
Step 3	Determine whether compensated or not compensated	• Compensation occurs in same direction • In case of primary metabolic acidosis (HCO_3 <24, $PaCO_2$ will be less for compensation) • Primary metabolic alkalosis (HCO_3 >24, $PaCO_2$ will get accumulated) • Primary respiratory acidosis ($PaCO_2$ >45, kidneys will retain HCO_3 and HCO_3 will be more) • Primary respiratory alkalosis ($PaCO_2$ <35, HCO_3 will decrease)
Step 4	Calculate PaO_2	
Step 5	Identify possible cause of acid–base imbalance	

Compensation in respiratory and metabolic disorders:

Disturbance	Response	Expected change
Metabolic acidosis		
↓ HCO_3	↓ $PaCO_2$	12 mm Hg/10 mEq↓HCO_3
Metabolic alkalosis		
↑ HCO_3	↑$PaCO_2$	8 mm Hg/10 mEq↑HCO_3
Acute respiratory acidosis		
↑$PaCO_2$	↑HCO_3	1 mEq/10 mm Hg ↑$PaCO_2$
Chronic respiratory acidosis		
↑$PaCO_2$	↑HCO_3	4 mEq/10 mm Hg ↑$PaCO_2$
Acute respiratory alkalosis		
↓ $PaCO_2$	↓HCO_3	2 mEq/10 mm Hg ↓ $PaCO_2$
Chronic respiratory alkalosis		
↓ $PaCO_2$	↓HCO_3	4 mEq/10 mm Hg ↓ $PaCO_2$

Example 1: A 900 g baby is born at 28 weeks of gestation and has respiratory distress at birth. Baby is put on nasal continuous positive airway pressure (CPAP) and the arterial blood gas (ABG) is pH 7.25, $PaCO_2$ 65, PaO_2 45, HCO_3 28, BE −3.

pH is 7.25 < 7.35 means acidosis and pCO_2 65 > 40 respiratory acidosis.

HCO_3—28, the rise of 4 is expected as compensatory rise and BE— −3 is within normal limits.

So, this is respiratory acidosis.

Since from the history we know it has been short duration since birth, it is acute respiratory acidosis; this highlights the importance of clinical history in interpreting blood gases. Using the acid–base map (which can be easily pasted in the ICU and act as a ready reference for interpretation) put a dot corresponding to pH 7.25 on the x-axis and HCO_3 28 on the y-axis, the dot will be there in the shaded area of acute respiratory acidosis. The pCO_2 65 line will also pass through this point.

Example 2: A 40-hour-old term baby develops respiratory distress, poor feeding, and seizures. There is history of two siblings' deaths and consanguinity. ABG shows pH—7.0, pCO_2—16, pO_2—95, HCO_3—4, BE— −30.

pH—7.0 means acidosis, HCO_3—4 means metabolic, and actual pCO_2—16.

As per compensation formula, pCO_2 should be 16 (for every 10 decrease is HCO_3, $PaCO_2$ decrease 12).

Interpretation: Compensated metabolic acidosis.

In Example 2, if pCO_2 would have been 40 with a pH 7.0 (it means CO_2 has not fallen which it should have done in case of normal lungs in a spontaneously breathing patient), it would be mixed metabolic and respiratory acidosis. If the CO_2 remains 40 with a HCO_3 4, the pH will drop to 6.6. This highlights the importance of compensation.

CLINICAL APPLICATION

- PaO_2 in blood gas in a baby with respiratory distress can tell us about severity of lung disease by calculating gradient of partial pressure of oxygen between alveoli (PaO_2) and arterial blood (PaO_2). At sea level, the atmospheric pressure is 760 mm Hg and water vapor pressure is 47 mm Hg.

$$PaO_2 = FiO_2 * (Patm - pH_2O) - pCO_2/RQ$$
$$= FiO_2 * (760 - 47) - pCO_2 * RQ$$
$$(A\text{-}a)\ DO_2 = PaO_2 - PaO_2$$

Example 3: A neonate breathing room air is having PaO_2—80 mm Hg and $PaCO_2$—40 mm Hg. What is the alveolar arterial oxygen gradient?

$PaO_2 = FiO_2 * (760 - 47) - pCO_2/RQ = 0.21 \times 713 - 40/0.8 = 150 - 50 = 100$ mm Hg

$(A\text{-}a)\ DO_2 = PaO_2 - PaO_2 = 100 - 80 = 20$ mm Hg.

In newborns, gradient up to 40 mm Hg is normal due to physiologic shunts.

Example 4: A neonate breathing in 100% O_2 is having PaO_2—80 mm Hg and $PaCO_2$—40 mm Hg. What is the alveolar arterial oxygen gradient?

$PaO_2 = FiO_2 * (760 - 47) - pCO_2/RQ = 1.0 \times 713 - 40/0.8 = 713 - 50 = 663$ mm Hg.

This shows that the lungs of this baby are bad or there is cardiac problem. If there is hypoxemia with a normal gradient, it is because of a central cause with normal lungs.

ETIOLOGY OF METABOLIC ACIDOSIS

Anion gap (AG) can guide regarding this.

Anion gap = unmeasured anions – unmeasured cations = measured cations – measured anions
$$= (Na + K) - (HCO_3 + Cl).$$ Normal value is <16 mmol/L

Normal AG: When there is bicarbonate loss from body or rapid dilution of extracellular fluid (ECF). Chloride is proportionately increased in these conditions, e.g. diarrhea gastrointestinal tract (GIT) and renal loss of bicarbonate (renal tubular acidosis).

Increased AG: Addition of strong acid in system. For example lactic acidosis, organic acidemias.

Urinary anion gap (UAG) = (UA – UC) = $(Na^+) + (K^+) - (Cl^-)$

It is a rough index of urinary ammonium excretion. Ammonium is positively charged; so a rise in its urinary concentration will cause a fall in UAG.

Urinary anion gap differentiates between GIT and renal causes of a hyperchloremic metabolic acidosis. Remember GUT (ne GET ive), if UAG is negative the HCO_3 losses are from the GUT and if positive, the loss is from the kidneys.

KEY POINTS

➤ Keep clinical condition, previous ABG and therapeutic interventions in mind while interpreting the ABG report.
➤ As a dictum, if both pCO_2 and HCO_3 move in the same direction and are in the compensatory range, it is a simple disorder. If they move in the opposite directions, i.e. one is rising and the other is falling (or only one is changing), it is a mixed disorder.
➤ There is no need to supplement bicarbonate routinely in case of high AG metabolic acidosis. Instead correct underlying etiology like adequate ventilation and circulation in case of lactic acidosis due to hypoxia.

SELF ASSESSMENT

1. **A baby was born through meconium-stained amniotic fluid and was depressed at birth requiring tracheal suctioning. ABG is done and report is pH 7.25, $PaCO_2$ 40, HCO_3 18, BE –8. What is your interpretation?**
   a. Metabolic acidosis
   b. Compensated metabolic acidosis
   c. Metabolic alkalosis
   d. Mixed disorder

FURTHER READING

1. Rose BD, Post T, Stokes J. Clinical Physiology of Acid-Base and Electrolyte Disorders, 6th edition. New York: McGraw-Hill; 2015.

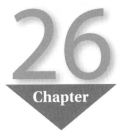

Retinopathy of Prematurity

26
Chapter

Harish Nayak, Kavitha Rao, Arvind Shenoi

INTRODUCTION

- Retinopathy of prematurity (ROP) is a potentially blinding, vasoproliferative disorder that affects the developing retinal vasculature of the premature infant.
- It is a complex disease that was reported by Terry in 1942, who named it retrolental fibroplasia, which represents the end stage of ROP with grayish white vitreous membranes and retinal detachment.
- It is entirely a disorder of the modern age, which is a consequence of the advances in medicine and technology that have helped to save increasingly premature infants.

INCIDENCE

- The incidence and severity of ROP varies remarkably with the main risk factors, gestational age, and birth weight.
- The large international landmark multicenter trials report an incidence of any ROP in infants under 1,250 g of around 66–70% and of serious ROP of 14–37%.

IMPORTANT RISK FACTORS

Risk factors known to be associated with ROP	Risk factors likely to be associated with ROP
• Gestational age • Birth weight • High exposure to oxygen for prolonged period • Sepsis • Respiratory distress syndrome • Multiple blood transfusion	• Apnea • Asphyxia • Jaundice • Intraventricular hemorrhage • Cardiac defects

PATHOGENESIS

Classically pathophysiology of ROP can be described in two phases:

- *Phase 1, Hyperoxic stage:* After birth, retinal vessels' growth slows or ceases. Cessation occurs largely as the result of a decrease in the level of growth factors, which is thought to be due to an increase in oxygen tension and low metabolic demand.
- *Phase 2, Hypoxic stage*: Retinal vessels proliferate in response to hypoxia of nonvascularized retina and increased metabolic demand. It is believed to be driven by increased growth

factors like vascular endothelial growth factor (VEGF) and insulin-like growth factor 1 (IGF 1). Initially, this process causes the formation of a visible tissue ridge (ROP stages 1, 2). As the disease progresses, vascular growth proliferates into the vitreous cavity (ROP stage 3). Eventually, there is involution of the blood vessels with cicatricial contraction, which can lead to tractional retinal detachment (ROP stage 4, 5).

- A particularly aggressive form of ROP called aggressive posterior ROP (APROP), which can progress very rapidly, cannot be explained by the classical pathophysiologic mechanism.

CLINICAL FEATURES

Retinopathy of prematurity is classified as its acute form and cicatricial (scarring)/involutional forms. Acute disease occurs in the initial phases of ROP. It can proceed through stages up to retinal detachment. Cicatricial disease follows occurrence of acute disease. It includes disease involution and regression, or tractional scar formation. The acute phase is seen between 30 weeks and 45 weeks, whereas cicatricial disease can start near term and can continue for months.

Classification

This is based on the International Classification of Retinopathy of Prematurity (ICROP) proposed in 1984 by the Committee for the Classification of Retinopathy of Prematurity. The severity of the acute disease is classified in stages 1–5 **(Table 1)**. The retina is divided into concentric zones I, II, and III to denote the location of the disease **(Table 1 and Fig. 1)**. The eye is classified into the highest stage present in any location and the most posterior zone affected by the disease. The retina is divided into 12 clock hours to classify the extent of each stage of disease.

Zones of ROP	The retina is divided into three concentric circles, each centered on the optic disc
Zone 1	Defined by a circle whose radius is twice the distance from the center of the optic disk to the center of macula (fovea)
Zone 2	Defined by a circle whose radius is the distance from the center of the optic disk to the nasal margin of the retina (ora serrata)
Zone 3	The remainder of the retina. This is crescent-shaped zone that largely involves temporal retina

Table 1: Staging of the severity of acute retinopathy of prematurity at the junction of vascular and avascular retina.	
Stage 1: Demarcation line	A flat, white line within the plane of the retina that separates the avascular retina anteriorly from the vascularized retina posteriorly
Stage 2: Ridge **(Fig. 2)**	A prominent line that has height and width and extends above the plane of the retina
Stage 3: Ridge with extraretinal fibrovascular proliferation **(Fig. 3)**	Extraretinal, fibrovascular proliferative tissue or neovascularization extends from the ridge into the vitreous
Stage 4: Partial retinal detachment	• Extrafoveal • Partial retinal detachment including the fovea
Stage 5: Total retinal detachment	Complete retinal detachment, mostly tractional and funnel shaped. The configuration of the funnel is described in anterior and posterior parts with an open or closed funnel

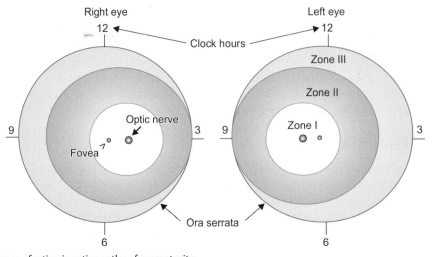

Fig. 1: Zones of retina in retinopathy of prematurity.

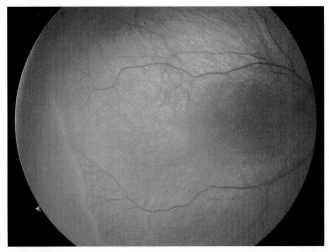

Fig. 2: Stage 2, Zone 2 retinopathy of prematurity.
Courtesy: Mr. David Clark, FRCOphth, Consultant Ophthalmologist, Aintree University Hospital, Liverpool, UK.

- Plus disease **(Fig. 4)** is said to exist when there is posterior venous dilation and arteriolar tortuosity of at least a photographically determined, minimum 2 or more quadrant. Iris vascular engorgement, poor pupillary dilatation (rigid pupil), and vitreous haze may also be present.
- Preplus denotes vascular abnormalities of the posterior pole that are insufficient for diagnosis of plus but more than normal.
- *APROP (Fig. 5)*: Aggressive posterior retinopathy of prematurity, previously called Rush disease is characterized by posterior location, rapidly evolving preplus and plus disease, and neovascularization that may be subtle or even intraretinal in nature. APROP is usually

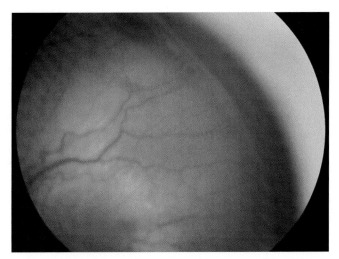

Fig. 3: Stage 3, Zone 2 retinopathy of prematurity.
Courtesy: Mr. David Clark, FRCOphth, Consultant Ophthalmologist, Aintree University Hospital, Liverpool, UK.

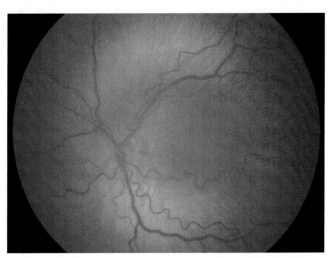

Fig. 4: Plus disease.
Courtesy: Mr. David Clark, FRCOphth, Consultant Ophthalmologist, Aintree University Hospital, Liverpool, UK.

seen in lowest birth weight infants, however, in India it has also been reported in bigger preterm infants commonly due to exposure to excessive oxygen in unblended form.

NATURAL HISTORY

The vast majority of patients with acute ROP undergo spontaneous regression:

- Regression may be heralded by the development of a clear zone of retina beyond the shunt, followed by the development of straight vessels crossing the shunt.
- Progression may occur to retinal detachment initially which can be exudative. Untreated there is a gradual cicatrization with variable degrees of fibrosis, contracture

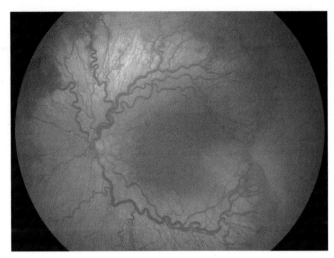

Fig. 5: Aggressive posterior retinopathy of prematurity .
Courtesy: Mr. David Clark, FRCOphth, Consultant Ophthalmologist, Aintree University Hospital, Liverpool, UK.

Box 1: Retinopathy of prematurity (ROP) National Neonatology Forum (India) screening guidelines.

Whom to screen?
- All babies born <34 weeks gestation age and/or <1,750* g birth weight
- Larger babies can also be screened till 34–36 weeks gestation age or 1,750–2,000 g birth weight if they have risk factors for ROP

When to screen?
- The first retinal examination should be done within first 4 weeks of age or 30 days of life in infants born ≥28 weeks of gestational age
- Smaller babies born <28 weeks gestation age or <1,200 g birth weight should be screened early, by 2–3 weeks of age, to detect APROP

(APROP: aggressive posterior ROP; ROP: retinopathy of prematurity)
*Universal Eye Screening in Newborns Including Retinopathy of Prematurity published by the Rashtriya Bal Swasthya Karyakram, Ministry of Health and Family Welfare, Government of India published June 2017 is similar to these except the birth weight cutoff is 2,000 g instead of 1,750 g.

---

of the proliferative tissue, vitreous and macular distortion, and finally tractional retinal detachment.

MANAGEMENT

Screening

The American Academy of Pediatrics recommends ROP screening for babies ≤1,500 g birth weight or ≤30 weeks gestational age and those infants >1,500 g or >30 weeks with an unstable clinical course or at high risk for ROP. In the United Kingdom, screening is recommended for those neonates that are <32 weeks gestation or have a birth weight of <1,501 g.

In India, the National Neonatology Forum (NNF) recommendations given in **Box 1** can be the basis for screening in any neonatal intensive care unit (NICU) in India.

- Examination is generally conducted by a retinal specialist or pediatric ophthalmologist experienced in ROP screening using an indirect ophthalmoscope or imaging device after pupillary dilation. This is done every week or once in 2 weeks depending on the location and severity of ROP.
- Screening is stopped when there is full retinal vascularization or entered Zone III without any previous ROP. Another criterion to stop screening is postmenstrual age of 50 weeks and no prethreshold disease/worse ROP is present. Documentation of the findings as in **Figure 1** with maintenance of records is an essential part of the care of the neonate with medicolegal implications.

PREVENTION

The measures undertaken to reduce ROP are listed in **Box 2**.

TREATMENT

Cryotherapy and Laser Photocoagulation

The landmark cryotherapy for retinopathy of prematurity (CRYO–ROP) trials established for the first time that ablation of the peripheral avascular retina as an effective form of therapy. The basis of this being the destruction of the avascular retina that stopped the angiogenic factors (VEGF, IGF1, etc.) from being produced leading to regression. The study described threshold ROP **(Box 3)** as a point to treat, which was the standard of care till the Early Treatment for Retinopathy of Prematurity (ETROP) trial where laser photocoagulation has replaced cryotherapy **(Fig. 6)**. The ETROP trial also determined the ideal point of treatment to be earlier which was defined as high-risk prethreshold ROP (also called type 1 ROP) given in **Box 4**.

Box 2: Measures that can be undertaken in the NICU to reduce ROP.

- Antenatal steroids for eligible mothers
- Ventilation and oxygenation measures
  - Early use of CPAP
  - Use of blenders and gentle ventilation
  - Mandatory pulse oximetry with targeting narrow oxygen saturation (90–93%)
- Prevention of sepsis
- Appropriate parenteral nutrition (especially in ELBW)
- Judicious use of blood transfusions

(CPAP: continuous positive airway pressure; ELBW: extremely low birth weight; NICU: neonatal intensive care unit; ROP: retinopathy of prematurity)

Box 3: Threshold and prethreshold retinopathy of prematurity (ROP) as defined by the CRYO–ROP study.

- Threshold disease signifies stage of retinopathy of prematurity with ROP of Stage 3 in Zone I or Zone II with extraretinal fibrovascular proliferations of at least 5 continuous or 8 cumulative clock hours with plus disease
- Prethreshold disease signifies ROP in Zone I of any stage; Zone II of Stage 2 with plus disease or Stage 3 less than threshold

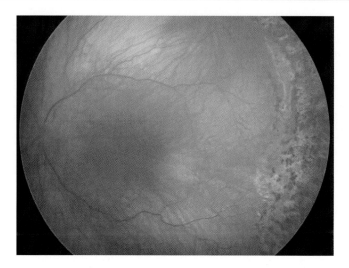

Fig. 6: Postlaser.
Courtesy: Mr. David Clark, FRCOphth, Consultant Ophthalmologist, Aintree University Hospital, Liverpool, UK.

Box 4: Prethreshold classification used for ETROP study.

- Type 1 (high-risk prethreshold, treat with peripheral retinal ablation)
- Zone I ROP of any stage with plus disease; Stage 3 without plus disease
- Zone II ROP Stage 2 or 3 with plus disease
- Type 2 (low risk, observe)
- Zone I ROP of Stage 1 or 2 without plus disease
- Zone II ROP of Stage 3 without plus disease

(ETROP: Early Treatment for Retinopathy of Prematurity)

Anti-VEGF Treatment

Intravitreal injection of anti-VEGF drugs, mainly Bevacizumab has shown great promise in blocking the neovascular response and permitting further vascularization of the retina in ROP. This can be beneficial in preservation of more of the peripheral retina (which is ablated in laser therapy) and possibly reduce the incidence of large refractive errors.

As there are significant concerns of possible long-term systemic complications primarily of brain development, it is not used routinely in ROP. Currently it is mainly used when laser photocoagulation is not possible or fails to cause regression, in cases of Zone I ROP (APROP) where even the macula is not fully vascularized and in retinal detachment with lot of vascularity to reduce intraoperative bleeding. The ideal dose to be administered by intravitreal injection is yet to be established with varying doses from 0.16 mg to 0.625 mg.

SURGERY

Eyes that develop ROP Stage 4 or 5 require surgical intervention. Surgery is usually scleral buckling or a lens-sparing vitrectomy to alleviate the vitreoretinal traction causing

> **Box 5:** Complications and sequelae of retinopathy of prematurity.
> - Refractive errors—myopia, astigmatism, anisometropia
> - Strabismus
> - Amblyopia
> - Cataract
> - Glaucoma—angle closure or pupillary block
> - Macular dragging
> - Tractional retinal detachment

retinal detachment. Eyes undergoing surgical intervention at Stage 4A have relatively more favorable outcomes.

FOLLOW-UP

Children born prematurely have significantly higher ocular morbidity if they have developed ROP **(Box 5)** and they need to have long-term eye care follow-up.

KEY POINTS

➤ Retinopathy of prematurity is a potentially blinding, vasoproliferative disorder of developing retinal vasculature of the premature infant.
➤ Standard screening protocol to detect ROP should be followed in premature infants.
➤ Peripheral ablation and/anti-VEGF should be offered in type 1 ROP.

SELF ASSESSMENT

1. **Which of the following cannot be explained by classical pathophysiology of ROP?**
   a. Preplus ROP
   b. ROP with plus disease
   c. APROP
   d. Type 2 ROP

2. **As per ETROP classification, type 1 ROP includes all except:**
   a. Zone II ROP, stage 2 with plus
   b. Zone I ROP, stage 1 with plus
   c. Zone I ROP, stage 3 without plus
   d. Zone II ROP, stage 3 without plus

FURTHER READING

1. Cryotherapy for Retinopathy of Prematurity Cooperative Group. Multicenter trial of cryotherapy for retinopathy of prematurity: ophthalmological outcomes at 10 years. Arch Ophthalmol. 2001;119(8):1110-8.
2. Good WV; Early Treatment for Retinopathy of Prematurity Cooperative Group. Final results of the early treatment for Retinopathy of Prematurity (ETROP) randomized trial. Trans Am Ophthalmol Soc. 2004;102:233-50.
3. National Neonatology Forum, India. Evidence Based Clinical Practice Guidelines. 2011. p. 253. [online] Available from: www.nnfpublication.org [Last accessed on September, 2019].

Neonatal Sepsis

Anita Singh

INTRODUCTION

Neonatal sepsis is responsible for 1 million deaths worldwide and accounts for more than 25% of all neonatal deaths.

DEFINITION

Neonatal sepsis is a clinical syndrome characterized by signs and symptoms of infection with or without bacteremia during first month of life.

CLASSIFICATION

Neonatal sepsis has been classified as early and late onset sepsis based on age of presentation. Early onset sepsis presents within 72 hours of life and late onset sepsis manifest after 72 hours of life. Early onset sepsis may be acquired from maternal genital tract and usually presents with pneumonia. On the other hand, late onset sepsis may be either acquired from the community or could be healthcare associated and commonly presents with septicemia, pneumonia, or meningitis.

Neonatal sepsis incorporates various systemic infections such as septicemia, pneumonia, meningitis, septic arthritis, osteomyelitis, and urinary tract infections (UTIs).

Probable sepsis: Clinical and laboratory findings consistent with bacterial infection without positive blood culture.

Proven sepsis: Clinical features along with isolation of pathogens from blood or cerebrospinal fluid (CSF) or urine or abscess or pathological evidence of sepsis on autopsy. It is also called bloodstream infection (BSI) and reported as episodes per 1,000 patient days.

Neonatal meningitis: Positive cerebrospinal fluid culture, Gram staining, or neutrophilic leukocytosis, with or without low sugar (less than 50% of plasma glucose level) and high protein content.

Central-line-associated bloodstream infection (CLABSI): Having a central line (umbilical or nonumbilical) for more than 24 hours before the day of onset of blood culture-positive sepsis. It is reported as number of episodes per 1,000 catheter days.

Ventilator-associated pneumonia (VAP): An episode of pneumonia in a patient who requires a device to assist or control respiration through a tracheostomy or endotracheal tube within 48 hours before the onset of the infection. It is reported as episodes per 1,000 ventilated days.

Bloodstream infection, CLABSI, and VAP are used as indices for audit and quality improvement for sepsis in neonatal intensive care units (NICUs).

INCIDENCE

According to National Neonatal Perinatal Database (NNPD) 2002–2003, incidence of:
- Neonatal sepsis is 30 per 1,000 live births
- Meningitis is 3 per 1,000 live births.

In a recent study from India, the incidence of sepsis was 14.3% and that of culture-positive sepsis was 6.2%. Early onset sepsis was two-thirds of total cases and gram-negative septicemia occurred in 64% of cases [Delhi Neonatal Infection Study (DeNIS) collaboration].

In another population-based study from India by Panigrahi P et al., the incidence of culture-positive sepsis was 6.7/1,000 births and gram-negative infections were the most common (51%). *Klebsiella pneumoniae* was the predominant organism. Gram-positive organism constituted 26% of positive cultures (mostly *Staphylococcus aureus*).

IMPORTANT RISK FACTORS

For early onset sepsis	For late onset sepsis
• Low birth weight (LBW) or prematurity	• LBW
• Febrile illness in mother with evidence of bacterial infection 2 weeks prior to delivery	• Preterm
• Foul smelling and/or meconium stained liquor	• Admission to neonatal intensive care unit
• Prolonged rupture of membrane >18 hours	• Mechanical ventilation
• Single unclean or >3 sterile vaginal examination during labor	• Central line
• Prolonged labor (sum of 1st and 2nd stage >24 hours)	• Prolonged parenteral nutrition
• Perinatal asphyxia (Apgar < 4 at 1 minute)	• Indiscriminate use of antibiotics
• Clinical chorioamnionitis	• Unhygienic feeding
• *Criteria of chorioamnionitis are*:	• Prelacteal/bottle feed
Maternal fever of >38 °C (100.4 °F) and at least two of the following criteria:	• Poor cord care
– Maternal leukocytosis >15,000 cells/cc	• Use of H2 blocker
– Maternal tachycardia >100 beats/minute	
– Fetal tachycardia >160 beats/minute	
– Uterine tenderness	
– Foul odor of the amniotic fluid	

ETIOPATHOGENESIS

As per NNPD 2002–03, amongst intramural births, *Klebsiella pneumoniae* was the most frequently isolated pathogen (32.5%), followed by *Staphylococcus aureus* (13.6%). Among extramural neonates, *Klebsiella pneumoniae* was again the most common organism (27%), followed by *Staphylococcus aureus* (15%), and *Pseudomonas* (13%). In the recent Delhi Neonatal Infection Study, *Acinetobacter spp* (22%), *Klebsiella spp* (17%), and *Escherichia coli* (14%) were the most common responsible pathogens.

Pathogenesis of neonatal sepsis is multifactorial. Factors directly attributable to the neonate include humoral, phagocytic, and cellular deficiencies. Underdeveloped immune systems, vertical transmission from maternal genital tract, disruption of neonatal host defense, and direct introduction of bacteria to neonatal blood from invasive procedures are important factors.

CLINICAL FEATURES

The manifestations of neonatal sepsis involve almost each system and can be summed up as below:

Generalized	Respiratory	Gastrointestinal	Central nervous system (CNS)
• Temperature instability • Refusal to feed • Bleeding/petechiae/purpura • Multiple pustules/sclerema/mottling • Umbilical redness and discharge. • Generalized edema/capillary leak syndrome • Direct hyperbilirubinemia	• Cyanosis • Respiratory distress • Apnea and gasping respiration *Cardiovascular* • Bradycardia/tachycardia • Low blood pressure • Poor perfusion • Shock • Decreased urine output	• Feed intolerance • Vomiting • Diarrhea • Abdominal distension • Paralytic ileus • Necrotizing enterocolitis *Metabolic* • Unexplained acidosis • Hyper/hypoglycemia	• Excess irritability/lethargy • Hypotonia, absent/weak neonatal reflexes • Bulging anterior fontanelle • High-pitched/poor cry • Seizures • Neck retraction/hypertonia

INVESTIGATIONS

Sepsis Screen

The components of sepsis screen include five parameters:

Component	Abnormal value
Total leukocyte count	<5,000/cc
Absolute neutrophil count	Low count as per Manroe's chart for term and Mouzinho's chart for very low birth weight infants **(Figs. 1 and 2)**
Immature/total neutrophil count	>0.2
Microerythrocyte sedimentation rate (in millimeter at the end of first hour)	>3+ age in days in the first week of life or >10 thereafter
C-reactive protein	>1 mg/dL
Presence of 2 or more components is considered as positive sepsis screen	

- Total leukocyte count, absolute neutrophil count, and immature-to-total leukocyte count are affected by several factors such as labor, maternal hypertension, perinatal asphyxia, and prolonged crying and therefore have significant limitation in the diagnosis of neonatal sepsis.
- *C-reactive protein (CRP):* It is an acute phase reactant which is synthesized by the liver. It takes 10–12 hours for CRP to change significantly after onset of infection. It has a half-life of 24–48 hours. CRP can be raised in several noninfectious conditions such as meconium aspiration syndrome, birth trauma or asphyxia, hemolysis, or chorioamnionitis. Repetitive

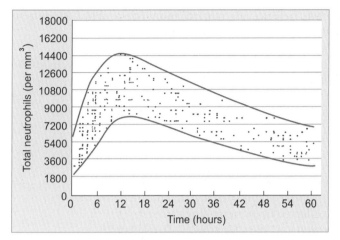

Fig. 1: Manroe's chart for absolute neutrophil count of term neonates.

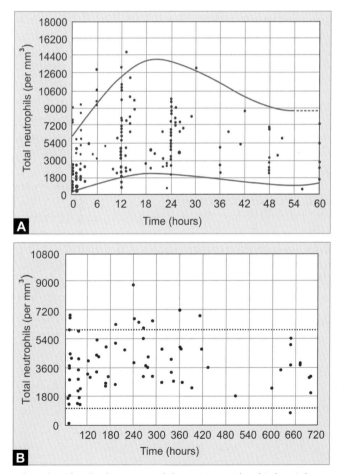

Figs. 2A and B: Mouzinho's chart for absolute neutrophil count in very low birth weight neonates.

normal CRP levels help to rule out infection. Sequential CRP determination to decide antimicrobial therapy cannot be recommended.

- In suspected early onset sepsis, sepsis screen is not helpful.
- Sepsis screen in neonates has a poor positive predictive value (<30%); however, a high (>99%), negative predictive value has been observed in many studies.
- Two consecutive sepsis screens repeated after 24–48 hours have 97% negative predictive value for sepsis.

Blood Culture

- Gold standard and definitive.
- Should be collected by sterile technique.
- Minimum 1 mL sample should be taken in culture bottle.
- Should not be collected from indwelling catheter.
- Should be observed for 7 days for growth of organism.
- BACTEC and BACT/ALERT system can detect even 1–2 colony forming units and within 12–24 hours.
- A new technology called matrix-assisted laser desorption ionization time-of-flight (MALDI-TOF) can help in early identification of the organisms from blood culture and helps in directed antibiotic therapy.

Cerebrospinal Fluid Examination

- Neonatal meningitis occurs in 0.3–3% of cases of neonatal sepsis.
- The indications of CSF analysis include late onset sepsis, blood culture-positive cases, and presence of neurological signs. In all cases, where empirical antibiotics are being started, ideally a CSF analysis should be done.
- In case a neonate is critically sick, it could be postponed.
- Cerebrospinal fluid is positive in 25% cases of blood culture-positive sepsis. Blood culture may be negative in 38% cases of meningitis.
- Cerebrospinal fluid should be sent for cell count total and differential, Gram stain/fungal stain, protein, sugar, and culture.
- Defining cutoffs for interpretation of meningitis is difficult as cell count, protein and glucose values of normal neonates is very variable. One cutoff has been suggested below for term and preterm babies. This cutoff is based on presumption of 5% prevalence of meningitis in hospitalized infants and best cutoff as per likelihood ratio and post-test probability.

Meningitis—indication for treatment	
Preterm neonate:	*Term neonate:*
Treat if:	Treat if:
• CSF WBC count ≥10 OR	• CSF WBC count >8 OR
• Glucose <24	• Glucose <20
OR	OR
• Protein >170	• Protein >120
Do not treat if:	
• CSF WBC count <25 AND	
• Glucose ≥25	
AND	
• Protein <170	

(WBC: white blood cell)

- If a neonate with meningitis shows inadequate clinical response to antibiotics after 48 hours of therapy, a repeat lumbar puncture (LP) should be done.
- Even if CSF contains blood due to traumatic LP, the CSF should be still sent for Gram stain and culture. In such scenario, a low CSF glucose may still be helpful for diagnosis of meningitis.
- Gram-negative bacteria usually take longer time to clear from the CSF (approximately 5 days) whereas gram-positive bacteria clear in much shorter time (approximately 36 hours) of appropriate therapy.

Urine Culture

- Low yield in early onset sepsis.
- Should be done in all cases of late onset sepsis.
- Obtained by suprapubic puncture or catheterization.
- High index of suspicion of UTI should be kept in:
  - Fungal sepsis
  - Very low birth weight (VLBW) infants
  - Poor weight gain
  - Known urinary tract abnormalities
  - Ongoing bladder catheterization
- Suprapubic aspiration is ideal method of sample collection in suspected UTI.
- UTI may be diagnosed in the presence of one of the following:
  - >10 WBC/cc in a 10 mL centrifuged sample.
  - $>10^4$ organisms/mL in urine obtained by catheterization and
  - Any single organism in urine obtained by suprapubic aspiration.

Newer Markers of Neonatal Sepsis

- *Procalcitonin:* It is an acute phase reactant produced both by hepatocytes and macrophages. It rises more rapidly than CRP (3–6 hours of infection) and plateaus after approximately 12–24 hours. Its level correlates well with severity. However, it can also be physiologically elevated during first 3 days of life, in neonates who required resuscitation at birth or who have history of maternal chorioamnionitis without evidence of neonatal infection.
- Cytokines such as interleukin 6, 8, and TNF-α usually peak early in cases of neonatal infections. However, levels of these cytokines become normal even if infection persists. Combination of these tests with CRP improves diagnostic accuracy.
- Other newer markers are:
  - Cell surface markers: CD 11β, CD64
  - Tumor necrosis factor α
  - Inter α inhibitor proteins (IAIP)
  - Polymerase chain reaction (PCR)—amplification of 16S rRNA.

Table 1 shows diagnostic accuracy of various markers in neonatal sepsis.

Other Tests should be Performed as Clinically Indicated

- Chest X-ray in case of suspected pneumonia.
- Abdomen X-ray in case of suspected necrotizing enterocolitis.
- Neuroimaging in case of meningitis.
- Coagulation profile in presence of bleeding.

Table 1: Diagnostic value of markers in neonatal sepsis.

Diagnostic test	Sensitivity (%)	Specificity (%)	PPV	NPV	Likelihood ratio (+)	Likelihood ratio (–)
WBC ≤ 5,000 or ≥25,000	44	92	36	94	5.5	0.60
I:T ratio >0.244	54.6	73.7	2.5	99.2	2.07	0.61
Platelets < 150,000 cells/cc	22	99	60	93	2.72	0.78
CRP > 1 mg/dL	70–93	78–94	7–43	97–99.5	3.18–15.5	0.07
PCT > 5.38 ng/mL	83.3	88.6	83.33	88.57	6.9	0.19
IL-6 > 100 pg/mL	87	93	76	97	12.42	0.14
IL-8 > 300 pg/mL	91	93	91	97	13	0.10
TNF-α > 13 pg/mL	75	88	67	51	6.25	0.28
IAIP ≤ 177 mg/L	89.5	99	95	98	89.5	0.11

(CRP: C-reactive protein; IAIP: inter-alpha inhibitor proteins; IL6: interleukin-6; IL8: interleukin-8; I:T ratio: immature to total neutrophil ratio; NPV: negative predictive value; PCT: procalcitonin; PPV: positive predictive value; TNF-α: tumor necrosis factor α; WBC: white blood cell)

MANAGEMENT

Management of neonatal sepsis can be summarized as.

Supportive

- Nurse in thermoneutral environment.
- Respiratory support should be in form of invasive or noninvasive ventilation. Oxygen saturation should be in target range.
- Fluid resuscitation and inotrope support to maintain tissue perfusion.
- Glucose infusion/insulin to take care of hypo/hyperglycemia.
- Blood components for anemia and bleeding.
- Correction of electrolyte imbalance.
- Optimization of nutrition (enteral/parenteral).

Antimicrobial Treatment

- No single recommendation can be made for all cases.
- Decision to start antibiotics depends upon clinical features and positive sepsis screen.
- Empirical antibiotic therapy should be unit-specific and based on the prevalent spectrum of etiological agents and their antibiotic sensitivity pattern. It should be reviewed periodically as per microbiological updates about organisms and sensitivity.
- De-escalation and escalation should be based on antibiotic culture sensitivity reports.
- Choice of antibiotics should be used according to organism and antibiotic sensitivity.
- A simplified algorithm for starting antibiotics in case of suspected sepsis is given in **Flowcharts 1 and 2**.
- Once the blood culture is available, antibiotic with narrower spectrum should be chosen depending on the sensitivity report.

Selection of antibiotic

Community-acquired sepsis:
- Ampicillin + Gentamicin/Amikacin (empirical)
- If evidence of *Staphylococcus*: Cloxacillin + Gentamicin/Amikacin
- If evidence of meningitis: Add Cefotaxime

Hospital-acquired infection:
- Antibiotic choice should be based on local guidelines and antibiotic sensitivity pattern of last few months

No clinical improvement in 48–72 hours or worsening status such as deranged perfusion/worsening respiratory status/need for ventilation—consider to change antibiotics as per culture/sensitivity report
- Piperacillin-tazobactam and aminoglycosides
- Carbapenems/aztreonam
- Colistin (should be reserved for multidrug resistant infections)

Flowchart 1: Algorithmic approach for antimicrobial treatment in asymptomatic neonates with risk factor for sepsis.

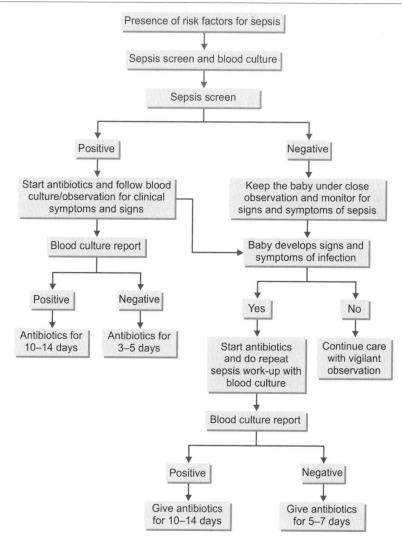

Flowchart 2: Algorithmic approach for antimicrobial treatment in symptomatic neonates with suspected sepsis.

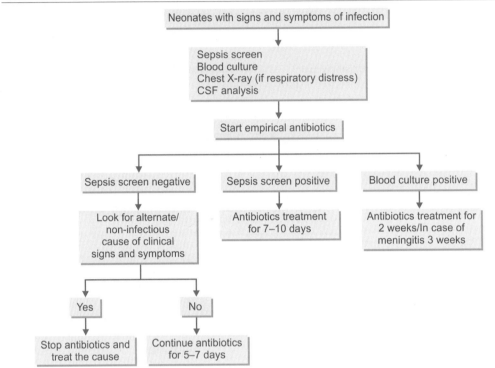

(CSF: cerebrospinal fluid)

- Generally a single sensitive antibiotic should be used except in case of *Pseudomonas* where two sensitive antibiotics should be used.
- Vancomycin should not be used for methicillin-sensitive *Staphylococcus aureus*.
- Duration depends upon positive blood culture, organism, and presence of meningitis.

Duration of antibiotic treatment	
Culture and sepsis screen negative but clinical course compatible with sepsis	5–7 days
Culture negative sepsis screen positive but clinical course consistent with sepsis	7–10 days
Blood culture positive but no meningitis	10–14 days (except in *Staphylococcus aureus* where 14 days is must)
Meningitis with or without positive blood/CSF culture	21 days
Urinary tract infection	7–14 days
Ventriculitis	6 weeks
Bone/joint infection	Up to 6 weeks out of which 4 weeks must be intravenous

Adjunctive Therapy

- Blood exchange transfusion (double volume) can be contemplated in cases of worsening clinical picture and presence of sclerema. The clinical condition should be good enough to allow the procedure.

- *Pentoxifylline*—recent evidence from some studies showed benefit in use of pentoxifylline as an adjunctive therapy to decrease mortality related to sepsis without any adverse effects. For practical use, more evidence is required from large studies.
- Current evidence does not support role of intravenous immunoglobulin, granulocyte infusion, granulocyte/granulocyte-macrophage colony stimulating factor (G/GM-CSF), probiotics, and lactoferrin as adjunctive therapy in neonatal sepsis.

A description of adjunctive intervention which has been tried in neonatal sepsis has been given in **Table 2**.

Table 2: Adjunctive intervention in neonatal sepsis.

Intervention	Prophylaxis/ treatment	Mechanism	Level of evidence	Conclusion
Exchange transfusion	Treatment	Remove toxins and harmful circulating cytokines, enhance immunoglobulins	Prospective cohort studies and RCTs	Has been found to improve survival
Pentoxifylline	Treatment	Xanthine derivative, phosphodiesterase inhibitor, increase adenylyl cyclase, decrease TNF-α, anti-inflammatory	Small RCTs	Has been found to improve survival in small studies
IVIG (Polyclonal)	Both prophylaxis and treatment	Provide opsonic activity, activate complement, and promote antibody-dependent cytotoxicity	Prospective cohort studies and RCTs	No significant benefit
IgM enriched IVIG	Treatment	Pentameric IgM confers superior toxin neutralization and bacterial agglutination	RCTs	No significant benefit
Granulocyte transfusion	Treatment	Enhance neutrophil numbers and function	Systematic review of RCTs	No benefit
G-CSF or GM-CSF	Treatment	Enhance neutrophil (G-CSF) or neutrophil and macrophage (GM-CSF) numbers	Systematic review of RCTs	• No difference • May improve survival in neutropenic babies
Antioxidants (selenium/ melatonin)	Prophylaxis	Component of glutathione peroxidase, antioxidant, and free radical scavenger	Systematic review	• No difference in mortality • May improve sepsis status
Glutamine	Prophylaxis	Anabolic for dividing immune and gut cells	Systematic review of RCTs	No difference in mortality or sepsis or disability free survival
Lactoferrin	Prophylaxis	Antimicrobial and anti-inflammatory	RCTs	Reduce late onset sepsis
Probiotics	Prophylaxis	Enhance local and systemic immunity, anti-inflammatory, suppress pathogenic organisms associated with NEC	Systematic reviews of RCTs	Reduce all-cause mortality and NEC

Contd…

Contd...

Intervention	Prophylaxis/ treatment	Mechanism	Level of evidence	Conclusion
Prebiotics	Prophylaxis	• Promote growth of beneficial bacteria and other probiotics in colon • Reduce growth of pathogens in gut	Systematic reviews of RCTs	No difference
Breast milk	Prophylaxis	Contains secretory IgA, cellular defenses, antimicrobial proteins and peptides	RCTs	Reduces sepsis
Broad-spectrum peripartum antibiotics	Prophylaxis	Reduce probiotic colonization in gut; down-regulate genes coding for antimicrobial products	RCTs and Cohort studies	Increases NEC and has poor neurodevelopment in follow-up

(G-CSF: granulocyte colony-stimulating factor; GM-CSF: granulocyte macrophage colony stimulating factor; IVIG: intravenous immunoglobulin; NEC: necrotizing enterocolitis; RCT: randomized controlled trial; TNF-α: tumor necrosis factor α)

PREVENTION OF NEONATAL SEPSIS

- Hand hygiene
- Promote breastfeeding and use of human milk
- Establishment of early enteral feeding in VLBW infants
- Proper disinfection and asepsis in neonatal intensive care units (NICUs)
- Antibiotic restriction and written policy for antibiotic usage
- Prevent overcrowding and understaffing of NICU
- Surveillance of neonatal infections.

KEY POINTS

- ➢ Neonatal sepsis is associated with high morbidity and mortality.
- ➢ Clinical signs are nonspecific and can involve any organ system.
- ➢ Blood culture is the gold standard for diagnosis.
- ➢ Supportive therapy and targeted antibiotic are the mainstay of treatment.
- ➢ Every unit should have a written antibiotic policy to prevent abuse of antibiotics.
- ➢ Good clinical practices should be adopted in units to prevent sepsis.

SELF ASSESSMENT

1. **Which of the following is false?**
   a. There is no role of sepsis screen in early onset sepsis.
   b. Lumbar puncture should be done in all cases of suspected sepsis in whom empirical antibiotic is being started except those based on risk factors for early onset sepsis.
   c. Lumbar puncture should only be done in cases of positive blood culture.
   d. Sepsis screen has high negative predictive value for sepsis.

2. **Which of the following is false?**
   a. Antibiotics should be upgraded in cases of deteriorating cardiorespiratory status in neonates with sepsis preferably after 48–72 hours of therapy and it should be based on culture and sensitivity report.
   b. Current evidence supports some role of pentoxifylline in late onset therapy as an adjunctive therapy.
   c. Intravenous immunoglobulin should be given in all cases of neonatal sepsis.
   d. Exchange transfusion is usually reserved in cases of sepsis with sclerema if the neonate can expectedly tolerate the procedure.

FURTHER READING

1. Dutta S, Kadam S, Saini SS. Management of neonatal sepsis. In: Kumar P, Jain N, Thakre R, et al. (Eds). Evidence Based Clinical Practice Guidelines. New Delhi, India: National Neonatology Forum of India; 2010.
2. Investigators of the Delhi Neonatal Infection Study (DeNIS) collaboration. Characterisation and antimicrobial resistance of sepsis pathogens in neonates born in tertiary care centres in Delhi, India: a cohort study. Lancet Glob Health. 2016;4(10):e752-60.
3. Panigrahi P, Chandel DS, Hansen NI, et al. Neonatal sepsis in rural India: timing, microbiology and antibiotic resistance in a population-based prospective study in the community setting. J Perinatol. 2017;37(8):911-21.
4. Shane AL, Sánchez PJ, Stoll BJ. Neonatal sepsis. Lancet. 2017;390(10104):1770-80.

Care of Extremely Low Birth Weight Infants

Chapter 28

Kumari Gunjan

INTRODUCTION

- Extremely low birth weight (ELBW) babies are those born with a birth weight of <1,000 g. These babies have special needs because of being physiologically immature.
- Extremely low birth weight infants are at high risk of morbidity and mortality and require tertiary intensive care for survival.
- Antenatal considerations include use of antenatal steroids, magnesium sulfate, antenatal counseling by neonatologist explaining the prognosis based on expected weight, gestation, singleton or multiple, sex and antenatal steroid coverage, delivery in a hospital with a well-equipped neonatal intensive care unit (NICU), and in-utero transport in case of expected preterm delivery that requires transfer to another unit.
- Standardized and protocolized care of ELBW infants should include prenatal consultation, delivery room (DR) management, optimizing ventilation strategies, fluid/electrolytes, nutritional management, providing cardiovascular support, management of patent ductus arteriosus (PDA), and stringent infection control policy.

CARE IN DELIVERY ROOM

National and institutional guidelines should be followed for limits of viability. Parents should be counseled in detail about anticipated outcomes and decision about resuscitation should be made before birth. ELBW infants need specialized care right at the time of birth. A team of neonatologists capable of performing all steps of neonatal resuscitation should be present at delivery. Current Neonatal Resuscitation Program (NRP) guidelines should be followed during resuscitation.

Cord Clamping

- Current neonatal resuscitation guidelines recommend delayed cord clamping (DCC) at birth (variably defined as delay >30 seconds or until pulsation is no longer detected) if baby does not require immediate resuscitation.
- Delayed cord clamping helps in providing additional 30% volume of blood in ELBW infants thereby improving pulmonary blood flow and increasing left ventricular preload.

- Compared with immediate cord clamping (ICC), DCC helps in improving short-term outcome in ELBW infants including higher blood pressure, hemoglobin on admission, reduced requirement of blood transfusion during NICU stay, decreased risk of intraventricular hemorrhage (IVH), and necrotizing enterocolitis (NEC).

Thermoregulation

- Extremely low birth weight infants are at high risk of developing hypothermia and active measures at birth include prewarming DR to 26°C, using warmed humidified resuscitation gases, occlusive wrapping, polyethylene caps, and warm transport to NICU.
- Both hypothermia and hyperthermia should be avoided and a temperature of 36.5°–37.5°C should be targeted. There is a dose-related risk of mortality with a rise of mortality by 30% for each degree fall in temperature from 36.5°C at admission.

Respiratory Support in Delivery Room

These neonates often require respiratory support at birth owing to pulmonary immaturity that includes surfactant deficiency and excessively compliant chest wall.

Continuous Positive Airway Pressure

- Routine use of DR continuous positive airway pressure (CPAP) has shown to decrease the need for intubation in preterm infants >24 weeks of gestational age.
- Recent meta-analysis of randomized controlled trials on use of CPAP versus prophylactic surfactant has shown that early use of CPAP in DR is associated with reduced risk of death or bronchopulmonary dysplasia (BPD).

Sustained Inflation

- Use of sustained inflation (SI) in DR has been reported to reduce intubation and mechanical ventilation, oxygen use, and incidence of BPD in NICU.
- However, Cochrane review did not show these benefits. Currently consensus on use of SI in DR is lacking and hence it is not recommended outside trials.

Oxygen use in Delivery Room

- Current neonatal resuscitation guidelines 2015 recommend initial resuscitation of preterm infant <35 weeks at birth with FiO_2 of 21–30% and titrate oxygen requirement as per recommended minute specific saturation targets. (Refer to Chapter 1—Neonatal Resuscitation)
- Beyond DR, oxygen saturation should be targeted in the range of 90–95%.

Use of Positive Pressure Ventilation, Intubation, and Use of Surfactant

- Extremely low birth weight infants at birth may have inadequate respiratory drive requiring positive pressure ventilation (PPV) or may have respiratory distress at birth requiring respiratory support. In spontaneously breathing infants, CPAP should be initiated early as it may decrease the need for intubation.

Table 1: Care of ELBW infants in delivery room (DR).	
Cord clamping	Delayed cord clamping—hematological benefits, decrease risk of IVH and NEC
Thermoregulation	• Both hypothermia and hyperthermia should be avoided • Additional measures such as occlusive wrap, polyethylene cap, warm delivery room, warm humidified resuscitation gases, and warm transport should be undertaken
Respiratory support	
Delivery room CPAP	• Maintains functional residual capacity (FRC) • Avoids intubation and mechanical ventilation
Sustained inflation	No consensus on its routine use
Oxygen use in DR	Follow NRP 2015 guidelines. In <35 weeks gestation, initiate resuscitation with 21–30% and follow target saturation guidelines
Positive pressure ventilation, intubation, and surfactant use in delivery room	• Use preferably T-piece device to deliver PPV • Early rescue with surfactant in infants who are intubated at birth or fail CPAP should be practiced • INSURE technique reduces subsequent need for mechanical ventilation • *MIST*: Minimally invasive methods of surfactant administration are under investigation and showed good initial results

(CPAP: continuous positive airway pressure; ELBW: extremely low birth weight; INSURE: intubation, surfactant, and extubation; IVH: intraventricular hemorrhage; MIST: minimally invasive surfactant therapy; NEC: necrotizing enterocolitis; NRP: Neonatal Resuscitation Program; PPV: positive pressure ventilation)

- Positive pressure ventilation at DR should be preferably provided by T-piece resuscitator providing optimum peak inspiratory pressure (PIP) and positive end expiratory pressure (PEEP). Infants who fail to achieve adequate respiratory drive despite PPV or CPAP may require intubation in DR. It is advisable to administer surfactant early in DR in case intubation is required. INSURE (Intubation, surfactant, and extubation) technique of administering surfactant has resulted in subsequent reduced rates of mechanical ventilation. Minimally invasive surfactant therapies (MISTs) are under investigation and reported to decrease the need for mechanical ventilation and BPD **(Table 1)**.

MAJOR PROBLEMS OF EXTREMELY LOW BIRTH WEIGHT INFANTS (TABLE 2)

Respiratory System

- Extremely low birth weight infants are likely to have surfactant deficiency, low functional residual capacity (FRC), decreased lung compliance, and increased chest wall compliance leading to respiratory distress syndrome and may require surfactant therapy.
- Delivery room CPAP has reduced the need for surfactant and mechanical ventilation. However, still a large proportion of these infants may require intubation, surfactant, and PPV leading to ventilator-associated lung injury (VALI), air leak syndromes, and BPD. These infants, in addition, are prone to have apnea of prematurity due to immature central nervous system and respiratory physiology.

Table 2: Major problems of extremely low birth weight infants.

System	Short-term problem	Long-term problem
Respiratory system	• Surfactant deficiency disorders • Air leaks • Apnea of prematurity • Intermittent hypoxemia • Ventilator-associated lung injury • Bronchopulmonary disease	• Chronic lung disease • Reactive airway disease in childhood
Gastrointestinal system	• Feed intolerance • Necrotizing enterocolitis • Growth failure	• Extrauterine growth retardation • Osteopenia of prematurity
Immunologic function	• Immature cellular and humoral immunity • Exposed to multiple risk factors for early onset sepsis	RSV, pertussis and other viral/bacterial infections
Central nervous system	• Intraventricular hemorrhage • Periventricular white matter disease	• Cerebral palsy • Neurodevelopmental delay • Hearing loss
Ophthalmologic	Retinopathy of prematurity	• Blindness • Retinal detachment • Refractive errors, astigmatism, myopia and strabismus
Cardiovascular	Hypotension, patent ductus arteriosus	Hypertension and coronary artery disease in adulthood
Fluid and electrolyte imbalance	• Excessive fluid loss • Immature renal system • Renal tubular acidosis • Electrolyte imbalance	
Hematological	• Excessive phlebotomy losses • Frequent transfusion • Anemia of prematurity	
Endocrine	• Hypothyroxinemia of prematurity • Delayed TSH rise • Cortisol deficiency	Impaired glucose regulation; insulin resistance

(RSV: respiratory syncytial virus; TSH: thyroid stimulating hormone)

Gastrointestinal System

- Feed intolerance in the form of vomiting and abdominal distension is frequent finding in ELBW neonates owing to immaturity of the gut physiology.
- Integrity and function of gastrointestinal system often gets compromised in ELBW neonates owing to prematurity, altered gut microbiota, increased susceptibility to infection and ischemia predisposing them to NEC. Exclusive breast milk feeds have been shown to reduce the incidence of NEC.

Immunological Function

- Extremely premature infants have immature adaptive immunity and immunological memory.

- Hypogammaglobulinemia and low complement activity have also been reported in premature infants.

Central Nervous System

- Data from different centers across the world suggest improved survival of ELBW neonates; however, survival has been associated with risk of neurological morbidity.
- Intraventricular hemorrhage, periventricular leukomalacia (PVL), seizures, NEC, and long-term ventilation are significant risk factors for adverse neurological outcomes.
- Intraventricular hemorrhage can occur in 20–30% of ELBW infants, owing to fragile and highly vascularized germinal matrix and disturbance in cerebral blood flow.

Ophthalmological

- Birth weight and gestational age are major risk factors for retinopathy of prematurity (ROP).
- Extremely low birth weight infants have increased risk of severe ROP and need for treatment. Prolonged ventilation, shock, sepsis, growth failure, and blood transfusion are known risk factors for ROP.

Cardiovascular System

- Patent ductus arteriosus is very common with incidence as high as 80% in ELBW infants.
- The presence of hemodynamically significant PDA is associated with increased morbidity, NEC, BPD, and neurodevelopmental impairment. Definitive management is still controversial (refer to Chapter 13—Patent Ductus Arteriosus in Preterm Infants).

Fluid and Electrolyte Imbalance

- Extremely low birth weight neonates are prone to fluid and electrolyte imbalance owing to increased transepidermal loss and immature renal system.
- This leads to contraction of extracellular fluid compartment and hypernatremia. Electrolytes should be evaluated at least once in 24 hours in first few days of life for maintaining optimum fluid and electrolyte balance.

Hematological System

Physiological anemia of infancy is exaggerated in ELBW infants due to reduced life span of RBC, excessive phlebotomy losses, diminished erythropoietin response, early postnatal drop in Hb (4–6 weeks of age) and lower nadir (7–8 g/dL).

MANAGEMENT IN NEONATAL INTENSIVE CARE UNIT (TABLE 3)

Weight Measurement

During first week, weight pattern should be followed closely to titrate fluid prescription. Once these infants have regained birth weight, documentation of weight pattern helps in identifying growth failure at an earlier stage.

Table 3: Management in neonatal intensive care unit.

Weight measurement	• At admission, thereafter at 8–12 hours interval in the first few days to guide fluid management • Later daily for growth assessment
Surfactant administration	Administered if indicated
Vascular access	• Early insertion of UAC and UVC as indicated • Replace after 7–10 days after replacing with peripherally inserted central catheters
Skin care	• Avoid use of alcohol or chlorhexidine • Apply minimal adhesive tapes • Hydrocolloid/pectin based tapes preferred • Use of warm cotton ball and emollient to remove adhesion
Fluid and electrolyte	• Initial fluid requirement—started at the rate of 100 mL/kg/day • Increment—guided as per weight and serum sodium values • Use of warm humidified incubators • Serum electrolyte and blood sugar monitoring
Ventilation	• Early use of CPAP—start with PEEP of 6–8 cm of water and titrate FiO_2 as per saturation • Heated humidified high-flow nasal cannula may be an acceptable alternative to CPAP (easy to use, less nasal trauma, better comfort but variable pressure delivery) • In case of failure of CPAP such as PEEP more than 8 cm of water and FiO_2 >0.5, recurrent apneas or severe respiratory acidosis, mechanical ventilation may be indicated • Lowest pressures required to deliver optimum tidal and maintain adequate oxygenation should be used • Volume targeted ventilation versus pressure limited ventilation—reduced risk of death, BPD, air leak, combined outcome of PVL and grade III and IV IVH • Avoid hypoxia and hyperoxia—target saturation between 90% and 95% • Minimal ventilation—initial pCO_2 target of 45–55. Higher pCO_2 may be acceptable in CLD • Rescue high frequency ventilation may be as a rescue therapy or in those with air leak syndromes as lung protective strategy • Use of periextubational caffeine and postextubation use of CPAP decreases extubation failure
Nutrition	• Early parenteral nutrition as soon as possible • Early administration of amino acid—to prevent catabolism • Early human milk feeding • Use of human milk fortifiers
Management and prevention of infection	• In case of perinatal risk factors for sepsis, screen for sepsis and start antibiotics empirically and discontinue promptly at 48 hours of negative growth • Increased risk of late onset sepsis—start antibiotics empirically if indicated • In NICUs with high incidence of sepsis, fluconazole prophylaxis can be started at a dose of 3–6 mg/kg twice weekly • Minimal handling and preventive strategies for infection should be applied

(BPD: bronchopulmonary dysplasia; CLD: chronic lung disease; CPAP: continuous positive airway pressure; IVH: intraventricular hemorrhage; NICUs: neonatal intensive care units; PEEP: positive end expiratory pressure; PVL: periventricular leukomalacia; UAC: umbilical arterial catheters; UVC: umbilical venous catheters)

Fluid and Electrolytes

- Fluids requirement increases exponentially in ELBW infants with decreasing gestation due to increased insensible losses owing to poor skin maturity, large head-to-body ratio, and renal immaturity.
- Use of humidified incubators can decrease transepidermal fluid loss and lead to lesser requirements of fluids.

Vascular Access

- Umbilical arterial catheters (UACs) and umbilical venous catheters (UVCs) may be placed especially in those infants requiring mechanical ventilation or those with hemodynamic instability.
- Central arterial lines are generally retained for 7–10 days and then may be replaced by a peripheral line if required. UVCs should be removed by 14 days and percutaneous insertion of a central catheter (PICC) lines can be inserted if required.
- Long lines are associated with complications such as bleeding, thrombosis, sepsis, effusion, and dislodgment. Utmost care should be taken to maintain asepsis during insertion and maintenance of these central lines to prevent central line-associated blood stream infection.

Skin Care

- Skin care of ELBW babies is extremely fragile due to nonexistent stratum corneum. There is greater risk of epidermal stripping with use of adhesives. These factors are responsible for susceptibility to infection and delayed wound healing.
- Use of chlorhexidine and alcohol is not recommended in this population to avoid burns. Emollient application and use of wet cotton balls to remove adhesive may help to reduce excessive stripping.

Ventilation

- Use of noninvasive ventilation in the form of nasal CPAP and noninvasive mechanical ventilation (NIMV) not only helps in maintaining FRC for adequate gas exchange but also avoids endotracheal intubation.
- Despite all efforts to avoid invasive ventilation approximately 60% of the ELBW babies will eventually need mechanical ventilation. The main goal of lung protective strategies in intubated preterm infants can be achieved by minimizing volutrauma (volume targeted ventilation), atelectotrauma (lung recruitment, by use of surfactant and providing PEEP; open lung concept, high frequency ventilation), and oxygen toxicity by titrating FiO_2 to saturations targets.
- Frequent assessments for readiness of extubation may avoid both prolonged ventilation and premature extubation. Periextubational use of caffeine and postextubation use of nasal CPAP may reduce rates of extubation failure.

Nutrition

- Due to premature delivery, ELBW infants are born with limited nutrient stores. It is often difficult to establish enteral feeds owing to immature gut and enzymes and decreased motility. Inadequate nutrition is responsible for growth failure which in turn has neurodevelopmental consequences.

- Parenteral nutrition may act as a safe means to meet nutrient requirements during initial week of life till enteral nutrition can be fully established. Prolonged parenteral nutrition may result in line-related sepsis, cholestasis, and osteopenia of prematurity. Gradual introduction preferably with human milk (mother's own milk/donor human milk) followed by progressive advancement is advisable.
- Breast milk has shown to be protective in reducing incidence of NEC but unfortified human milk often results in extrauterine growth retardation. Human milk fortifiers (dose as per manufacture's recommendation) should be added to meet the caloric and protein deficit of ELBW infant.

Infection

- In preterm births with peripartum risk factors for sepsis, workup including blood culture should be sent and empirical antibiotics should be started. Antibiotics should be discontinued once blood culture is documented to be negative.
- Extremely low birth weight infants are vulnerable to develop late onset sepsis due to risk factors such as prolonged IV access, parenteral nutrition, and mechanical ventilation. A high index of suspicion should be kept due to initial nonspecific manifestation which, if not addressed timely, results in catastrophic deterioration. Invasive procedures should be minimized and if at all needed should be carried out in full aseptic precaution.
- Hand washing is the most effective intervention to prevent cross infection among this vulnerable population. Auditing hand hygiene practices, minimizing duration of mechanical ventilation, early enteral feeds preferably human milk, removal of central lines once not required are some of the good practices that can reduce the risk of hospital acquired infections.
- The preventive management for major complications of ELBW infants is summarized in **Table 4**.

RECOMMENDATION FOR SCREENING

Intraventricular Hemorrhage

- The risk of IVH increases with decreasing gestational age due to structural fragility and cerebral blood flow instability. Additional risk factors include chorioamnionitis, lack of antenatal glucocorticoid exposure, neonatal transport, hypotension, sepsis, and aggressive ventilation. Majority of IVH occurs in first 72 hours of life.
- In all ELBW infants, screening for IVH should be done by cranial ultrasonography (USG) at 7 days and later USG is to be repeated at 36–40 weeks of postmenstrual age. Also it should be done at any point of time when there is abnormal clinical signs suggestive of IVH.

Retinopathy of Prematurity

- As stated above, prematurity and low birth weight are strongest risk factors for ROP requiring treatment. In addition prolonged ventilation, sepsis, shock, transfusion, low

Table 4: Preventive management for major complications of ELBW.

Complication	Prevention
IVH	• Minimal handling, avoid rapid changes in BP or ventilator settings, avoid rapid IV boluses/avoid use of hyperosmolar solutions such as bicarbonate
Bronchopulmonary dysplasia	• Vitamin A supplementation: 5,000 IU intramuscular thrice weekly • *Caffeine*: Early use of caffeine • Cautious use of systemic corticosteroids • *Nutrition*: Fluid restriction and increased calorie density • Gentle ventilation, use of noninvasive ventilation, and lung protective strategies • Prevention and prompt treatment of systemic infections
Retinopathy of prematurity	• Judicious use of oxygen • Maintain target saturations 90–94% in NICU • Prevention and early treatment of infection • Optimum nutrition to achieve adequate growth
Necrotizing enterocolitis	• Use of human milk (either mother's own milk or donor milk) • Protocolized feeding policy
Acute kidney injury	• Maintain fluid and electrolyte balance • Avoid use of nephrotoxic drugs

(BP: blood pressure; ELBW: extremely low birth weight; IVH: intraventricular hemorrhage; NICU: neonatal intensive care unit; IV: intravenous)

caloric intake, hyperglycemia all of which occur frequently in ELBW infants also are known to be independent risk factors for ROP.

- First screening in ELBW neonates is recommended earlier at 2–3 weeks of postnatal age to reduce the risk of missing aggressive posterior ROP. Guidelines for screening and treatment of ROP are discussed in Chapter 13—Retinopathy of Prematurity.
- Timely recognition of this entity will result in prompt treatment by laser photocoagulation and off lately by anti-VEGF (vascular endothelial growth factory) and prevent blindness due to further progression to retinal detachment.

Hearing Loss

- Extremely low birth weight neonates are at increased risk for hearing impairment due to associated risk factors such as sepsis, exposure to ototoxic drugs (antibiotics and diuretics), and prolonged ventilation/hospital stay.
- Early intervention approach calls for an early screening (not before 34 weeks) and to be repeated at 3 months to take a decision for initiating early intervention/s at 6 months.

KEY POINTS

➢ Special stress should be given on thermoregulation of ELBW neonates to prevent hypothermia.

➢ Use of noninvasive ventilation and avoiding invasive ventilation would help to reduce risk of VALI and BPD.

➢ In case of intubation in DR or at admission to NICU, early surfactant therapy is desirable followed by extubation as soon as feasible.

> Extremely low birth weight neonates are very vulnerable to excessive fluid loss and subsequent dyselectrolytemia. Fluids and electrolyte homeostasis need to be maintained with frequent monitoring and adjustments.
> Aggressive parenteral nutrition should be initiated from the very first day followed by establishment of enteral nutrition preferably with human breast milk (mother's own milk or donor human milk).
> Prevention, early detection, and treatment of sepsis are of utmost importance to prevent morbidity and mortality.
> Routine screening protocols for IVH, ROP, PVL and hearing should be followed for timely detection and early intervention.

SELF ASSESSMENT

1. **What is the most appropriate DR temperature?**
   a. 21–23°C
   b. 23–24°C
   c. 25–26°C
   d. 29–31°C

2. **Delayed cord clamping is associated with all except**
   a. Reduced risk of IVH
   b. Reduced risk of NEC
   c. Reduced risk of BPD
   d. Reduced need for transfusion

FURTHER READING

1. Gleason C, Juul S. Avery's Diseases of the Newborn, 10th edition. US: Elsevier; 2017.
2. Nosherwan A, Cheung PY, Schmölzer GM. Management of Extremely Low Birth Weight Infants in Delivery Room. Clin Perinatol. 2017;44(2):361-75.

29 Chapter

Transport of the Sick Neonate

Anurag Fursule

INTRODUCTION

- Sick neonates may require transport for further care to another healthcare facility. Although in-utero transport remains the safest mode of transfer, it may not be feasible always necessitating the need for ex-utero transport of neonates.
- Neonatal transport is continuously evolving and has become the backbone of modern perinatal medicine.
- Unorganized transport may lead to hypothermia, hypoglycemia, and hemodynamic disturbances therefore increasing the risk of neonatal morbidity and mortality. Organized transport is challenging yet rewarding aspect of neonatology.
- The transport scenario in India is still primitive. However, progress has been made in some government initiatives and private sectors. Many private institutions have their own transport systems responsible for transfers to their centers only. On the other hand, government has implemented transport services in some part of the country. An example is transport services in the model of public–private partnership (PPP) established by Government of Andhra Pradesh.

INDICATIONS OF TRANSPORT

The indications of transport in neonates are listed below:

• Very low birth weight infants especially below 1,250 g	• Seizures
• *Prematurity*: Gestational age <32 weeks	• Multiorgan involvement
• Respiratory distress or apnea	• Sepsis with signs of systemic infection
• Requiring supplemental oxygen	• Jaundice with potential for exchange transfusion
• Apnea requiring bag and mask ventilation	• Active bleeding from any site
• Cyanosis persisting despite oxygen therapy	• Infant of diabetic mother or hypoglycemia unresponsive to recommended treatment
• Hypoxic ischemic encephalopathy	• Surgical conditions
• Requiring intubation and assisted ventilation	• Congenital heart disease (antenatal diagnosis or suspected)
• Suspected metabolic disorder	• Heart failure or arrhythmia
• Severe electrolytes abnormalities	• Infants requiring special diagnostic and/or therapeutic service

TYPES OF TRANSPORT

Types of transport
• Home to hospital
• Intrahospital transport (including delivery rooms, operation theaters, for neuroimaging and special procedures)
• Facilitation of specialist management of the neonate (movement to a regional center for cardiac, neurological, renal or surgical opinion)
• Retrieval from a peripheral hospital for ongoing intensive care (example—when mothers deliver prematurely without warning)
• Returning infants to local neonatal units following care elsewhere (either locally or long distance)—reverse transport

MODES OF TRANSPORTATION

Types of vehicle	Distance	Advantages	Disadvantages
Ground ambulance	10–200 km	• Less prone to weather changes • Transport vehicles may be better equipped • Better patient access due to spacious interiors	• Slowest mode of transport • Need to secure neonatal incubator and other equipment physically inside the transport vehicle
Rotor wing aircraft	50–300 km	Less time taken for patient retrieval	• Requires a landing space near the hospital • Adverse weather conditions may lead to grounding of the aircraft • Costlier • Patient intervention is difficult due to noisy environment and high vibration levels • Restricted patient access during flight
Fixed wing aircraft (airplane)	>250 km	• Economical due to relatively low fuel costs over long distance • Patient access is better	• Adverse weather conditions may lead to grounding of the aircraft • Needs an airport for take-off and landing • Ground transfer may require additional time

PROBLEMS WITH AIR TRANSPORT

Air leaks	It may become worse since air expands at higher altitudes and so even small leaks should be drained before transport. Cabin pressure should be set to that of sea level in case of meconium aspiration syndrome and pneumothorax
Low partial pressure of oxygen	At high altitude, partial pressure of oxygen becomes lower even after cabin pressurization, i.e. oxygen becomes rarer. A neonate requiring very high $FiO_2 > 80\%$ may not be fit for air transfer and should be stabilized first. Care should be taken to minimize hypoxia
Risk of intraventricular hemorrhage (IVH)	Risk of IVH may increase during taking off and landing (sudden acceleration and deceleration)
Temperature	As altitude increases, there is drop in temperature (drop of 2°C for every 300 m of altitude). Thermoneutral environment should be maintained with help of transport incubator, transwarmer mattresses, hats or phase changing material
Noise and vibration	Vibrations may dislodge tubings and lines thus a close watch is advisable. In order to minimize artifacts use of pulse oximeter with Masimo technology is recommended

NEONATAL TRANSPORT SYSTEM COMPONENTS

Human resource	The traditional neonatal transport team includes doctor, nurse/paramedical staff

Vehicle	• A minivan/SUV or a VAN can be used/modified to neonatal transport needs
	• Ambulance used should have:
	  – Source of compressed gases—air and oxygen
	  – Power source—battery connected to appropriate adapters useful for connecting incubators, syringes, and monitor
	  – System for secure fixation of incubators

Communication and family support	• Communication before transport parents should be communicated regarding:
	  – Bed availability at the receiving center
	  – Clinical condition of the baby before transport
	  – Any necessary procedure before transport (e.g. endotracheal intubation, central line insertion)
	  – Severity and duration of illness
	  – Cost of care
	  – Implications of transport on baby (e.g. risk of IVH during transport, etc.)
	• Communication during transport—can be maintained by mobile phones. Live tracking of the transport vehicle can be done remotely
	• After transport to the treating hospital—the transport team should brief about demographic details and clinical status of the baby

Documentation and consent forms	All transport calls should be documented accurately including details of transport times (call received, dispatch notified, transport commenced, length and various other time parameters) and team members involved in the transport. Patient history, condition of the patient, and management should be duly noted

Equipment	*Thermal support*	*Respiratory support*	*Suction*	*Monitoring*	*Parenteral infusion*	*Medications*
	• Transport incubator • Thermometer • Plastic wrap/ insulating blanket	• Oxygen/Air cylinder • Flow meter • Oxygen tubing • Oxygen hood • Pulse oximeter • Mechanical ventilator with backup circuit and battery • Endotracheal tube • Laryngoscope • Tape to secure	• Mucus suction trap • Suction regulator • Feeding tube • Sterile glove • Sterile water for irrigation	• Stethoscope • Pulse oximeter • Glucometer	• IV catheter • Syringes • Splint • Adhesive tape • Stopcock • Microdrip set • Syringe pumps • Transparent dressing	• Calcium gluconate 10% • Epinephrine • Dopamine • Dobutamine • Morphine • Midazolam • Normal saline • Phenobarb • Surfactant

STEPWISE APPROACH TO NEONATAL TRANSPORT HAS BEEN LAID DOWN BY NNF

Assesment: Assess the baby

Temperature: Correct hypothermia, utilize KMC/incubator/phase-changing material/warm clothing

Airway: Check for secretion, clear airway

Breathing: Assess respiratory distress, ventilatory need

Circulation: HR, pulse, urine output, CRT, BP

Sugar: Manage hypoglycemia with 10% dextrose

Transport personnel: ASHA/paramedic

Equipment: Ambulance

CARE DURING TRANSPORT

Monitor	Temperature, breathing, perfusion, oxygen saturation
Feeds	Sick babies are kept nil per oral, stable babies can be fed
Procedures	Avoid performing any procedure in moving vehicle
Clinical deterioration	In case of clinical deterioration, transport vehicle should be stopped and stabilization/resuscitation should be started

TRANSPORT IN SPECIFIC CONDITIONS

Conditions	Specific instructions
Respiratory distress syndrome	Babies with respiratory distress should be managed with appropriate modality of ventilation. Oxygenation and perfusion should be maintained throughout the transport
Air leak syndromes	Pneumothorax may worsen during the transport. Chest tube should be placed before transportation and fixed firmly to avoid dislodgement
Esophageal atresia	To prevent pulmonary aspiration, a continuous suction should be done with the help of two catheters (one attached to suction and the other left open to air)
Meningomyelocele	A gauze piece soaked in normal saline should be used to cover the exposed swelling on the back. Avoid putting the baby on the back and preferably lateral position should be adopted during transport

MODELS/SCORING SYSTEM IN TRANSPORT

Prior to transport and during transport stabilization of the neonate should be a priority. Some of the models are mentioned here. Certain scores can be used following transport for assessment of the baby such as MINT or TRIPS.

Pretransport stabilization models	Predicting mortality post-transport
TOPS: Temperature, oxygenation, perfusion and sugar	*MINT:* Mortality index for neonatal transportation
STABLE: Sugar, temperature, airway, blood pressure, laboratory work, and emotional support	*TRIPS:* Transport risk index of physiological stability
PSSAT: Pretransport stabilization self-assessment tool	

MEDICOLEGAL ISSUES DURING TRANSPORT

Majority of medicolegal issues during transport occur as a consequence of the poor communication and provision of inadequate information.

If the baby deteriorates or dies during transport:

- The ambulance should be stopped immediately and cardiopulmonary resuscitation (CPR) should be initiated as per Neonatal Resuscitation Program (NRP) guidelines.
- If baby dies on the way, he/she should be first taken to the nearest health facility.
- Casualty admission should be done. Parents should be explained and updated about baby's condition.
- Transporting team is responsible for making death certificate of baby.

QUALITY MANAGEMENT

Quality assurance is now an important aspect of patient care in medicine. Quality management programs should assess all aspects of transport including manpower, management of vehicle, training, operational and safety issues. Audits should be done to ensure quality assurance of transport systems.

KEY POINTS

- ➢ Neonatal transport services are still in developmental phase in India and remain a challenge.
- ➢ Organized neonatal transport constitutes trained personnel, equipment, logistics, and quality improvement program.
- ➢ Pretransport care and stabilization for maintaining temperature, oxygenation, perfusion, and blood sugars are important aspect of transport.

SELF ASSESSMENT

1. **What kind of suction is required during transport of a baby with esophageal atresia?**
    a. Continuous suction with one catheter.
    b. Continuous suction with two catheters.
    c. Continuous suction with two catheters with one left open to air.
    d. Continuous suction with two catheters with both open to air.

2. **For every 300 m of altitude, there is a drop in temperature by:**
   a. 1°
   b. 2°
   c. 3°
   d. 4°

3. **At high altitude, the need for oxygen in a baby may increase/decrease?**

FURTHER READING

1. Kler N, Thakur A. Neonatal transport: Systemic disorders and social pediatrics. In: Gupta P, Menon PS, Ramji S, Lodha R (Eds). PG Text Book of Pediatrics, Volume 3. New Delhi: Jaypee Brothers Medical Publishers; 2017.
2. National Neonatology Forum. Evidence Based Clinical Practice Guidelines. India: National Neonatology Forum; 2010. pp. 253-64.

30 Chapter

Pain Management in Neonate

Arun Soni, Ajoy Kumar Garg, Aakriti Soni

INTRODUCTION

It was a common belief that neonates do not perceive pain and till late 1980s even neonatal surgery was conducted under minimal anesthesia. But this myth came to end when various neurophysiological studies indicated that the anatomic and physiologic systems for pain perception are adequately developed by as early as 18–20 weeks of gestation.

- At around 8th week of gestation, cutaneous sensory receptors first appear in the perioral region. By 18th week of gestation, they are present in nearly all mucous surfaces.
- During 6th week of gestation, synapses between peripheral sensory fibers and dorsal horn interneurons begin to appear in the spinal cord and are mature by 20 weeks of gestation.

NEONATAL RESPONSE TO PAIN

- Neonates respond to noxious stimuli by release of stress hormones like catecholamines, glucocorticoid, growth hormones, and other stress hormones. This brings about nonspecific physiological, behavioral, and biobehavioral response. The lack of verbal skills, immature, behavioral, and nonspecific physiological response makes pain assessment in neonates quite difficult and challenging.
- Self-reporting using validated scales which is the gold standard of pain assessment cannot be applied to neonates. Healthcare providers must rely on nonspecific physiologic, behavioral, and biobehavioral indicators as a surrogate for self-reporting as illustrated in **Table 1**.

Table 1: Physiologic, behavioral, and biobehavioral response to pain.		
Physiologic/autonomic response	*Behavioral response*	*Biobehavioral response*
Fluctuations in heart rate, blood pressure, oxygen saturation, respiratory rate, intracranial pressure, color change, pallor, flushing	Crying, facial expressions, body movements, change in tone, fist clenching, changes in sleep-wake cycles, activity levels, fussiness or irritability	Increase in catecholamine, growth hormone and endorphins, cortisol, glucagon, and aldosterone and decrease in insulin secretion leads to increased serum glucose, lactate, and ketones

ASSESSMENT OF PAIN IN NEONATES

Using above clues, various pain scoring tools have been developed. More than 40 discrete scoring tools exist till date to assess pain in neonates but only few neonatal pain scales have undergone rigorous psychometric testing. But it is important to know, understand, and train the nursing staff on scoring systems which will be practical in day-to-day practice for the individual unit. Common tools for assessing pain in neonates are outlined in **Table 2**.

Table 2: Commonly used neonatal pain scoring tools.

Assessment tools	Physiologic indicators	Behavioral indicators	Gestational age tested	Nature of pain assessed
PIPP: Premature infant pain profile	Heart rate, oxygen saturation	Brow bulge, eyes squeezed shut, nasolabial furrow	28–40 weeks	Acute procedural and postoperative pain
CRIES: Crying, Requires Oxygen Saturation, Increased Vital Signs, Expression, Sleeplessness	Heart rate, oxygen saturation	Crying, facial expression, sleeplessness	32–36 weeks	Postoperative pain
NIPS: Neonatal Infant Pain Scale	Respiratory patterns	Facial expression, cry, movements of arms and legs, state arousal	28–38 weeks	Procedural pain
N-PASS: Neonatal Pain Agitation and Sedation Scale	Heart rate, respiratory rate, blood pressure, oxygen saturation	Crying, irritability, behavior state, extremities tone	0–100 days of age	Ongoing and acute pain and sedation
NFCS: Neonatal Facial Coding System	None	Facial muscle group movement	Preterm and term till 4 months of age	Procedural pain
PAT: Pain Assessment Tool	Respirations, heart rate, oxygen saturation, blood pressure	Posture, tone, sleep pattern, expression, color, cry	Neonates	Acute pain
SUN: Scale for Use in Newborns	Central nervous system state, breathing, heart rate, mean blood pressure	Movement, tone, face	Neonates	Acute pain
EDIN: Échelle De La Douleur Inconfort Nouveau-Né (neonatal pain and discomfort scale)	None	Facial activity, body movements, quality of sleep, quality of contact with nurses, consolability	25–36 weeks (preterm infants)	Prolonged pain
BPSN: Bernese Pain Scale for Neonates	Heart rate, respiratory rate, blood pressure, oxygen saturation	Facial expression, body posture, movements, vigilance	Term and preterm neonates	Acute pain

MODALITIES OF PAIN PREVENTION AND MANAGEMENT

The pain management in neonate can be broadly classified as nonpharmacological or pharmacological interventions.

Nonpharmacological Interventions

Best nonpharmacological modality of pain management is avoidance of unnecessary painful procedure by planning all nonemergent sampling and laboratory investigations. It includes bundling of procedures with blood sampling, placement of central line or arterial line if prolonged intravenous access or frequent sampling is required, use of noninvasive or minimal invasive modalities for monitoring of blood gas, electrolyte, hemoglobin level, bilirubin level wherever possible. There are various nonpharmacological pain relieving modalities available, which are effective in reducing pain from minor procedures in neonates. These include use of oral sucrose/glucose, breastfeeding, expressed breast milk, non-nutritive sucking, kangaroo mother care, facilitated tuck, swaddling, soothing music therapy, vocalization, perfumes, gentle massage therapy, and developmental care designed to alter environmental and behavioral components. Non-pharmological interventions are more effective when used in combination.

Pharmacological Interventions

These include use of topical, local, systemic analgesic, and anesthetic agents. Most common used in combination with nonpharmacological modalities for alleviating moderate-to-severe pain in neonate. Choice of therapy depends upon procedure, gravity of the pain, and its potential adverse effects. **Table 3** gives the various pharmacological interventions along with its doses.

*Optimal approach to neonatal pain management should include (**Table 4**):*
- Reducing the frequency of painful procedures.
- Reducing environmental stressors.
- Facilitating development supportive care.
- Determining the best technique to minimize the pain and stress associated with procedures.
- Delegating responsibility for pain assessment and treatment to the bedside nursing staff.
- Using a balanced multimodal approach to pain control.
- When pharmacologic intervention is necessary for pain control, use the least amount of drug that controls the pain.

Long-term effect of pain in neonates:
- Frequent pain and stress during the neonatal period are linked to adverse long-term outcomes.
- Biochemical responses to pain like elevations of the levels of cortisol, catecholamines, lactate and glucose instability, and physiological changes like hypertension, tachycardia, respiratory instability, and changes in cerebral blood flow affect developing organs including brain.
- Pain and stress experienced by developing brain during early infancy is associated with altered pain perception, abnormal cortisol responses to stress in later infancy and at school age. It has potential deleterious effects on long-term memory, social and cognitive development, and neural plasticity.

Table 3: Pharmacological intervention along with its doses which will help managing pain in neonates.

Drugs	Doses	Comments
Opioid analgesics		
Morphine	Loading dose: 0.05–0.1 mg/kg IV in 60 minutes; Infusion dose: 0.01–0.04 mg/kg/hr	Respiratory, central nervous system depression, hypotension constipation, nausea, urinary retention
Fentanyl	Loading dose: Fentanyl 0.5–3 µg/kg IV in 30 minutes; Infusion dose: 0.5–3 µg/kg/hr	Advantages over morphine: • More potent than morphine • Causes less histamine release • Reduce pulmonary vascular resistance Rapid infusion can cause chest wall rigidity so it must be administrated over a minimum of 3–5 minutes
Alfentanil	Loading dose: 5–10 µg/kg IV; Infusion dose: 0.5–1 µg/kg/hr IV	Advantages: • Fast acting • Unaffected by liver metabolism Used in ventilated neonates only
Nonopioid analgesics		
Paracetamol	10–15 mg/kg (IV/oral)	Doses interval: 6–8 hourly <32 weeks: 7.5 mg/kg
Ibuprofen	5–10 mg/kg po	Every 12–24 hours
Sedatives		
Midazolam	Loading dose: 0.1 mg/kg Maintenance dose: 0.05–0.1 mg/kg/hr	No analgesic effect Used as adjuvant to analgesia as sedative
Lorazepam	0.02–0.1 mg/kg IV	
Dexmedetomidine	Bolus doses for short procedural sedation 1–3 µg/kg or continuous IV infusion 0.25–0.6 µg/kg/hr	Selective α-2-adrenergic receptor agonist Advantage: Does not produce significant respiratory depression
Chloral triclofos sodium	30–50 mg/kg po/per rectal	Used for sedation without analgesia caution in preterm and young term neonates
Topical and local anesthetics		
Lidocaine 1%	2–4 mg/kg buffered with sodium bicarbonate 1:10	Maximum dosage 5 mg/kg
Oxybuprocaine 0.4% and tetracaine 1% eye drops	1 drop per eye	
Eutectic mixture of local anesthetic (EMLA cream) lidocaine (2.5%) and prilocaine (2.5%)	Single 0.5 g (Max 1 g) dose applied for 1 hour	Applied 1 hour before the procedure on the area where anesthesia is desired and then cover with an occlusive dressing Not effective for heel lance

Table 4: Common procedure in NICU and their pain managements.

Source of pain	Management of pain	Comments
Routine care	Nonpharmacologic measures	Development supportive care Nonpharmacological modalities are used for all procedure
Heel stick	Use of mechanical lance	Venipuncture is more efficient, less painful; local anesthetics, acetaminophen, heel warming does not reduce heel stick pain
Venipuncture	Use topical local anesthetics	Requires less time and less resampling than heel stick
Arterial puncture	Use topical and subcutaneous local anesthetics	More painful than venipuncture
IV cannulation	Topical local anesthetics	—
Central line placement	Topical local anesthetics Low-dose opioids or deep sedation based on clinical factors	Some centers prefer using general anesthesia
Subcutaneous injection	Topical local anesthetics if procedure cannot be avoided	Avoid if possible
Intramuscular injection	Topical local anesthetics	—
Lumbar puncture	Topical local anesthetic, lidocaine infiltration, careful positioning	Use IV analgesia/sedation, if patients are intubated and ventilated
Peripheral arterial line	Topical local anesthetic, lidocaine infiltration, consider IV opioids	—
Circumcision	Topical local anesthetic, lidocaine infiltration, IV/PO acetaminophen before and after procedure	Lidocaine infiltration for distal, ring, or dorsal penile nerve blocks (DPNB); liposomal lidocaine is more effective than DPNB
Suprapubic bladder aspiration	Topical local anesthetic, lidocaine infiltration, consider IV fentanyl (0.5–1.0 µg/kg)	—
Arterial or venous cutdown	Topical local anesthetic, lidocaine infiltration, IV fentanyl (1–2 µg/kg), consider deep sedation	Most arterial or venous cutdowns can be avoided, consider referral to interventional radiology
Peripherally inserted central catheter (PICC)	Topical local anesthetic, lidocaine infiltration, consider IV fentanyl (1 µg/kg) or IV ketamine (1 mg/kg)	Some centers prefer using deep sedation or general anesthesia
ECMO cannulation	Propofol 2–4 mg/kg, ketamine 1–2 mg/kg, fentanyl 1–3 µg/kg, muscle relaxant as needed	—
Mechanical ventilation	Morphine, fentanyl remifentanil, alfentanil, sufentanil	Not used routinely
Intercostal drains	IV opioid, adequate local analgesia (lidocaine), or both	

Contd...

Contd...

Source of pain	Management of pain	Comments
Tracheal intubation	Give fentanyl (1 µg/kg) or morphine (10–30 µg/kg), with midazolam (50–100 µg/kg), ketamine (1 mg/kg), use muscle relaxant only if experienced clinician, consider atropine	All newborns should receive analgesic premedication for endotracheal intubation except for emergency intubations during resuscitation or newborns in whom instrumentation of the airway is likely to be extremely difficult; superiority of one drug regimen over another has not been investigated
Retinal examination and surgery for retinopathy of prematurity	Sucrose, anesthetic drops opiate-based pain relief	Shield the eyes for 4–6 hours and decrease sources of light
Gastric tube insertion	Consider local anesthetic gel	Perform rapidly, use lubricant, avoid injury
Chest physiotherapy	Gentle positioning, fentanyl (1 µg/kg) if a chest tube is present	Avoid areas of injured or inflamed skin, areas with indwelling drains or catheters
Removal of intravenous catheter	Solvent swab, consider nonpharmacologic measures	
Wound treatment	Use topical local anesthetics, consider low-dose opioids, or deep sedation based on extent of injury	
Umbilical catheterization	IV acetaminophen (10 mg/kg), avoid sutures to the skin	Cord tissue is not innervated, but avoid injury to skin
Tracheal extubation	Use solvent swab for tape, consider nonpharmacologic measures	
Dressing change	Topical local anesthetic, consider deep sedation if extensive	
Postoperative analgesia		
Nonventilated	Morphine:10–50 µg/kg IV bolus over 15 minutes with formal pain/comfort scoring at 5-minute intervals until analgesia is optimal; maintenance: 0–20 µg/kg/hr IV Regular paracetamol (caution after 48 hours)	
Ventilated	Morphine: 50–150 µg/kg IV bolus as required; maintenance: 0–40 µg/kg/hr IV Fentanyl 0.5–10 µg/kg IV bolus until analgesia is optimal 2.5–10 µg/kg/hr for IV maintenance; regular paracetamol (caution after 48 hours)	

(ECMO: extracorporeal membrane oxygenation; NICU: neonatal intensive care unit; IV: intravenous; PO: per oral)

CONCLUSION

All neonates like adults feel pain. Developing brain undergoing neuronal organization, synaptic plasticity and myelination are influenced by neurotransmitter and neuroendocrine milieu. Painful experiences during these periods, may effect brain development which can have short- and long-term implication. Therefore, the clinician must develop methods of assessing pain and formulate standing order procedure to adequately and effectively deal with it. Children may not recall painful experiences from their NICU stay but they may demonstrate altered behavioral states resulting from painful experiences that were not well managed. Every effort should, therefore, be made to offer optimal pain management to each and every neonate.

KEY POINTS

➢ Studies suggested that the anatomic and physiologic systems for pain perception are sufficiently developed by 18–20 weeks of gestation.
➢ Pain activates physiologic stress responses in neonates.
➢ Pain and stress during early infancy has potential deleterious effects on long-term neurological outcome.
➢ There are number of pain assessment tools but each unit should adopt a tool which is well validated and doable by frontline healthcare provider.
➢ Unit should use combination of pain management modalities to avoid adverse effect of drugs.

SELF ASSESSMENT

1. **Which of the following statement(s) is/are false?**
   a. Cutaneous sensory receptors first appear in the perioral area during the 8th week of gestation and are present in nearly all mucous surfaces by the 18th week of gestation.
   b. Cutaneous sensory receptors first appear in the perianal area during the 8th week of gestation and are present in nearly all mucous surfaces by the 18th week of gestation.
   c. Synapses between peripheral sensory afferents and dorsal horn neurons in the spinal cord appear early in the second trimester and are mature by 20 weeks of gestation.
   d. Synapses between peripheral sensory afferents and dorsal horn neurons in the spinal cord appear early in the first trimester and are mature by 20 weeks of gestation.

2. **Which of the following statement(s) is/are false?**
   a. Pain activates physiologic stress responses, which are associated with the release of catecholamines, cortisol, and other stress hormones.
   b. All newborns should receive analgesic premedication for endotracheal intubation except for emergency intubations during resuscitation or newborns in whom instrumentation of the airway is likely to be extremely difficult.
   c. In ventilated patients, postoperatively morphine or fentanyl can be used as analgesia.
   d. Morphine is 80-fold to 100-fold more potent than fentanyl and causes less histamine release.

FURTHER READING

1. Hall RW, Anand KJ. Pain management in newborns. Clin Perinatol. 2014;41(4):895-924.
2. Kumar P, Denson SE, Mancuso TJ; Committee on Fetus and Newborn, Section on Anesthesiology and Pain Medicine. Premedication for nonemergency endotracheal intubation in the neonate. Pediatrics. 2010;125(3):608-15.
3. Vanhatalo S, van Nieuwenhuizen O. Fetal pain? Brain Dev. 2000;22(3):145-50.

Discharge Planning

Chapter

31

Arpita Gupta, Harish Chellani

INTRODUCTION

Discharge of newborn from the neonatal intensive care unit (NICU) is a time of mixed emotions for the family including excitement and anxiety. Discharge planning of high-risk NICU graduates depends primarily on baby's medical and physiological condition but also includes ability of family to provide appropriate care to the newborn at home.

DISCHARGE READINESS

- Discharge preparedness is a process of facilitating discharge readiness to successfully make the transition from NICU to home.
- American Academy of Pediatrics has classified high-risk infants into four categories—(1) the preterm infant, (2) the infant with special healthcare needs or dependence on technology, (3) the infant at risk because of family issues, and (4) the infant with anticipated early death.
- Discharge readiness includes attainment of technical skills and knowledge, emotional comfort, and confidence with infant care by the primary caregivers at the time of discharge.

Since there are differences in the outcome of high-risk NICU graduates and other newborns, it is vital to keep this in mind while discharging the baby. Factors deciding newborn discharge readiness are shown in **Box 1**.

DISCHARGE PREPARATION

When planning a high-risk discharge, it is important to consider the baby's relative fragility and complexity of care needs. Infants with specialized needs require a complex, flexible, and ongoing discharge plan. As medications, special formulas, and/or dietary supplements may be challenging for the parents to obtain, the need for these items should be identified early, so that they can be obtained as soon as possible to optimize discharge teaching opportunities. **Table 1** summarizes the essential elements of discharge planning.

- According to Government of India guidelines, low birth weight or a high-risk baby if discharged early because of financial constraints or lack of beds should have a provision of being closely monitored by ASHA worker or healthcare worker by prompt home visits.
- In case of any emergency, the baby should be referred and taken to appropriate medical facility (e.g. community health center). This step is taken to decrease the post-discharge neonatal mortality as much as possible.

Box 1: Factors to consider at discharge.

- Ability to maintain temperature in an open environment (e.g. Crib).
- On full feeds without any respiratory compromise.
- Three consecutive day weight gain of 15 g/kg/day (in preterm and term LBW/VLBW babies) on breast/direct feeds.
- Demonstrate maturity of respiratory control without episodes of apnea and bradycardia. (The length of time before discharge that an infant should be free from apnea and bradycardia is controversial. However, 5–8 days of observation after discontinuation of caffeine therapy probably offers a sufficient margin of safety).
- Appropriate supplements started (iron, vitamin D).
- Immunized as per schedule according to National Immunization schedule or Indian Academy of Pediatrics.
- Newborn screening done as required.
- Primary caregiver taught and confident about the feeding and dangers signs.
- Review of the hospital course has been completed, unresolved medical problems have been identified, and plans for follow-up monitoring and treatment have been instituted.
- An individualized home-care plan has been developed with input from all appropriate disciplines.

(LBW: low birth weight; VLBW: very low birth weight)

Table 1: Elements of discharge planning.

Assessment of family	• Identification of primary caregiver, mostly mother, if possible • Any health issue in the family requiring treatment • Any psychological or mental health issue in the family that may have impact on caretaking ability • Their cultural beliefs that may have an impact on the infant feeding and health
Home environment preparation	• Supplies for baby care—feeding related equipment like breast pump, paladai, etc. diapers, thermometer, crib (safety approved), and infant clothes • Providing a realistic and practical idea of their home life in immediate and long-term period (potential infant developmental and growth-related issues) • Providing information about use of hand washing/sanitizer to prevent infections and room thermometer for maintaining thermal controlled environment at home
Discharge teaching/ advice	• Teaching the mother and making her confident about feeding the baby by making her practice the skills in front of a medical person • Providing specific, practical information with examples that are meaningful to the family's everyday experience (e.g. massage and bath of the baby) • Providing information about danger signs (e.g. lethargy, refusal to feed, difficulty breathing, fever, cold to touch, etc.) • Providing information about making the baby sleep in supine position and avoiding use of stuff toys in the cot to reduce the chances of respiratory compromise
Newborn screening (high-risk newborn)	• USG head—all babies with gestational age <32 weeks, all babies who were critically ill • Audiology screening—all babies being discharged from NICU • Ophthalmologic screening—refer to Chapter 26—Retinopathy of Prematurity
Follow-up visits (high-risk newborn)	• Follow-up protocol should include assessment of growth, nutrition, development, vision, hearing, and neurological status of all high-risk newborns • All newborns with unresolved medical issue, e.g. bronchopulmonary dysplasia, congenital heart disease should be closely followed up

(NICU: neonatal intensive care unit; USG: ultrasonography)

CONCLUSION

- It is imperative to mention that on one hand, if shortening the length of stay of a preterm newborn may help in decreasing adverse effect on parenting and hospital-related morbidities, it may lead to increase in morbidity and mortality related to physiological immaturity.
- It has been seen that there is a higher rate of hospital readmission and mortality during the first year of life in low birth weight and preterm newborns as compared to healthy term babies appropriate for gestational age.
- According to a study, the overall re-hospitalization rate in these babies is 22.72% during the first year of life, which is 20% higher than the rate among healthy term newborns (2.3%).
- Careful preparations for discharge and good follow-up after discharge may reduce these risks.

KEY POINTS

➢ Comprehensive discharge planning can decrease the risk of morbidity and mortality because of premature discharge and at the same time prevent unnecessary hospital stay of infants fit for discharge.

➢ The essential component of discharge planning includes assessment of neonatal medical readiness, parental readiness, assessment of family and home environment, and integrated follow-up.

SELF ASSESSMENT

1. **The following are criteria to assess readiness of discharge except:**
   a. Ability to maintain temperature in an open environment (e.g. Crib).
   b. On full feeds without any respiratory compromise.
   c. Three consecutive days weight gain of 5 g/kg/day.
   d. Demonstrate maturity of respiratory control without episodes of apnea and bradycardia and at least 5 days of caffeine therapy.

2. **All of the following are recommended predischarge screens for preterm very low birth weight infants except:**
   a. Neuroimaging
   b. Audiological screen
   c. Ophthalmologic screen
   d. Expanded metabolic screen

FURTHER READING

1. American Academy of Pediatrics Committee on Fetus and Newborn. Hospital discharge of the high-risk neonate. Pediatrics. 2008;122(5):1119-26.
2. Chaudhari S, Kulkarni S, Pandit A, et al. Mortality and morbidity in high risk infants during a six year follow-up. Indian Pediatr. 2000;37(12):1314-20.
3. Follow up of High Risk Newborn. Evidence Based Clinical Practice Guidelines. National Neonatology Forum; 2010. pp. 218-46.
4. Hulsey TC, Hudson MB, Pittard WB 3rd. Predictors of hospital postdischarge infant mortality: implications for high-risk infant follow-up efforts. J Perinatol. 1994;14(3):219-25.

32 Chapter

Developmentally Supportive Care

Naveen Jain

INTRODUCTION

- Developmentally supportive care (DSC) is a clinical care model that looks beyond ensuring improved vitals and survival of sick babies in intensive care unit. DSC model understands that the baby is an individual and the baby's family is a critical component of baby's world. The sick/preterm baby's brain is extremely vulnerable. It is dependent on sensory inputs. Abnormal inputs from care processes that are not baby friendly can result in development and psychological problems.
- Developmentally supportive care addresses care processes beyond medications and procedures [feeding, position, sleep time, touch, pain control, neonatal intensive care unit (NICU) light and sound, etc.] that the baby experiences and that influence the baby's developing brain.

NEONATAL INTENSIVE CARE UNIT ENVIRONMENT

- The NICU environment is very different from the in utero world of the baby. The NICU has very bright lights and is noisy most of the "day and night" with alarms and activities of the unit. Loud conversations of busy doctors and nurses add to the stress.
- The preterm baby spends many days in postures not conducive for development; the fact that the baby's postures have an impact on development of tone of the baby seldom crosses the minds, except when in DSC workshops.
- Many painful procedures are part of the NICU care, like checking blood sugars; varying sensitivity exists on decreasing painful procedures and nonpharmacological/pharmacological analgesia.

HINDRANCE TO DEVELOPMENTALLY SUPPORTIVE CARE

- Sick babies spend many days in NICUs separated from their parents. Parents are "allowed to visit" their own baby for only during visiting hours so that infections may be reduced, and baby's safety is not compromised!! It is not difficult to figure out who is safer—parents or healthcare workers, and who poses greater risk of cross-infection.
- Family-centered DSC has still not impressed the "evidence based" medicine model of care; it is amazing that it requires a randomized trial to prove that a gentle mother's touch, a quiet environment, allowing baby to sleep, etc. are good for a baby.

- Most often the process of caregiving simply requires just the presence of parents. DSC has often been made to appear complicated—special nurses to understand the baby and multiple charts to decide if baby is in the right state or position. This has led to evaluating the worth of investing in resources and interfering with critical care to support physiology of a sick baby.
- Kangaroo care (KC), nonnutritive sucking, and massage are well known good practices, but often take back seat, as everybody is busy with X-rays, blood gases, fluids and antibiotics decisions. Most NICUs fear accidental displacement of endotracheal tubes, central lines or nasal prongs if handled.

The guiding principles may be borrowed from many programs that have researched and evaluated the DSC model. This chapter will evaluate various domains/caregiving processes that are evidently beneficial to a sick baby in NICU that will decrease the stress of baby and the family.

PRINCIPLES OF DEVELOPMENTALLY SUPPORTIVE CARE

- Family-centered care
- Neonatal intensive care unit environment—light and noise
- Care beyond technology and pharmacotherapy
    - Pain management and procedural support—recognizing stress cues
    - Positioning
    - Cue-based feeding
    - Skin-to-skin (Kangaroo) care
    - Massage.

Family-centered Care

- Parents and the family must not be separated from the sick baby. Family-centered NICUs allow parents/family unlimited access to the baby. Some request parents to wait when invasive procedures are performed, sometimes restrict parent involvement if baby is unstable and critically ill. A few units restrict parent entry at unit handover time.
- Parents must be informed periodically and completely about baby's healthcare plans and must be a part of decision-making. Their cultural (religious) values, perception of disease, and healthcare must be respected. Efforts must be made to help the parents cope with stressful situations; avoid ambiguous messages, educate about care plans in advance and involve counselors as necessary.
- Parents must participate in care of the sick baby. They must hold the baby's hands, tuck the baby and provide comfort, perform KC, gently stroke and massage the baby. Under supervision, units have involved parents in orogastric feeding, change of diapers and many other care processes like taking weight of the baby. Parents' participation in the care of sick babies leads to early discharge from hospital and better transition from NICU to home. Occasionally parents are overwhelmed and report physical and mental exhaustion.
- The way forward is couplet care or single-family room concept. The sick baby would be nurtured with the mother and the family living with the baby in the same room throughout the period of hospitalization. The room would be customized as per family traditions and culture. Baby would be mostly nursed by parents under medical supervision.

Neonatal Intensive Care Unit Environment—Light and Noise

- Neonatal intensive care unit light should be dimmed except when skilled procedures are performed. Day night cycling is expected to help baby's behavior maturation.
- Alarms should be muted once addressed, their volumes be reduced.
- Avoid loud conversations. Many good developmentally supportive units have improved the designs of NICU by using sound absorbing floors and walls.

Care beyond Technology and Pharmacotherapy

Pain Management and Procedural Support—Recognizing Stress Cues

- Painful procedures must be minimized; e.g. clubbing of blood tests that are not urgent can decrease painful pricks. For example, lancet pricks are less painful than needle pricks. Tucking the baby, talking to the baby, and holding hands have all shown to decrease pain. Breast milk and sucrose decrease pain of procedures.
- Topical anesthetics, paracetamol, and opioid analgesia may be required when more painful procedures are planned.
- One must recognize infant behaviors that suggest stress like rapid breathing, change in skin color, stop sign of hand, etc.

Positioning

- Placing the baby "frog legged" for prolonged periods in NICU results in external rotation at shoulder and hips. Gravity acting on forearms and legs (not present in utero) results in unequal lengthening of flexors and extensors and causes tone abnormalities.
- Babies must be nursed with head in midline, hands brought to midline, toward the mouth. Legs and arms must be flexed, supported by boundaries. The baby must be contained in a nest, like in utero.
- Practice tummy time, i.e. keeping baby prone for some time when baby is alert.

Cue-based Feeding

- Most NICU feed babies by the clock, e.g. every 2–3 hours. The baby may be sleeping when the nurse starts giving an orogastric feed. It is recommended to wait for baby cues that baby is waking up from sleep to decide the right time to feed. Nurses and parents are often concerned that feeds may be missed or delayed and hence, parental involvement is critical to implement cue-based feeding.
- Even procedures considered routine like diaper change and cleaning of baby can cause unpleasant experiences to baby and must be planned based on babies' state of wakefulness.

Skin-to-skin (Kangaroo) Care

- Kangaroo care has been the most understood DSC in the last decade. Scientific evaluation has demonstrated better sleep, saturations, heart rates, weight gain, exclusive breast-feeding rates, decrease in infections, and early hospital discharge.
- Although long durations of KC are recommended, translation to practice requires counseling and education of family members. Hospitals should be able to provide support for the family to stay long hours, provide comfortable chairs and privacy to perform KC.

Massage

- Massage reduces behavioral and physiological response to pain and reduces cortisol levels. Better weight gain is demonstrated. Bonding to mother improves.
- Maturation of electroencephalogram (EEG) was shown to be better and development scores were also better in a study. Most studies enrolled stable preterm or term babies and performed massage for 15–20 min/day.

IMPLEMENTATION OF DEVELOPMENTALLY SUPPORTIVE CARE

Translation of the concept of care principles that support healthy development to practices requires many changes.

- Written policies on DSC
- Training of doctors, nurses, occupational therapists, and speech language therapists
- Parent participation
- Integration of DSC with clinical care (rather than a parallel service run by a specialist nurse or physiotherapist)
- Engineering changes of NICU structure.

KEY POINTS

- ➤ Developmentally supportive care is a clinical care model that looks beyond ensuring improved vitals and survival of sick babies in intensive care unit.
- ➤ Hindrances to DSC in NICU include lack of awareness of its implementation, preoccupation of clinicians with intensive care of sick infants, fear of dislodgement of lines and tubes, fear for requirement of special nurses and complex charts and barrier to family-centered care.
- ➤ Components of DSC include family-centered care, control of NICU environment—light and noise, pain management and procedural support—recognizing stress cues, positioning, cue-based feeding, skin-to-skin (Kangaroo) care, and massage.

SELF ASSESSMENT

1. **Which of the following statement is false?**
   a. Scientific evaluation of KMC has demonstrated better sleep, saturations, heart rates, weight gain, exclusive breastfeeding rates, decrease in infections, and early hospital discharge.
   b. Massage reduces behavioral and physiological response to pain and reduces cortisol levels.
   c. Practice tummy time, i.e. keeping baby prone for some time when baby is alert.
   d. Feeding should be scheduled in NICU every 2–3 hours as a part of DSC.

FURTHER READING

1. Esser M, Dore S, Fitzgerald F, et al. Applying Developmentally Supportive Principles to Diapering in the NICU: What We Know. Neonatal Netw. 2018;37(3):149-54.
2. Schiavenato M, Holsti L. Defining Procedural Distress in the NICU and What Can Be Done About It. Neonatal Netw. 2017;36(1):12-7.
3. Westrup B. Family-centered developmentally supportive care: the Swedish example. Arch Pediatr. 2015;22(10):1086-91.

Follow-up Care for High-risk Infants

Chapter 33

Suman Rao PN, Shridevi S Bisanalli

INTRODUCTION

Advances in perinatal intensive care have been associated with improved survival of high-risk neonates but have resulted in increased morbidity and adverse outcomes. These neonates have high risk of feeding problems, growth failure, neurosensory impairment (blindness and deafness), developmental, cognitive, and learning disabilities, behavioral problems like attention deficit hyperactivity disorder (ADHD), and other chronic medical illness.

- Timely and regular follow-up care is essential for better long-term outcomes of high-risk neonates. They need close monitoring and special care for timely detection of various morbidity and early intervention to achieve optimal results.
- It requires a multidisciplinary approach involving a team of pediatricians, child psychologist, pediatric neurologist, ophthalmologist, audiologist, otorhinolaryngologist, physiotherapist, occupational therapist, medical social worker, lactation specialist, and a dietician. Prior to discharge, the follow-up of the high-risk graduate requires proper planning.

DISCHARGE PLANNING

Discharge preparedness and planning is vital to ensure a good follow-up. A predischarge checklist is helpful.

- Documentation of biological risk factors and therapies (postnatal steroids or lack of antenatal steroids/magnesium sulfate)
- Neurological examination at discharge (Hammersmith/Amiel-Tison)
- Documentation of growth, particularly head circumference during neonatal intensive care unit (NICU) stay
- Neuroimaging (as indicated)
- Screen for congenital hypothyroidism and metabolic screen
- Hearing screening
- Retinopathy of prematurity (ROP) screening
- Initiation of early intervention
- Assessment of parent understanding, coping, and home environment.

In addition, the family must have a good understanding of the continued care for the neonatal problems, e.g. continuing kangaroo mother care for low birth weight infants, antibiotic prophylaxis for hydronephrosis, etc.

High-risk Infant

A high-risk infant is defined as any newborn or young infant who has a high probability of manifesting in childhood a sensory or motor deficit or mental handicap.

The following groups of high-risk infants need neurodevelopmental follow-up as given in **Box 1** (customize as per unit policy).

Structured follow-up protocol is needed to implement and improve compliance for follow-up.

The follow-up protocol involves:

- Monitoring of growth and nutrition
- Thyroid screen/metabolic profile
- Neuromotor assessment
- Neurodevelopmental assessment
- Neurosensory examination (vision and hearing)
- Neuroimaging assessment
- General movements assessment
- Immunization
- Early intervention therapy when indicated
- Anticipatory guidance to parents
- Record keeping

Follow-up Schedule

A usual recommended schedule is as follows:
- First visit within 7 days of discharge.

Box 1: High-risk infants who need neurodevelopmental follow-up.

- Babies with birth weight 1,800 g or gestation <34 weeks
- SGA (<3rd centile) and LGA (>97th centile)
- Perinatal asphyxia—Apgar score 3 or less at 5 minutes and/or hypoxic ischemic encephalopathy stage 2 or stage 3
- Seizures
- Mechanical ventilation for more than 24 hours
- Metabolic problems—symptomatic hypoglycemia and hypocalcemia
- Infections—meningitis and/or culture positive sepsis/NEC
- Shock requiring inotropic/vasopressor support
- Major morbidities such as chronic lung disease, intraventricular hemorrhage, and periventricular leukomalacia
- Infants born to HIV-positive mothers
- Twin with intrauterine death of co-twin
- Twin-to-twin transfusion
- Hyperbilirubinemia >20 mg/dL or requirement of exchange transfusion
- Rh hemolytic disease of newborn
- Major malformations
- Inborn errors of metabolism/other genetic disorders
- Abnormal neurological examination at discharge

(HIV: human immunodeficiency virus; LGA: large for gestational age; NEC: necrotizing enterocolitis; SGA: small for gestational age)

- Subsequent visits—at term (corrected age), 6 weeks, 3 months, 6 months, 9 months, 12 months, 18 months, 2 years, 3 years, 4 years, and 5 years. Neonatal follow-up clinic (NFC) can be held once or twice a week.

Concept of corrected age: To assess growth and development, age needs to be corrected/adjusted to the age for prematurity.
Corrected age = Chronological age – No. of weeks born prematurely
That is a 3-month-old baby (chronological age) who is born 6 weeks prematurely is actually 6 weeks old (corrected age). Appointment dates as per corrected age must be given on discharge itself.

GROWTH AND NUTRITION

- Premature infants are more prone to extrauterine growth restriction. Inadequate nutritional support leads to energy and protein deficits and hence growth failure which is implicated in poor neurodevelopmental outcomes and long-term morbidity. Optimal nutrition is paramount for optimal growth outcomes.
- Anthropometric measures like head circumference, length and weight should be plotted according to gender and age (adjusted until age 2 years) on growth charts in every visit. The current recommended growth charts are the INTERGROWTH 21st charts that integrate with the WHO growth charts and Fenton's growth chart.
- Other measures of growth used include skinfold thickness, calculated measures of weight-to-length ratio, growth velocity, protein and caloric intake, energy expenditure, and bone density.

NEUROMOTOR ASSESSMENT

- From 28 weeks to 40 weeks of gestation, the acquisition of muscle tone and motor functions spreads from the lower extremities in the direction of the head and is caudocephalic. Maturation is so rapid between 28 weeks and 40 weeks gestational age (GA) that it is possible to describe changes by 2-week intervals. After term, the process is reversed and is cephalocaudal for the next 12–18 months. Progressive caudocephalad development of muscle tone between 28 weeks and 40 weeks GA, is linked with myelination progressing in a caudocephalic direction for descending motor pathways. In the first year of life, the progressive cephalocaudal development of active tone in the trunk is probably linked with the progress in maturation of the corticospinal tract, which proceeds rostrocaudally from the midbrain to the lumbosacral levels.
- Passive tone develops first in flexor muscles while active tone develops earlier in the extensor muscles of the axis than in the flexor muscles between 28 weeks and 40 weeks GA. In the first year, for passive tone, flexor tone of the extremities decreases starting with the upper extremities proceeding to the lower extremities to result in physiological hypotonia typically seen at 8 months **(Fig. 1)**. Differential development of tone in extensor and flexor muscles correlates with the successive myelination of medial subcorticospinal, lateral subcorticospinal, and corticospinal pathways **(Fig. 2)**.
- The upper limbs begin to relax and acquire skills before the lower limbs. In the axis, head control appears first, followed by the ability to sit, stand, and finally walk by 12–18 months. The timing of this sequence is subject to wide individual variations in addition to familial and ethnic influences, but the order is constant in all normal individuals.
- Both passive and active tones are assessed. Tone can be identified as normal/hypotonia/hypertonia.

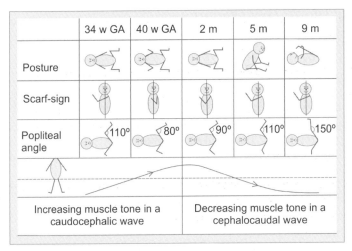

Fig. 1: Passive tone in upper and lower extremities.

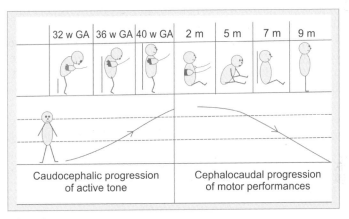

Fig. 2: Active tone in the axis.

Various assessment methods can be used to evaluate the neurological status and tone in newborns and infants including:

- The Amiel-Tison method
- Vojta's neurokinesiologic method
- Infant Neurological International Battery (INFANIB)
- Milani-Comparetti and Gidoni method.

NEUROSENSORY ASSESSMENT

- *Ophthalmic examination:* Indirect ophthalmoscopy till retinal vascularization is complete. Subsequently high-risk babies need to be evaluated annually by an ophthalmologist.
- *Auditory evaluation:* Hearing screening by auditory brainstem response (ABR). Confirmation of any hearing deficit should be done by 3 months and rehabilitation by 6 months.

GENERAL MOVEMENTS ASSESSMENT

- General movements (GM) are a reliable tool in early identification of infants at risk of neuromotor deficits.
- These are generated by a neural network, the central pattern generators (CPGs), which are most likely located in the brainstem and modulated lending variability.
- Reduced modulation of the CPGs results in less variable (i.e. abnormal) movements and indicates fetal or neonatal compromise. Abnormal GMs during preterm and term age are classified as poor repertoire, cramped synchronized, and chaotic.
- Fidgety movements are tiny movements of the neck, trunk, and limbs in all directions and of variable acceleration.

Age	1 month	3 months
Normal	Normal writhing movements	Normal fidgety movements
Abnormal	Poor repertoire Cramped synchronized Chaotic	Absent

- Abnormal GM in very preterm infants, particularly at 3 months post-term, is predictive of worse neurodevelopment at ages 2 years and 4 years. Abnormal GM especially at 3 months has 95–100% sensitivity and 90–95% specificity to predict cerebral palsy (CP). Among all the tests to predict CP, GM has the same sensitivity and almost the same specificity as magnetic resonance imaging (MRI). In fact a combination of GM at "fidgety age", i.e. 3 months and MRI at term equivalent age (TEA) has highest sensitivity and almost 100% specificity in predicting CP among extreme preterm babies **(Fig. 1)**.
- Minor abnormality in GM is associated with minor neurologic dysfunction, poorer functional outcome, memory, ADHD, and aggressive behavior at later age.
- Other neuromotor assessment tools such as test of infant motor performance (TIMP) and neurosensory motor development assessment (NSMDA) have a wide range of sensitivity (43–81%) and specificity (67–93%) for predicting abnormal outcome.

NEUROIMAGING

- All preterm babies born before 32 weeks and <1,500 g birth weight must undergo screening neurosonograms at 1–2 weeks after birth and 36–40 weeks postmenstrual age (PMA).
- Babies with ventriculomegaly and cystic periventricular leukomalacia (PVL) have increased risk of CP as compared to normal ultrasonographic finding.
- *Application of MRI:* Conventional MRI is effective for detecting developmental abnormalities of the CNS and PVL virtually any time after birth. Diffusion magnetic resonance methods are used as an early indicator of brain injury becoming sensitive 2–5 days after injury in infants. Functional MRI is used to assess the cortical reorganization associated with injury and recovery. Electroencephalogram (EEG) is done as indicated.

NEURODEVELOPMENTAL ASSESSMENT

Developmental Screening Tools

There are several tests available for screening of infants and toddlers. The commonly used ones as follows:

				Sensitivity and
Tool	Purpose	Domains measured	Time taken	specificity
Baroda development screening test	Assess motor and mental development of infants	Motor and mental	Quick	Sensitivity 95% Specificity 65%
Developmental Assessment Tool for Anganwadis (DATA)	Identify children with developmental delay	Gross motor; fine motor; cognitive; personal; social; expressive language; receptive language	Short	Not available
Disability screen test	To screen major disabilities	Physical, motor, sensory, and mental retardation	Around 5 minutes	Sensitivity 89% Specificity 98%
Trivandrum Screening Chart (TDSC)	Assess mental and motor development	Mental; motor development; hearing and visual functions	Around 5 minutes	Sensitivity 66% Specificity 78%
Parents' Evaluation of Developmental Status (PEDS)	Assess parents' concerns on child's learning, development and behavior	Learning; development and behavior	Short	Sensitivity 61% Specificity 65%

Table 1: Development screening tools for low-middle income countries.

Bayley Infant Neurodevelopment Screen

This test identifies the child who requires a complete assessment by Bayley Scale for infant development (BSID III) for diagnosing developmental delay and planning intervention strategies.

Denver Developmental Materials II (Formerly DDST)

The DENVER II is designed to reflect the development of a broad range of heterogeneous skills in a minimum amount of time.

This is a surveillance and monitoring tool used by professionals or trained paraprofessionals to determine if a child's development is within the normal range. The results are not diagnostic.

Ages and Stages Questionnaire

Ages and Stages Questionnaire (ASQ) is used to screen infants and young children for developmental delays during the first 5 years of life. The assessment covers five key developmental areas—communication, gross motor, fine motor, problem solving, and personal-social skill.

The above screening tools are developed in the western world. However, there are many tools developed for the low-middle income countries (LMIC) **(Table 1)** but none of them have a high sensitivity and specificity.

Development Assessment Tests

An infant/child who fails a screening test should be evaluated by a detailed development assessment. The two well-accepted development assessment tools are as follows:

1. *BSID III—Bayley Scale of Infant and Toddler Development III:* Bayley III, originally developed by psychologist Nancy Bayley, is used to assess the development of infants and toddlers 1–42 months. It has separate cognitive, gross motor, fine motor, receptive and expressive language, and social and behavior scales. These can be administered separately but are needed to provide the development quotient.
2. *DASII—Development Assessment Scale for Indian Infants:* DASII is the Indian adaptation of BSID II. It is conducted for infants between 3 months and 2.5 years of age, and it assesses both the motor development and mental development. A motor and mental developmental quotient is provided at the end.

IMMUNIZATION

Immunization should be ensured according to chronological age. Parents should be offered the option of using additional vaccines such as pneumococcal vaccine, etc.

EARLY INTERVENTION

- It implies a system of programs that works with an infant and his or her family to prevent or minimize adverse outcomes in the child.
- Principle—Hebb rule—"Neurons that fire together wire together". It is this neuroplastic principle which forms the basis for the early stimulation.
- Stimulate the child in all sectors of development—motor, cognitive, neurosensory, and language.
- Developmentally appropriate—stimulate to achieve the next "mile-stone" rather than age-based.
- Early stimulation—preventing active inhibition of the central nervous system (CNS) pathways due to inappropriate input and supporting the use of modulating pathways during highly sensitive period of brain development.
- Physical stimulation—passive exercises to prevent development of hypertonia.
- Avoid over-stimulation (different modes of stimulation all at once).
- Vision—bold patterns with strong contrast (newborn's eyes examine the edges and learns to process simple visual information). Making faces and moving objects stimulate visual tracking.
- Hearing—playing classical strains helps development of spatial reasoning pathways and connections within the auditory system. Talking to the baby, reading books, and singing rhymes.
- Touch—massage—gentle firm strokes to be used, at least 12 strokes to each area.
- Home—parent participation in decision making and actual hands-on experience in caring for their child is essential and key to successful developmental intervention.

ANTICIPATORY GUIDANCE TO PARENTS

- Parents are made to understand the problems of babies, treatment required, importance of follow-up, and prognosis.
- Immunization.
- Nutrition—reemphasis on exclusive breastfeeding till 6 months, complementary feeds to be started at 6 months, and breastfeeding to be continued till 2 years.
- Other aspects of neonatal care.

RECORD KEEPING

All babies in follow-up are given special high-risk discharge cards with follow-up number. Documentation of the multidisciplinary follow-up is important.

KEY POINTS

- ➤ Neonatal intensive care unit graduates are at greater risk for abnormal neurological outcomes. They need a multidisciplinary follow-up to monitor growth and development and provide early intervention therapy.
- ➤ Neuromotor assessment is very reliable in infancy.
- ➤ There are various tools for developmental surveillance, screening, and formal assessments. Formal development assessment by BSID III or DASII is indicated once in all the high-risk infants.

SELF ASSESSMENT

1. **Which of the following is false about maturation of tone?**
   a. From 28 weeks to 40 weeks of gestation, the acquisition of muscle tone and motor functions spreads from the lower extremities in the direction of the head and is caudocephalic.
   b. Maturation is so rapid between 28 weeks and 40 weeks GA, that it is possible to describe changes by 2-week intervals.
   c. After term, the process of acquisition of muscle tone and motor functions is reversed and is cephalocaudal for the next 12–18 months.
   d. Passive tone develops first in extensor muscles while active tone develops earlier in the flexor muscles of the axis than in the extensors muscles between 28 weeks and 40 weeks GA.

2. **Which of the following is not abnormal GM during preterm and term age?**
   a. Poor repertoire
   b. Cramped synchronized
   c. Chaotic
   d. Writhing

FURTHER READING

1. Bliss TV, Collingridge GL. A synaptic model of memory: long-term potentiation in the hippocampus. Nature. 1993;361(6407):31-9.
2. Hadders-Algra M, Groothuis AM. Quality of general movements in infancy is related to neurological dysfunction, ADHD, and aggressive behaviour. Dev Med Child Neurol. 1999;41(6):381-91.
3. Pandit A, Mukhopadhyay K, Suryawanshi P. Follow up of High Risk Newborn: NNF Clinical Practice Guidelines. Delhi: NNF; 2010. pp. 217-52.
4. Prince A, Groh-Wargo S. Nutrition management for the promotion of growth in very low birth weight premature infants. Nutr Clin Pract. 2013;28(6):659-68.
5. Spittle AJ, Doyle LW, Boyd RN. A systematic review of the clinimetric properties of neuromotor assessments for preterm infants during the first year of life. Dev Med Child Neurol. 2008;50(4): 254-66.

ANSWERS TO SELF ASSESSMENT QUESTIONS

Chapter no.	Question 1	Question 2	Question 3	Question 4
1	A	B	B	B, C
2	B	D		
3 Glucose	C	D		
3 Calcium	C	D		
4	C	C	B	
5	B	C	B	
6	C	B		
7	C	A		
8	C	C		
9	C	D		
10	D	A		
11	D	B		
12	B	A	C	
13	B	D		
14	D	A	D	B
15	C	D		
16	D	D		
17	D	D		
18	C	C		
19	D	B		
20	D	78 mL		
21	B	C		
22	A	A	B	
23	C	D		
24	B	D		
25	A			
26	C	D		
27	C	C		
28	C	C		
29	C	B	Increase	
30	B, C	D		
31	C	D		
32	D			
33	D	D		

INDEX

Page numbers followed by *b* refer to box, *f* refer to figure, *fc* refer to flowchart, and *t* refer to table.